Essays in Drama Therapy

*of related interest*

**Persona and Performance**
The Use of Role in Drama, Therapy and Everyday Life
*Robert J Landy*
ISBN 1 85302 230 6

**Introduction to Dramatherapy**
Theatre and Healing – Ariadne's Ball of Thread
*Sue Jennings*
*Foreword by Clare Higgins*
ISBN 1 85302 115 6

**Practical Approaches to Dramatherapy**
The Shield of Perseus
*Madeline Andersen-Warren and Roger Grainger*
ISBN 1 85302 660 3

**Theory and Practice of Action and Drama Techniques**
Developmental Psychotherapy from an Existential-Dialectal Viewpoint
*Leni Verhofstadt-Deneve*
*Preface by Hubert Hermans*
ISBN 1 85302 803 7

**Making a Leap – Theatre for Empowerment**
A Practical Handbook for Creative Drama Work with Young People
*Sara Clifford and Anna Herrmann*
ISBN 1 85302 632 8

**Rebels with a Cause**
Working with Adolescents Using Action Techniques
*Mario Cossa*
ISBN 1 84310 379 6

**Sambadrama**
The Arena of Brazilian Psychodrama
*Edited and translated by Zoltán Figusch*
*Forewords by Adam Blatner and José Fonseca*
ISBN 1 84310 363 X

# Essays in Drama Therapy
## The Double Life

*Robert J. Landy*

*Foreword by Gavin Bolton*

Jessica Kingsley Publishers
London and Philadelphia

First published in the United Kingdom in 1996
by Jessica Kingsley Publishers
116 Pentonville Road
London N1 9JB, UK
and
400 Market Street, Suite 400
Philadelphia, PA 19106, USA

*www.jkp.com*

Copyright © Robert J. Landy 1996
Foreword Copyright © Gavin Bolton 1996

Printed digitally since 2005

**Library of Congress Cataloging in Publication Data**
Landy, Robert J.
 Essays in drama therapy: the double life / Robert Landy.
 p. cm
 Includes bibliographical references and index.
 ISBN-13: 978-1-85302--322-1 (alk. paper)
 ISBN-10: 1-85302--322-1 (alk. paper)
 1. Psychodrama. I. Title.
 RC489.P7L33 1995
 616.89'1523--dc20                                    85-32057
                                                          CIP

**British Library Cataloguing in Publication Data**
Essays in Drama Therapy : Double Life
I. Landy, Robert J.
616.891523

ISBN-13: 978 1 85302 322 4
ISBN-10: 1 85302 322 1

# Contents

Acknowledgements viii

Foreword by Gavin Bolton ix

1. Training the Drama Therapist: A Four-Part Model (1982) 1

2. The Use of Distancing in Drama Therapy (1983) 13

3. Conceptual and Methodological Issues
of Research in Drama Therapy (1984) 28

4. Puppets, Dolls, Objects, Masks, and Make-up (1984) 44

5. The Image of the Mask:
Implications for Theatre and Therapy (1985) 54

6. Reflections Upon Training:
The Making of a Drama Therapist (1987) 70

7. One-on-One:
The Role of the Drama Therapist
Working with Individuals (1990) 84

8. The Concept of Role in Drama Therapy (1991) 99

9. A Taxonomy of Roles:
A Blueprint for the Possibilities of Being (1992) 111

10. A Research Agenda for the Creative
Arts Therapies (1993) 137

11. The Child, the Dreamer, the Artist and the Fool: In Search of
Understanding the Meaning of Expressive Therapy (1993) 140

12. Three Scenarios for the Future of Drama Therapy (1993) 159

13. The Dramatic World View: Reflections on the Roles
Taken and Played by Young Children (1993) 169

14. A Short-term Model of Drama Therapy
Through the Role Method (1994) 190

15. Isolation and Collaboration in the Creative Arts Therapies:
The Implications of Crossing Borders (1994) 202

16. In Search of the Muse (1995) 207

17. The Double Life:
A Case of Bipolar Disorder (1995) 216

References 252

Index

## List of Figures

| | | |
|---|---|---|
| 4.1 | Story dramatization through make-up | 52 |
| 5.1 | Ragged Dick, from *Rags to Riches* | 55 |
| 5.2 | The Rich Banker, from *Rags to Riches* | 56 |
| 5.3 | The Policeman, from *Rags to Riches* | 57 |
| 5.4 | Boy with Mask, from *Still Lives* | 59 |
| 5.5 | E, from *Still Lives* | 60 |
| 5.6 | A.D. 1952 | 63 |
| 17.1 | Mondo Wiley – The Silent Scream of the Hippo | 219 |
| 17.2 | Schmarty | 234 |
| 17.3 | Havel | 235 |
| 17.4 | The Hero | 236 |

For Katherine, Georgie, and Mackey

# Acknowledgements

I would, first, like to acknowledge my dear friends and colleagues in Britain who have been a constant source of inspiration throughout the years in which these essays were written – most especially Sue Emmy Jennings and Alida Gersie. Both Sue and Alida have provided the dialogue and refreshing wells that I needed to drink from in order to remain connected to the field of drama therapy.

I would further like to express my appreciation for the extended community of European creative arts therapists whose fellowship has also provided a reason to be constant and committed.

I am proud to have discovered in Jessica Kingsley a publisher of vision who believes that the creative arts therapies are essential means of signifying and healing, and who is willing to champion many worthy volumes to that effect. I feel especially honored that Jessica is supporting this collection of my essays.

My appreciation goes to Ken Brannon, my graduate assistant at New York University, for his help in preparing the manuscript. And I sound a note of deep gratitude to Sylvia Halpern, the managing editor of *The Arts in Psychotherapy*, for her many years of support, camaraderie, kindness, and professional excellence.

I remain forever indebted to my students and clients who have allowed me a glimpse into their role systems and an opportunity to see in ways I never thought possible over these 15 years. I end with a special thanks to Sam, who taught me the meaning of the double life and provided the courageous example of how to live it.

## Acknowledgement of Previous Publications

I wish to thank Elsevier Science for permission to reprint a number of articles which first appeared in *The Arts in Psychotherapy*: Training the drama therapist: A four-part model; The use of distancing in drama therapy; Conceptual and methodological issues of research in drama therapy; The concept of role in drama therapy; A Taxonomy of roles: A blueprint for the possibilities of being; A research agenda for the creative arts therapies; The child, the dreamer, the artist and the fool: in search of understanding the meaning of expressive therapy; Three scenarios for the future of drama therapy; and Isolation and collaboration in the creative arts therapies: The implications of crossing borders.

The author and publisher thank *The Journal of Mental Imagery* for permission to reprint the articles: Puppets, dolls, objects, masks, and make-up; and The image of the mask: implications for theatre and therapy. I would also like to thank Routledge Publishers for permission to reprint the book chapters: One-on-one: the role of the drama therapist working with individuals, in Sue Jennings (ed) *Dramatherapy – Theory & Practice 2*; and The dramatic world view – Reflections on the roles taken and played by young children, in Sue Jennings (ed) *Dramatherapy with Children and Adolescents*.

Finally, 'A short-term model of drama therapy through the role method' originally appeared in Alida Gersie (ed) *Dramatic Approaches to Brief Therapy* published by Jessica Kingsley Publishers.

# Foreword

These essays, collected from Robert Landy's recent published and unpublished writings, represent a densely told story of the history of drama therapy, a hybrid form of one-to-one and group healing, derived from theatre and psychotherapy and to some extent superseding earlier approaches such as psychodrama and remedial drama. The story is, in part, a personal one, giving some insight into Landy's own struggle to establish a new genre of therapy, but the main purpose of this collection is to provide a firm theoretical base for a practice that uses a wide, flexible and seemingly limitless range of techniques. We are given striking glimpses of some of those techniques as they arise creatively from the clinical context Landy is describing, but for us to understand why they were chosen, why at that time and why handled in just that way, requires us to grasp the underlying rationale which this book so effectively explores.

In the first chapter Landy is at pains to give the field some validity by drafting out an inter disciplinary scheme of training in drama therapy. In 1982 his own course at New York University was already established and available as a model for other centres. We see in this chapter the beginnings of Landy's search for a vocabulary that will uniquely define his subject and the corresponding competences required of its leaders.

'Distancing' is to become a critical concept which he expands and consolidates in subsequent chapters. Drawn from performance theorists such as Bullough and Brecht, it suits Landy's purpose to conceive of 'distancing' as both an interpsychical and intrapsychical phenomenon which in its most healthy state achieves a balance between closeness and separation.

One of the book's intriguing threads traces Landy's changing conception of 'Self' (with a capital 'S'). At first accepting Sarbin's aphorism that 'The Self is what a person "is", the Role is what a person "does"', Landy gradually overrides this dualism by positing an image of 'a dramatic world view' peopled by a wide range of characters. Such a model frees him to work out a new central tenet of his theory and practice: that the healthy person can live with the tension of conflicting roles, leading 'a double life' of paradox and ambiguity.

Robert Landy is an acknowledged leader in the field of drama therapy. This book confirms him as a key figure in defining that field through sharp theoretical exposition and honest reporting of illuminative practice. He is aware, perhaps painfully aware, of the responsible position in which he is placed. He, of course, draws our attention to the need for hard research, indicating some of the directions it might take, but his concern necessarily extends to institutional problems, that is, to the place, in a diminishing world market, of drama therapy as reflected by its association of professional practitioners. The future viability of drama therapy as a recognized form of healing may be in part dependent on its choice of kinship. Historically linked with both the theatre and psychology, it may now be time to honour its implicit interpendence with expressive and creative arts therapies. In his practice Robert Landy demonstrates how drawing or modelling or music-making have a legitimate place in a role-playing scenario. 'Can you draw your anger?' might well be a natural first step towards expressing that emotion dramatically. For the drama therapist is operating first and foremost as an artist, inviting the client to find the artist in him/herself; in discovering (as for any other artist) something anew, the 'client/artist' may begin a process of self-healing.

That journey may be a long one, as illustrated in Landy's last chapter giving a penetrating account of sustained drama therapy over a period of three years, but drama therapy may also be effective as a medium or even short-term process. Its proven flexibility marks it as a form of therapy unparalleled in the healing profession. This dynamic collection of essays, written with such perception, clarity and passion, goes a long way to establishing its unquestionable stature.

*Gavin Bolton*
*University of Durham, England*

Look how men live, always precariously
Balanced between good and bad fortune.

*Sophocles*

In the midst of their prosperity
Florence and Dodger will never forget
the time when they were adrift in New York.

*Horatio Alger*

Without contraries is no progression.

*William Blake*

Let me call myself, for the present,
William Wilson.

*Edgar Allan Poe*

Call me Ishmael.

*Herman Melville*

# CHAPTER 1

# Training the Drama Therapist
## A Four-Part Model

As a field, drama therapy is a hybrid. It refers most obviously to two disciplines – drama/theatre and psychotherapy, implying principles and techniques that are common to both. After a brief discussion of the interdisciplinary nature of this relatively young field, I would like to present a four-part model of training the drama therapist. This approach will emphasize the need for the drama therapist to be skilled in drama/theatre and psychotherapy as these processes are applied to work with various disabled populations.

Before I proceed, let me try to clarify a few terms. When I speak of drama/theatre as a field, I am referring to an entire range of activities that vary according to form and purpose. I will use the term 'drama' to refer to more informal, improvisational enactments. Drama is both indigenous to human behavior, as we see in the play of children, and consciously applied to the education, recreation and therapy of individuals. Theatre on the other hand, refers to an actor's presentation of a script to an audience within a performance space. Although it can well serve an educational purpose, theatre generally is performed to entertain and/or to enlighten.

Psychotherapy refers to a range of verbal and action-oriented techniques of treating clients with psychological problems. Counseling implies a similar process, although counselors may see clients for a variety of reasons, vocational as well as personal. The larger academic field within which therapy and counseling subsist is that of psychology.

There is a long history of interrelationship between drama/theatre and psychology. Often, therapists and theatre artists share the same language. Role, for example, originally referred to an object upon which a portion of the text of a play was written. Today, theatre artists commonly use the term to refer to a character in a play. And in describing characteristics of everyday behavior, sociologists and psychologists also speak of behaviors in role. In the early twentieth century, the social scientists, Charles Cooley and George Herbert Mead, later to be known as symbolic interactionists, spoke of role-taking, the assimilation of roles from one's social environment, as an essential factor in determining self-concept.

The term 'mask' originally applied to religious then theatrical contexts, has also been used by therapists to describe a change in behavior or role in response to certain social circumstances. C.G. Jung used the term 'persona' to describe this phenomenon. This is another term borrowed from theatre, as we see in *dramatis personae* or cast of characters.

The brief passage in Aristotle's *Poetics* referring to catharsis has led to an abundance of psychotherapeutic theorizing and experimentation in the work of Freud, J.L. Moreno and scores of their followers.

Since the establishment of psychotherapy as a profession and academic discipline, theatre artists have routinely used the terms subconscious, ego, projection and repression to refer to aspects of actor training and dramatic criticism. Reading Stanislavski's *An Actor Prepares* (1936) is, in some ways, like reading the journal of a man experiencing psychoanalysis for the first time. The writings of such performance theorists as Jerzy Grotowski, Julian Beck and Antonin Artaud are replete with psychotherapeutic jargon and imagery. In referring to the cathartic potential of the theatre, Artaud (1958) writes:

> The theatre...releases conflicts, disengages powers, liberates possibilities... The action of the theatre, like that of the plague, is beneficial, for, impelling men to see themselves as they are, it causes the mask to fall, reveals the lie, the slackness, baseness and hypocrisy of our world. (p.31)

Of his actor training, Grotowski (1968) writes:

> I am talking of the method, I am speaking of the surpassing of limits, of a confrontation, of a process of self-knowledge and, in a certain sense, of a therapy. (p.131)

Psychotherapists and drama/theatre practitioners not only share a common rhetoric, but also share common objectives and techniques. The range of therapeutic and dramatic aims can be seen in terms of the following: cognitive aims, concerning understanding and insight; affective aims, concerning values and feelings; psychomotor aims, concerning body image and fluency of move-ment; aesthetic aims, concerning sensation, form and appreciation; and thera-peutic aims, concerning the development of healthy functioning and a change in behavior or consciousness.

Most drama educators would agree that all these aims apply to their work in schools and community organizations. Many of the standard educational drama texts, such as Winifred Ward's *Playmaking with Children* (1957), Peter Slade's *Child Drama* (1954) and Brian Way's *Development through Drama* (1967) explicitly re-state these aims.

Performance theorists and actor trainers also subscribe to these aims, although the emphasis can vary substantially. Bertolt Brecht, for example, bases his notion of epic theatre upon a cognitive perspective and a corresponding devaluation of empathy. His contemporary, Stanislavski, initially stressed affective objectives above all else, then discovered that psychomotor aims were equally important in training his actors. However, in practice, Brecht did create characters with whom actors and audiences could empathize. And Stanislavski did develop actors and productions of great intelligence. The point is that in spite of philosophical differences actor trainers have exemplified a confluence of aims through their work.

Some drama educators and theatre artists deny that they aim toward therapeutic goals, stating that they are not trained to deal with emotional problems. Although it is true that they are not trained therapists, it is equally true that they have chosen a profession concerned with the expression of feelings, with empathy, with catharsis and with the revelation of character. Even the most intellectual of Brecht's Lehrstücke (learning plays), such as *The Measures Taken*, concerns man's struggle to recreate a more sane, reasonable world. Brecht (1965) writes:

> Sink down in the filth
> Embrace the butcher
> But change the world: it needs it! (p.96–97)

Although actor trainers are not therapists, then, they do work toward therapeutic aims to help the actor achieve a fully functional representation of a character and to help the audience envision the possibilities for a healthier world.

Most therapists work toward a combination of affective, cognitive and psychomotor aims. Again, given certain perspectives, there is much variation. Behavioral therapists would be unlikely to speak of affective aims. Gestalt or primal therapists might de-emphasize cognition. And many therapists are uncomfortable with aesthetic aims. Yet some therapists proceed like a director of a play and aim toward helping their clients enact representations of their everyday lives. Psychodramatists actually call themselves directors. Some work with theatrical props and lighting to create a theatricalized environment in which to treat clients.

In the area of techniques, there are also many interrelationships. Psychodramatists use improvisation and role-playing. Stanislavski-oriented 'method' trainers use techniques of free association and affective memory. Drama techniques have become accepted means of training counselors. One training group, Performing Arts in Crisis Training (PACT), located in Manhattan, uses structured improvisations as their primary means of training mental health professionals to deal with crises within communities. Also, as drama educators have begun to work more frequently with disabled populations, they have sought out training in counseling and special education.

In spite of the great variation in frames of reference within each field and between the two fields, then, basic commonalities do exist as both explore the human dilemma of individuals struggling with crucial issues of their existence.

Anthropological concerns are also important in understanding the interdisciplinary nature of drama therapy. In 1975, David Cole wrote a convincing book, *The Theatrical Event*, analyzing performance from the point of view of the ritual and magical practices of the shaman, a spiritual healer, and the hungan, or one possessed by a spirit. Since theatre appears to have developed from early shamanic and religious practices which exemplified interrelated elements of performance and healing, then an understanding of these practices might well further our conceptualization of drama therapy.

There are many other interrelated sources that contribute to our understanding of drama therapy. We must know something of the function of play as it affects child development. We must understand the natural tendency for human beings to engage in identification, impersonation and role-play. We can also look to the work of the action-oriented psychotherapists such as Moreno and Perls who viewed the spontaneous moment as the crucial one in uncovering a client's deepest concerns.

Underlying all these sources is a most fundamental understanding of both the dramatic and the therapeutic process. It is called, variously, transference, representation and acting 'as if.' Both the therapeutic session and the dramatic enactment occur in a place removed from the actor/client's everyday environment. He comes to this isolated, safe place to create or re-create a representation of his everyday experience so that it can be explored and understood. As in psychoanalysis, he might transfer significant characteristics of his father, for example, onto his therapist. Or as in psychodrama, he might choose another in the group to represent the character, Father. Or he, himself, might be asked to act 'as if' he were the father in a particular scene.

Representation is a dramatic means of representing or re-enacting an incident that has already occurred or that might occur in the future. As a method it applies equally to shamanic and other religious practices, to the dramatic play of children, to fantasies and dreams, to the process of rehearsal and performance in theatre and to the act of healing through psychotherapeutic means. It is a basic dramatic process that implies two realities – the everyday and that removed from the everyday by means of a change in environment or consciousness. And it is within that representational environment where the client re-enacts roles and scenes from his everyday or fantasy life in order to understand them better and to learn how to integrate them back within his everyday environment.

The interdisciplinary nature of drama therapy and its underlying method of representation has many implications for training. I would like to propose a model for training the drama therapist that focuses upon four areas:

1.  The self, involving the development of personal creativity and psychological awareness;

2. The client, involving an understanding of various disabled groups;

3. The techniques, involving a range of interdisciplinary practices;

4. The theory, involving interdisciplinary principles and philosophical considerations.

Anyone contemplating a career in drama therapy might well begin with a self-evaluation of interests and competencies. Some people involved in drama/theatre as educators, artists or viewers may recognize that their attention is focused upon the more psychological aspects of acting, directing, writing, designing or viewing. These people might view psychological issues as more important than aesthetic ones. Or conversely, people involved in the mental health field might recognize a need to work through more dramatic means.

Having identified an interest to combine drama/theatre with therapy, one can then begin to evaluate one's competencies in both areas. Drama/theatre competencies include: the ability to engage in role-play and improvisation, to tell a story, to play, to work with masks and puppets and other projective techniques, to move flexibly and creatively, to use one's voice creatively, to develop and lead creative dramatic experiences, to create and perform scripted material and to help others do the same. Therapeutic competencies include: the ability to listen, to support and challenge others, to analyze issues, to interpret behavior and infer motivations, to feel comfortable dealing with a wide range of emotional and mental disorders, to appreciate individual differences and to develop strategies for change. If such descriptions are accurate statements of an individual's competencies, then he would be an excellent candidate for training as a drama therapist.

The first area of training concerns the development of personal creativity and psychological awareness. Many students who enter drama therapy programs do so with a background in theatre performance. These students should be encouraged to continue their creative work in the theatre, either through actual performing or taking further performance-oriented classes. To balance out their theatre training with work in informal, spontaneous drama, students should be exposed to courses in creative drama, improvisation and drama in education. Those with a solid educational drama background should, in a like manner, be encouraged to study and to experience theatre performance from the point of view of the actor, director, designer and/or writer.

Another important area in developing personal creativity is that of play. Through coursework, students can explore their spontaneity or inhibitions to play and the relationship between play and human development. Through courses and experiences in the related arts of music, dance and visual arts, students can further develop their personal creativity.

In training the drama therapist, it is not enough to simply expose students to these creative experiences. We must also provide a means for them to reflect upon their experiences and relate them to both their general psychological well-being and to that of others with whom they might work.

In developing psychological awareness, the student should also experience a process of therapy. This can occur through a student's private therapy and through classroom experiences in drama therapy, counseling and group process. Within classroom courses, students can work through simulation not only to develop their skills as therapists, but also to examine their own needs and behaviors. Coursework should include group counseling practices as well as individual counseling practices. Even though some drama therapists will never work with individuals, it is important that they develop an awareness of their personal style of counseling and of their fears and needs, strengths and weaknesses that affect interactions with others.

The second area of training concerns an awareness and understanding of various disabled groups. Drama therapists have generally worked with the following populations: the emotionally disturbed, the physically disabled – including deaf and blind groups – the developmentally disabled, the sociopathic, groups of incarcerated or ex-offenders, the language-impaired, the gifted and the elderly. Some drama therapists work with non-disabled individuals who are in crisis or in need of exploring certain confusing aspects of their lives. Even if the demand for drama therapists was to become as great as the demand for computer programmers, which is highly unlikely, practitioners still must be able to work competently with several populations. Although the few advertised positions might specify the need for a creative arts therapist to work with an outpatient psychiatric population or to develop a drama program at a residential center for the developmentally disabled, there may be great discrepancies between diagnostic labels and individual behavior.

We live in a time of specializations within specializations, but in some cases there are fewer jobs for specialists. I think it imperative that we train the drama therapist who is, after all, a specialist, to be able to work with the range of disabled and non-disabled groups. To do this, it is important, when teaching principles and techniques of drama therapy, to discuss and demonstrate their application to several populations.

Some students will take courses in the education and counseling of special populations. All should study normal human psychological development and abnormal psychology. Further, through fieldwork experiences, students should both observe and lead drama groups comprised of several populations.

As an adjunct to this area, it is also important for students to become familiar with the environments within which disabled people live, work and receive treatment. The types of environments as well as the quality of life there will vary considerably. Therefore, it is of added importance to encourage fieldwork placement at a variety of sites including city and state operated hospitals and special schools, private clinics and nursing homes, and any of a number of other community recreational and therapeutic centers. As it becomes evident that there are all too few organizations where drama therapy is consistently used as a method of treatment, students might be encouraged to design their own programs centered in such organizations as the YMCA, the church and various institutions for the elderly. These designs might be hypothetical, as beginning students research a selected population in a selected environment and write out a plan of treatment, or, with advanced students at the level of internship, a design might be implemented with, of course, the cooperation and support of a relevant community organization.

A drama therapy training program should include a practicum or internship component. Not only would students study the etiology, behavior and needs of disabled populations, but also work with them in the field for an extended period of time. At the graduate level, an internship in drama therapy might include approximately 20 hours per week for a period of two semesters or 30 weeks.

The third area of training concerns a competence in applying interdisciplinary techniques of drama therapy to treatment. My assumption is that with the knowledge and technical skill of both drama/theatre and psychotherapy, the student will be well prepared to practice drama therapy. In reality, most drama therapists come from either one or the other discipline. Few psychodramatists, for example, come from a strong background in drama/theatre. The leading figures in this country tend to be sociologists, clinical psychologists and other mental health professionals. Likewise, many professional theatre artists or drama educators who work with disabled populations have little formal training in psychotherapy or minimal academic study of psychology. Of this group, some may call themselves drama therapists. Others refer to their work as drama or theatre practiced purely for recreational, educational or aesthetic purposes.

The actual techniques used by drama therapists will be based essentially in the area of drama/theatre. In the case of such therapeutic practices as psychodrama and Gestalt therapy, we find that therapists not only work through drama techniques, but also base their entire theoretical perspective upon the representational nature of dramatic action.

The basic dramatic techniques available include: short-term drama exercise in sensory awareness, movement, pantomime and creative speech; dramatic play; storytelling and story dramatization; role-playing; puppetry and mask work; simulation and improvisation; and extended dramatizations as practiced by Dorothy Heathcote and Gavin Bolton. These techniques do not exist in isolation of each other. For example, puppetry work may also include storytelling. In essence, all of the above techniques are improvisational in nature. It is important for the student to experience these techniques as participant and as leader. He must become aware, too, of the strengths and weaknesses of each technique and of its relevance to treating a specific disabled population within a specific environment and time frame. A student might be expert in the use of storytelling and verbal games, but, given a nonverbal group of profoundly disturbed children, such a treatment strategy would be inappropriate. Likewise, emphasizing pantomime and game-playing with certain groups of elderly people can also prove inappropriate, especially if they are mistrustful of any recreational experience they perceive as childish or demeaning.

Further, a student might be trained to work in an ongoing group, but finds himself in an internship or job situation with a short-term group of outpatients that is never consistent from week to week. Again, all techniques should be learned and viewed in relation to various environmental, human and bureaucratic realities.

The technique that is most widely practiced and in some ways most insufficiently examined, is theatre performance. In looking at the groups who practice drama/theatre with the disabled in this country, we find an overwhelming emphasis upon performance. These groups include The National Theatre of the Deaf, The National Theatre Workshop of the Handicapped, Theatre Unlimited and The Rainbow Theatre, among others.

On the one hand, these groups are not in the business of drama therapy, nor would they claim to be so. However, they are concerned with the therapeutic goals of building positive self-concept, group identity and a public awareness as to the cultural experiences of the disabled. When the therapeutic goals become secondary to more theatrical goals of pleasing audiences and presenting commercially-viable, slick products that can compete with Broadway fare, then the therapeutic aspect of the experience will be compromised. In my opinion, this is the greatest threat of using theatre with disabled groups.

It might very well be that all human beings have the inherent dramatic need to perform and to be applauded for their performance. In process-oriented drama therapy work, we try to explore this need through helping the client discover that his actions are worthy of positive self-regard, that he can become a competent performer in everyday life. It is more difficult to make the case for theatre in that the goal for many involved is an unrealistic one – to become a star. The performance art of theatre is not necessarily for everyone. The expressive art of spontaneous drama is for all, as we are all performers in everyday life. Drama therapy, I think, can also be a form of treatment for all people, regardless of their inherent theatrical abilities.

I do not mean to imply, though, that theatre has no place in treatment. It does. It has worked very effectively with groups of prisoners and ex-offenders, for example, who needed a positive creative outlet and tight structure through which they could express themselves cooperatively. But if groups begin to compete with commercial theatre, a myriad of problems develop – financial, artistic and psychological. Prison plays were very much in vogue eight years ago during the successful run of Miguel Piñero's *Short Eyes*. At that time, federal funding was available. Now, as federal funding is minimal and the public is interested in other 'diversions', theatre-in-prisons organizations have disbanded or are in severe financial difficulties.

The implication for training in all this is that the student needs to be able to distinguish between theatre as therapy and theatre that aims toward commercial viability. When groups such as the National Theatre of the Deaf go commercial and compete for money with high-powered commercial producers, they must make many compromises that more often than not diminish their identity and effectiveness in raising consciousness as to the deaf cultural experience.

The student of drama therapy, though, should become well acquainted with the basics of theatre production – how to build and light a set, how to act, direct and write dramatic pieces. The main reason is that he will probably be asked to produce a play in a hospital or other community setting. Administrators want plays. Patients want plays. When most people think of drama, they think of plays. Theatre can be a most positive therapeutic experience, but only if all involved are willing to confront the hard philosophical and psychological issues of performance. We all want to be stars; we all want recognition. Some have such overwhelming needs for recognition that they develop emotional problems and seek treatment. Drama therapists can deal with this kind of therapeutic issue. But often in their zeal to get a show up on stage that looks 'professional' and to prove that the disabled can sing and dance and act, they lose sight of the therapeutic issues.

A drama therapy program should, then, provide training in the techniques and aesthetics of performance, but should also encourage continual exploration of the therapeutic issues inherent in performance.

There is another dramatic technique relevant to training that bridges the gap between drama and theatre. It is called theatre-in-education or TIE. TIE originated in England during the mid-1960s as a method of teaching aspects of the curriculum often avoided in schools. TIE programs have dealt with sexuality, racism, violence and any of a number of political, social and historical issues. The TIE team is comprised of people trained as actors and teachers who develop a script around a central issue, present it to a group of students who often participate in the dramatic action, then follow up their work through discussion or relevant curricular tie-ins. Through training in TIE, the student of drama therapy can learn to build scripts around concerns of the disabled and develop programs to work with disabled students or clients through a process of viewing, participating in and reflecting upon the issues presented. To my knowledge, TIE has not as yet been adapted for use in drama therapy.

The student of drama therapy would also be trained in individual and group counseling techniques. As mentioned above, it is important for students to participate in group and individual counseling sessions as clients. It is also imperative that they acquire experience in leading such sessions. Through simulation and laboratory experiences, students can develop appropriate skills.

There are a wide variety of counseling and therapeutic orientations. Gestalt therapists work very differently than psychoanalysts. Behavioral therapists work very differently than Rogerian therapists. In group counseling, there also exists a variety of approaches. Tavistock groups, encounter groups, psychodrama groups, among others, imply particular technical knowledge.

Students of drama therapy should become aware of the various therapeutic perspectives and techniques applied to treatment. Each one is valuable for diagnostic and evaluative purposes, as well as for providing a model for understanding human behavior. However, their practical training will focus upon those techniques that are dramatic in nature or adaptable to drama therapy. Special attention should be focused, therefore, in the most obviously dramatic of therapies, that of psychodrama. The problem in training the student in psychodrama is deciding how much training is sufficient. The American Society of Group Psychotherapy and Psychodrama specifies that a certified director of psychodrama will have completed in excess of 700 hours of training. In a three or four credit university course, the student will normally receive 30–45 hours of training. Therefore, those students seeking certification as psychodramatists would complete their training privately with a qualified director.

Many will not invest the time in such extensive training. In fact, most students will acquire a *mélange* of technical knowledge rooted in diverse therapeutic and dramatic practices. Some of this technical knowledge may be rather superficial. A 30-hour course in psychodrama or in improvisational techniques for psychiatric populations will certainly not provide sufficient training. However, students will acquire those skills that relate to their personal styles of working. Through their classroom training and internships, that style will be developed and refined.

The techniques of drama therapy exist in relationship to each other. Psychodrama can be enacted with puppets. Theatre rehearsal can be conducted improvisationally. The psychodramatic technique of the double can be used in pantomime. The technical connections are endless. Through training drama therapists in technique, then, we are helping them to understand the range of representational practices available and develop means of adapting these prac-tices in ways consistent with their psychological and creative strengths and consistent with the needs of specific disabled populations.

The fourth and final area of training is that of theory. Given a series of relevant techniques and aware, creative leaders to implement them with various populations, the question still arises – why? Why is drama therapy important? What principles of drama therapy exist to justify its use as a valid treatment strategy? These are certainly crucial questions. There are few existing jobs. Few jobs are advertised. Sources of federal and state funding available for research are shrinking by the day. Most people have never heard of drama therapy. Those that have generally are suspicious of theatre people dabbling in 'medical concerns' or psychologists dabbling in theatre.

Why, then, go on? Because we must. Because we intuit that the dramatic process of representation is essential to all human development; that the child's cognition and affect develop through drama and play; that a severe limitation in the adolescent or adult's ability to play a role in everyday life or to engage in a diversity of role behaviors can lead to alienation, loneliness and violent or self-destructive behavior.

There has been much significant research in diverse fields to justify these statements. In sociology, we can look to the work of the symbolic interactionists and role-theorists, like Goffman, Mead and Cooley. In anthropology, we can look to the studies of ritual, play and cross-cultural practices in the work of Margaret Mead, Johan Huizinga and Geza Roheim. In psychology, we can look to the studies of play, symbolic thinking and human development in the work of Jean Piaget, Sigmund Freud and Erik Erikson. In educational drama, we can look at the work in developmental drama, dramatic play and creative drama as developed by Peter Slade, Richard Courtney and Winifred Ward. In theatre and performance theory, we can look at Stanislavski's notion of affective memory, Brecht's notion of alienation, Artaud's notion of theatre as a primal event, Grotowski's notion of *via negativa*, of theatre as a laboratory for confrontation and self-knowledge. In philosophy, we can look at the work of John Dewey, Martin Buber and Suzanne Langer in clarifying the process of human develop-ment through aesthetic and dialogical means. And in the area of the language arts, we can look to the work of James Britton, who sees language as a way of re-presenting our world views, and James Moffett, who sees drama as the most essential mode of human discourse.

This interdisciplinary perspective can provide the theoretical foundation for graduate study in drama therapy. Principles of drama therapy and appropriate research methodologies can be developed from these interrelated perspectives. But the process of delineating principles and research methods must be carefully conceived and subject to much discussion and experimentation. Students need to realize the difficulties inherent in studying a new field that is essentially a hybrid. Definitive definitions and lists of objectives, principles and research methods are premature. Students of drama therapy need to be encouraged to wrestle with the hard theoretical issues – What is drama therapy? Why is it valuable? How does one collect and analyze data to research its effectiveness? And as trainers, we must not pretend to have firm answers to these questions, as we, too, must explore the same issues.

This four-part model for training drama therapists is based in a university setting and is designed for students at the graduate level. It is an attempt to respond to four questions – What must the leader of a drama therapy group know about himself? Who are the clients in a drama therapy group? What techniques must the drama therapy leader master in order to effectively treat his clients? Why is this form of treatment valuable? A fifth and larger question that has really been present throughout this chapter is – What is the nature of drama therapy?

It will take many years of training and research before we can approach answers to these questions. As my personal background is interdisciplinary and I am a trainer of drama therapists, I have naturally adopted an interdisciplinary perspective. I see training as essentially a study of the techniques and principles of drama/theatre, psychology, counseling, play, anthropology and the related areas of special education, recreation and interrelated arts therapies.

There are several academic and individual training programs in drama therapy at various stages of development. The most prominent training center for psychodrama is the Moreno Institute in Beacon, New York. Undergraduate drama therapy programs are underway at California State University in Los Angeles and Loyola University in New Orleans. At New York University, an MA and PhD specialization in drama therapy within the Program in Educational Theatre is developing. Other programs in the formative stages include those at Avila College in Kansas City and Antioch College in San Francisco. Various courses in drama therapy are taught regularly by Dr Eleanor Irwin at the University of Pittsburgh and Dr Barbara Sandberg at William Patterson College in Wayne, New Jersey. Professor Gertrud Schattner of New York City and Dr David Johnson of New Haven regularly train private students.

Drama therapy has been incorporated within interrelated creative arts therapy programs such as the Expressive Therapies Program at Lesley College in Cambridge, Massachusetts, and Media and Arts for Social Services (MASS) at the University of Connecticut at Storrs.

New training programs have also been developing in England. Examples include SESAME, a private institution specializing in movement and drama work, and several colleges, such as The College of Ripon and St John in York and Kingsway Princeton College in London.

Further, two professional organizations have developed – The National Association for Drama Therapy in the United States, and The British Association for Dramatherapists in England.

Those of us who are presently creative arts therapists or educators and those of us who are studying to become professionals in the field have a particularly important responsibility. At a time in our political history when the arts are most desperately needed to reveal the absurdities of armaments and pollution, of violence and greed, of loneliness and personal misery, political officials are withdrawing their support. We must work together to make a strong case that drama in relationship to all the arts is essential as a means of making meaning, of restoring equilibrium and health within individuals and families, among communities and societies.

Before countries engage in war, they rehearse their soldiers through the dramatic technique of war games. We, too, have a battle to fight that is quite difficult and risky. Through our research, our dialogue, our further development of training programs, we must prepare for the business of helping people, all people, live their lives as fully as possible.

# CHAPTER 2

# The Use of Distancing in Drama Therapy

Drama therapy as a discipline is still very much in its formative stages of development. Being an interdisciplinary form, it borrows its concepts and techniques freely from drama/theatre, sociology, psychology, psychotherapy and psychodrama. However, drama therapists have neither clearly specified nor sufficiently researched which concepts and techniques are most relevant to the development of a theoretical base and to the treatment of specific populations. This chapter will examine one such concept, that of distancing, which has been explored in some detail in the fields of drama/theatre, sociology and psychology.

All human interactions can be characterized by the degree of distance therein. Distancing is a means of separating oneself from the other, bringing oneself closer to the other, and generally maintaining a balance between the two states of separation and closeness. The distance can be physical, as in maintaining a space of so many feet from another in a face-to-face conversation; or it can be emotional, as in choosing whether or not to empathize with another's personal dilemma; or the distance can be intellectual, as in choosing to analyze rather than empathize with another's problem. In actuality, distancing is a confluence of physical, emotional, and intellectual elements.

Distancing, however, does not only refer to a person-to-person interaction. It is also an intrapsychic phenomenon, as individuals identify closely with certain roles they play and separate themselves from other roles. One might make a strong identification with one's professional role, for example, but remove oneself from one's family roles, e.g. son or husband. This might express itself behaviorally in viewing the person as self-assertive, positive and energetic at work, yet passive, negative and sluggish at home.

Furthermore, at the intrapsychic level, one can remove or create distance from one's own feelings, thoughts and physical self-image. For example, an individual feeling a sense of alienation might perceive his image in a mirror as being somewhat disconnected from himself.

The concept of distancing is particularly relevant to drama therapy since the drama therapist draws upon a wide range of psychodramatic and projective

13

techniques that implies a variation of relationship between self and role, self and other. Some dramatic media, such as puppetry and mask, imply a projection of the self and, thus, a certain kind of intrapsychic and interpersonal distancing.

Also, inasmuch as the drama therapist characteristically plays a more active and flexible role than a psychoanalyst, for one, and at times becomes a player in the client's drama, he needs to become aware of the implications of his interactions with clients, of his closeness to and separation from them, of the issues of transference and countertransference that arise given his active participation.

Furthermore, distancing is relevant to drama therapy in that the therapist bases much of his work in examining the dialectics of actor and observer, self and role, one role and another role; and it is in exploring the degree of separation and closeness within these relationships that the therapist realizes his therapeutic goals. These goals include enhancing the client's ability to differentiate between roles, to gain further mastery of a single role, or to expand his repertory of roles. More specifically, the drama therapist might aim toward helping clients distinguish between behavior appropriate to themselves and behavior appropriate to characters who are not themselves. A most important therapeutic goal might also be to help clients find the proper balance between participation in a dramatic action and observation of that action, that is, a balance between self as subject and self as object.

Throughout this chapter, I will argue that distancing is a central concept and tool in the dramatic treatment of clients and that the drama therapist can be more effective in his treatment if he can understand the dimensions of distancing as applied to his choice of techniques, the needs of his clients, and his relationship to his clients.

Before looking directly at the application of distancing to the practice of drama therapy, I will examine its use as a concept in the fields of drama/theatre, psychology and sociology. I will draw upon Bertolt Brecht's theatrical notions of the alienation effect, then look at a social-psychological model as specified by the sociologist and therapist, Thomas Scheff. Distancing as a theatrical concept is to a great extent centered in the metaphor of the world as stage or the stage as world. The actor and the spectator in the theatre are removed from the everyday world, but paradoxically recreate that world through an identification with and participation in the fictional reality of the characters and scenes presented. All is artifice in the theatre. The performers play characters who are not themselves; the set and props merely represent real rooms and real objects; lamps and spotlights represent a variety of natural light and darkness. Yet within the fiction, there is truth to the extent that both actors and viewers suspend their disbeliefs and participate physically, emotionally and intellectually in the dramatic actions. If the world is not a stage, but, rather, like a stage, then one could manipulate and study the distance between the stage and the world for a variety of aesthetic and therapeutic purposes.

Viewers of theatre are constantly shifting between participant and observer roles. As they relive an experience stimulated by a dramatic action, they can be so underdistanced that they believe it is they, rather than the actors, who are having an experience. Conversely, the dramatic action might be so alienating that they remain safely aloof, looking in. In balancing the dual roles of participant and viewer, the audience member is engaging in an unconscious act of distancing.

The director and designer of a play are more conscious manipulators of distance. They often choose the extent to which they want their actors and viewers to identify with and participate in the action (underdistance) or the extent to which they want them to separate themselves from the action (overdistance) in order to see more of the universal aspects of the drama. Their methods are based in a choice in style of acting and design, whether highly stylized, as in the *commedia dell'arte* and more modern expressionistic forms, or rather naturalistic, as in the forms influenced by Stanislavski's methods (1936) and the derivative Actor's Studio in America.

Bertolt Brecht is regarded as a modern master of theatrical distancing. His model for a distanced theatre, epic theatre, stood in marked contrast to the more traditional dramatic theatre of the early twentieth century. The epic theatre for Brecht was one where narrative had supremacy over drama, where the spectator became an observer of the action, rather than a participant in the action, and was encouraged to face a certain situation and make decisions, rather than become involved in a situation and luxuriate in it. The epic theatre presented a circular rather than linear structure where each scene was meaningful and whole in itself, rather than one scene leading directly, consecutively, and chronologi-cally into another. In the epic theatre, reason played the primary role; feeling was secondary (Willett 1964).

Brecht's epic theatre, at least in theory, was one dependent upon an emotional overdistancing. His Verfremdungs-Effect or alienation-effect implied a separation of actor from role and of spectator from a reliving of the dramatic events presented. It was Brecht's notion that if the actors and spectators could overdistance, then they would be liberated from expected and conventional responses to the drama. According to Brecht, this liberation was possible only if the rational, analytic part of the spectator and actor was not superseded by the irrational, feeling part that led one to an easy identification with characters and restimulation of experiences.

Brecht achieved his overdistancing effects in many ways. By calling his theatre a narrative theatre, he attempted to transform the dramatic first personal form into the narrative third personal form. In rehearsal, he asked his actors to view their characters as 'he' and 'she' rather than 'I,' and to demonstrate through their actions the contradictions within their characters. In readings of the text during early rehearsals, Brecht would ask his actors to include readings of the stage directions, again stressing the narrative nature of his aesthetic. During performance, spectators would see frequent use of slides, titles, and placards, stating settings of scenes, historical facts and quotations underlining moral and political points. Further, Brecht used music as a device of overdistancing. Rather than having his music reveal a character's sentiments and inner thoughts and proceed directly from the dramatic action, Brecht set his songs apart from the flow of the action and through irony and commentary used them as a way to elucidate a political or moral issue.

Other epic theatre devices of overdistancing included the use of puppets and masks, oversized props, and highly stylized gestures and blocking, all intended to help the actor and spectator see beyond the individual case to the universal condition.

As a model of distancing, however, Brecht's theory is incomplete. In that his concern was primarily for overdistancing, he did not take into consideration the human need for a balance of attention. Ironically, Brecht has been successful to the extent that his theory was not realized on the stage. That is, actors and viewers did identify with the characters. Tears were shed when Kattrin died in *Mother Courage* and even when Mac the Knife was about to be hanged in *The Threepenny Opera*. When an authentic epic theatre production of a Brecht play is staged today, some 63 years after the writing of *Baal*, Brecht's first major work for the theatre, audiences are often baffled and unsatisfied because they do experience too much aesthetic distance. It is, of course, difficult to define what an 'authentic' epic theatre production is, although Brecht and his collaborators have left behind model books of various productions, including photographs and stage directions. Even the most 'authentic' production would be very much dependent upon the director's and others' interpretation of Brecht's dramaturgy.

In shifting from a theatrical to a therapeutic context, let us look at another model of distancing that attempts to address the human need for a balance of attention. The model, developed by Thomas Scheff, goes beyond Brecht in accounting for an aesthetic distance that is midway between overdistance and underdistance. In that Scheff's model is psychotherapeutically-based and derivative from psychological sources (Freud and Breuer 1966; Jackins 1965), it is not directly comparable to the theatrically-based Brechtian model. Yet, Scheff's conceptual thinking about distancing includes a discussion of dramatic criticism and an analysis of levels of awareness of characters in and viewers of classical drama (Scheff 1976, 1979). Furthermore, Scheff uses the central concept of catharsis to characterize the balance of attention between overdistance and underdistance, borrowing the term from theatre, as Aristotle was the first to formally speak of dramatic catharsis in his *Poetics* (1954). In fact, the concept of catharsis has been used historically by psychotherapists and theatre artists alike with some frequency (Freud and Breuer 1966; Moreno 1946, 1959; Aristotle 1954; Nichols and Zax 1977; Boal 1979). The originator of psychodrama, J. L. Moreno, bridged the natural gap between psychotherapy and improvisational drama by basing his work in both fields and speaking of catharsis from both the dramatic and psychotherapeutic points of view.

In Scheff's model (1981), catharsis occurs when the participant or viewer relives emotions, but is not overwhelmed by them. That is to say, there is a balance between overdistance, which Scheff refers to as a state of repression, and underdistance, which he calls the return of repressed emotion. Overdistancing becomes a cognitive process of remembering the past; underdistancing, an affective process of reliving or reexperiencing a past event. At aesthetic distance, the two extreme states are in balance, and the participant/observer is able to return to the past safely, that is, through both remembering and reliving a past event.

Remembering implies a more passive observer role, as one looks back over time at oneself or at specified events. Reliving implies a more active participant role as past events are restimulated and the individual plays them out again in his mind or in action. At aesthetic distance, the individual plays both roles of participant and observer simultaneously; or he is able to move fluidly from one role to another, as appropriate. The appropriateness of the role choice would depend upon the individual's need for distance. For example, at a holiday dinner with the family, there are many levels of distancing in effect. If one feels threatened by the demands or criticisms of one's relatives, one might move into an observer role to create the proper safe distance. Conversely, if one becomes too overdistanced thus feeling alienated from the family, one might shift into a more active participant role through direct interaction with the family. In this particular example, the drama associated with the family gathering is dependent upon a restimulation of past experiences with the family. For the individual family member to achieve a proper balance of attention, he must have access to both observer and participant roles so that he has a sense of history and connectedness with the family as well as a sense of himself as an independent person in relationship to them in the present.

Scheff takes his discussion of distancing further by stating that at aesthetic distance a central paradox of repressed emotion is resolved. That paradox, stated in the form of a question, is: If the reason we repress emotion is because it is too painful to bring to consciousness, then how can we be able to bring ourselves to a conscious awareness of that painful state? An example of the paradox is the common fear: 'If I would ever allow myself to get mad at person X, that is, consciously express my anger and rage toward X, I would certainly kill him.' The answer to the above question, according to Scheff, is that we can handle painful repressed emotion through manipulating distance, through simultaneously playing participant and observer roles. If the emotion becomes too unbearable, we can achieve a margin of safety in the observer role. By in fact standing outside ourselves, by watching ourselves enact an episode of severe anger through screaming and gesticulating, for example, where we fear that we might kill the object of our anger, we create enough distance to feel somewhat in control.

One drama therapy student recently reported an episode where he expressed severe anger and hostility toward his parents. He acted out his rage by screaming, sobbing, cursing, banging his fists on the table and verbally attacking them, all behaviors he had never demonstrated before. As he was acting out his anger and feeling quite out of control, he nevertheless reported an awareness that he would not go too far because he became aware of seeing himself performing his actions as they were occurring. That is, in order to safeguard himself from the fear of losing control and committing an act of physical violence against his parents, he assumed, unconsciously, an observer role to provide a safe margin of distance.

In a psychotherapeutic context, it is the therapist who modulates distance, or rather the therapist helps the client to achieve a balance of distance. The assumption here is that the therapist perceives balance of distance as a desirable goal. In Scheff's terms, the therapist would help the client reach catharsis through moving him to a point of aesthetic distance, a balance between overdistance and underdistance, between remembering and reliving, between participating and observing.

Scheff mentions four choices that the therapist can make in managing aesthetic distance. They include: the use of present time events vs. past time events; fictional or fantasy events vs. reality events; a rapid reviewing of past events vs. a detailed recollection of the past; and the enactment of positive emotions vs. the enactment of negative or unpleasant ones. Generally speaking, the use of present time, fiction or fantasy, rapid review and positive emotions provide the client with a means of overdistancing. The converse would lead the client toward an underdistanced enactment.

Like most listings of polarities, Scheff's notions are not intended to be prescriptive in an absolute sense. Rather, they are intended to provide a range of choice for the actual client whose needs for both over- and underdistance vary with great frequency. Further, Scheff emphasizes the importance of training the therapist to be flexible in choosing modes of distancing to suit the needs of a client, instead of depending upon a fixed conception of either underdistance or overdistance.

There are many techniques of distancing in drama therapy that can be drawn from Brecht, Moreno, Scheff and from many other theatre artists, educational drama specialists, sociologists and psychologists. The choice of technique would depend upon three basic factors: the quality of distance inherent in the technique, the special need of a client at a given moment in the therapeutic process, and the therapeutic goals of the therapist. Generally speaking, diagnostic categories of clients and therapeutic goals, like specific techniques, can be seen as implying a specific degree of distancing. However, the use of distancing in drama therapy often is situationally based and dependent upon the changing needs of the client or therapist and the flexible quality of a given technique.

Techniques of distancing in drama therapy include: the use of narrative or storytelling; projective techniques such as dolls, puppets, masks, makeup and videotape; psychodramatic techniques such as role-reversal and doubling; sociodramatic techniques such as caricature and social group rather than individual role-playing.

Storytelling has a function in the overdistanced epic theatre that is different from its use in the dramatic theatre. In the latter, the story of a past event told by a character must point to a present dramatic situation that is emotionally based. Hamlet asks the players to enact the story of the murder of Gonzago so that he might 'catch the conscience of the king' at the present moment. The characters in Eugene O'Neill's *Long Day's Journey Into Night* tell their long narratives in order to affect each other in the present and to purge themselves of endless years of guilt and anger.

In the epic theatre, however, the story functions as fable and has a 'once upon a time' quality. The narrative of what happened stays within the confines of a past that might be historically-based, as in *Galileo*, or mythically-based, as in *The Good Woman of Szechwan*, and does not necessarily lead to the classic dramatic structures of hamartia, anagnorisis, catastrophe, and catharsis. Because the play is enacted as a story, as events which have occurred in the past, the spectator is not led to believe that the events dramatized are happening now, and thus is able to maintain a psychic distance from the action.

In drama therapy, storytelling is used frequently. Play therapists often ask children with emotional problems to tell stories based upon dolls or objects they have been manipulating. Psychodramatists direct clients of all ages and with varying degrees of emotional problems in enacting stories from their lives. Storytelling has become increasingly popular with groups of elderly (Perlstein 1981).

The use of storytelling in drama therapy can be conceptualized along a continuum. At one pole is the most underdistanced kind of psychodramatic enactment where the client tells a story from his own life, reexperiences emotion from the past or previews emotion associated with the future. Through catharsis, the client releases tension in tears, laughter, shaking, blushing, etc. At the other pole is the most overdistanced form of storytelling, based in the epic theatre model, where clients create a story that does not relate overtly to their own lives. The story may be set in an imaginary land inhabited by fictional characters. These epic stories might be narrated verbally, enacted dramatically, or com- posed on a moving story board, used often by Brecht. The story board is also known as a crankie, because a handle or crank moves the scroll, upon which the story has been composed, forward. In working with a crankie, clients are not only exposed to a dramatic experience in creating a story, but also to an art experience as the story is drawn in words and images on long sheets of paper.

The easiest way to construct a crankie is to take a roll of adding machine paper and ask the client to create a story on it by drawing pictures and using words. Then both ends of the paper are attached to pencils. When the story is presented, two people hold the pencils and wind the paper from one side to the other, as if unwinding a scroll.

Either extreme of psychodramatic storytelling or epic theatre style storytelling may be indicated for specific clients in need of over- or underdistancing. A group of verbal elderly clients might work comfortably with underdistanced autobiographical material, while a group of psychotic children would need further distancing in working with story material. In most cases, though, the drama therapist is likely to move between the two poles as he discovers the proper balance necessary to lead the client to aesthetic distance.

The use of such projective devices as dolls, puppets, masks, and makeup is also valuable in facilitating distance within a drama therapy session. Dolls and puppets have become a mainstay in most forms of play therapy. As projective devices, they allow most clients a safe margin of overdistance. Although there have been several articles and books written about puppetry in therapy (Philpott 1977; Irwin and Shapiro 1975), little actual research has uncovered the therapeutic potential of this powerful projective device.

In observing drama therapy sessions, this author has noted that some clients react in an underdistanced way when confronted with puppets and/or masks. Masks especially can be frightening to severely emotionally disturbed clients, because their sense of their own face and body is rather precarious. As imaginative, representational extensions of the face and the body, masks, dolls and puppets can be both underdistancing, to the degree that the client is unable to make a separation between self and inanimate object; and overdistancing, to the degree that the client is able to make that distinction and endow the inanimate object with human characteristics, that is, to project himself onto the object.

In working with puppetry as a way to achieve aesthetic distance, the drama therapist might begin with a relatively nonthreatening, overdistanced kind of enactment. This might take the form of asking the client to build a puppet, or choose a puppet, that represents a character quite removed from oneself and create a story or dramatic action with the puppet as the central character. The balance of distance can be altered by encouraging the client to conceive the puppet as closer to himself, or to create a new puppet figure that represents a part of himself. At a more underdistanced level, the therapist might ask the client to build a puppet that represents a hidden part of himself and create a scene where that part is revealed.

In working with severely emotionally disturbed clients, the therapist might aim toward helping them recognize the difference between self and puppet. He would thus work toward moving from an underdistanced posture to an overdistanced one. His approach might be different with a less severe group of withdrawn, emotionally repressed adolescents who need to move from emotional overdistance to underdistance in order to demonstrate an affective response within the drama.

The building of puppets, like the construction of the crankie, is an experience in drama and art. The value of creating one's own puppet as opposed to using a prefabricated one is that it brings the client into a closer relationship with the character he is creating.

Masks are generally less distancing than dolls and puppets. For one, the client in mask is altering his own face rather than manipulating an object apart from his actual body. The mask is separate from the body, yet part of the body when it is worn on the face. The experience of building a mask to wear has a certain ceremonial and magical quality (Sorell 1974). And because masks are associated not only with ancient cultures engaged in hunting, battle, or burial activities, but also with contemporary images of muggers and psychopathic killers in horror movies, they can be rather frightening in their underdistancing qualities.

However, with proper use, masks can provide a balance of attention. As an example, one client was asked to create simple masks out of paper bags to represent the members of her family, herself included. Having set up a dinner table scene and placing the masks on selected members of the drama therapy group, she was asked by the therapist to wear the mask of each family member, one at a time, and engage in a dialogue with the others, in role. The therapist helped create overdistance in this scene, when necessary, by encouraging a fairly rapid changing of roles, humorous dialogue, and helping the client shift from participant to observer role. Conversely, he worked toward underdistance through encouraging more intense dialogue within a single role. Generally the therapist worked toward a balance of attention which in this case was achieved as the client experienced both laughter and tears, followed by a verbal expression of her ability to better understand the dynamics of the family's interactions.

At an even more underdistanced level, the drama therapist can work with makeup where the client is actually creating a character or part of himself on his own face. Work in this area has been demonstrated by Nancy Breitenbach, who practices drama therapy with emotionally disturbed children, primarily through the use of makeup, in Paris, France. Breitenbach (1979) has compiled a developmental scale that represents age ranges at which children create certain forms on their faces through the application of makeup.

The process of making oneself up has all the ceremonial and magical qualities of mask-making. It is potentially more underdistanced though, because there is no longer a separation of the face. The face becomes the mask; the mask becomes the face. In Breitenbach's work, the act of applying makeup is in itself a therapeutic process. Dramatic action in role does not necessarily follow. The object of the drama therapy in this instance is the creation of the role through making up the face. Of course, dramatic action in the form of improvisation could occur after the makeup has been applied. The client might be asked to look at himself in a mirror and speak a monologue or soliloquy in response to his own image, or he might be asked to engage in a dialogue with other characters. The therapist can manipulate the distance through helping the client conceive of his made-up character as close to or removed from himself. Too, through encouraging light or heavy enactments, present or past events, fantasy or real characterization, positive or negative feelings, participant or observer roles, the therapist will be balancing distance within the experience of applying makeup and acting in role of the made-up character.

The very least distanced dramatic technique based in a projection of body and/or face concerns a view of oneself as oneself, without the guise of puppet, mask, or makeup. This can be achieved through the use of a mirror or through the use of a video recorder and monitor that can record and playback one's actions. If the equipment is available, work in video can be quite powerful (Fryrear and Fleshman 1982).

In an experiment by this author, clients were instructed to sit in front of a video camera for five minutes without leaving the range of the camera. Following the sitting, the tape was played back to the client and he was asked to verbalize his reactions to the tape. This procedure was also videotaped. During the third part, the client watched the final videotape and verbalized and recorded his reactions in writing.

The distancing process proceeded from a very much underdistanced perspective of sitting in front of a camera with no specific objective, of acting without an action, of being fully oneself apart from a social context; toward an overdistanced perspective of being an observer of oneself, twice removed, of watching oneself watching. Within this one video experience, then, the drama therapist has available a range of distancing perspectives he can modulate to help the client achieve a balance of attention so that he may be able to more clearly see the face or faces or masks he fashions.

Psychodramatic techniques can also be used to balance distance. As implied above, psychodrama is basically a technique of underdistancing, as the protagonist usually plays the role of himself and is asked to relive experiences from his own life. The psychodramatic enactment often leads to catharsis, and many psychodrama directors aim toward an overt emotional release. Even when dealing with past or future events, the protagonist is encouraged to enact them in a present time frame, with all associated feelings. Negative feelings and detailed recall are often enacted in psychodrama, thus underlying its underdistancing quality. However, devices within the psychodramatic technique serve to overdistance the protagonist. For example, if the protagonist is at a point of being overflooded with emotion, he might be asked to reverse roles with the auxiliary ego, and thus move from a participant to an observer role. Through a carefully modulated series of role-reversals, the director is able to balance the distance, and thus move the protagonist closer to aesthetic distance and its corresponding catharsis. As psychodrama is the most overtly catharsis-oriented technique of drama therapy, Scheff's notion of aesthetic distance as a necessary condition for catharsis is most relevant. If this concept is valid, then the psychodramatic director should be skilled in modulating distance.

A second psychodramatic device of distancing is that of the double or alter ego of the protagonist. The double can serve the function of underdistancing as well as overdistancing. The more natural function, that of underdistancing, is to help the protagonist become more connected to his feelings. The protagonist might, for example, make analytical statements in a scene exploring anger toward his mother. The voice of the double might help him to express anger toward his mother, thus breaking through the overdistanced posture.

Through overdistancing, the double might also help the protagonist who is overflooded with feeling reestablish a sense of equilibrium. In the above example, the double might help the son come back from an underdistanced, emotionally charged response by speaking in a humorous voice, moving from reality to fantasy, moving from unpleasant experience to pleasant experience, or helping the protagonist shift from a participant to an observer role.

Many other psychodramatic techniques are regularly used to modulate distance. For one, the director at times interrupts the dialogue between protagonist and auxiliary ego and asks the protagonist to speak out a soliloquy or write a letter orally to a significant other. The switch from dialogue to monologue is a significant way to modulate distance. When interrupting the dialogue, the director can use both the monologue, wherein one speaker develops a thought or feeling at length in the presence of a listener, and/or the soliloquy, wherein the speaker verbalizes his innermost thoughts or feelings in depth, in the absence of any particular listener (Moffett 1968). The soliloquy form is less distancing than the monologue.

The director can also move from focus upon the protagonist to focus upon the group as a means of separating the protagonist from an intensity of feeling. This group sharing is generally part of the closure portion of the psychodrama. Closure, though, can also be cathartic for group members who have reexperienced their own feelings through an identification with the protagonist. The director, then, has to be aware of balancing distance for others in the group during closure to promote aesthetic distance.

Psychodrama has been used with many groups of emotionally disturbed clients, from mildly neurotic to severely psychotic. Although inherently underdistancing as a method, psychodrama, like puppetry and other projective techniques, can be used to overdistance and aid a psychotic client in distinguishing between reality and fantasy, between 'me' and 'not me.'

Sociodrama also provides many examples of distancing devices. For one, sociodramatic techniques are in essence more distancing than their psychodramatic counterparts in that the protagonist is no longer playing the role of self, but rather the role of a social group, e.g. women, men, blacks, whites. Although sociodrama as a technique was developed by J. L. Moreno and was based fully in his theory and practice of psychodrama, many others in the fields of drama/theatre, psychology, sociology and related areas have used drama as a means of exploring social and political issues (Goffman 1959; Shaftel 1967; Boal 1979; Gregoric 1982).

An example of a sociodramatic experience developed by this author, demonstrating the use of distancing devices, involves an exploration of male and female images and interrelationships. The experience began with a group of twenty adults, all of whom were asked to choose one gender and write the word male or female on a large piece of paper, which was then taped to their clothing, like a sign. Individuals were then instructed to begin a series of movements that represented their conceptions of the gender they chose. All were told they could be as stereotypical or caricatured in their movements as they wished. All participants worked with a partner. They were further instructed to respond to the movements of their partners.

During this initial warm-up part of the sociodrama, there was much overdistancing in evidence. Through the use of stereotype and caricature in movement, the participants were able to separate themselves from their roles. In that the role was a generalized one, a certain degree of overdistance was provided. As participants were not allowed to communicate verbally, overdistancing was also enhanced. However, there was also much evidence of catharsis through laughter. For some, then, there was a balance of attention present even in the warm-up. That is to say, even in portraying a stereotypical or caricatured social role, there may be enough affect associated with the role to balance out the overdistanced quality of the technique. For those to whom gender identity is an immediate issue, even the most overdistanced of techniques will be counterbalanced by a certain degree of underdistanced emotion.

Following the movements in role, the participants were asked to reverse signs and reverse roles with their partners. In those groups where each had chosen the same role, individuals were asked to find a different way of portraying the gender through movement.

The director then asked each individual to choose the gender he initially worked with and to write a five-minute piece on his sign, in first person, from the point of view of a specific male or female, specifying: Who am I (name, age, occupation, etc.)? Where am I? When am I there? What am I doing there? Participants were instructed not to censor themselves, but to write freely, without attending to the mechanics of writing, nonstop, for five minutes.

Through the writing, the director was providing both further distance from the former action, and removing distance as the individual prepared to move from a generalized enactment to a specific one.

During the next stage, two groups were formed. Group A, consisting of one partner in the dyad, became an inner circle. Group B, consisting of the other partner, became an outer circle. Members of Group A were asked, in turn, to speak a monologue or soliloquy in the role of their chosen character, using their written piece as a basis for their speech. The director stated that the purpose of the speech was to reveal an essential aspect of their character as male or female. The monologue/soliloquy could be in the form of a story or an improvised song. All were asked to enact the voice quality, body posture, and emotional tone of their character as much as possible. People in Group B were asked to observe the actions of their partners, as they would later comment upon their enactments.

Following the speeches, Groups A and B switched positions and those in B told their stories while A observed. During the storytelling, most participants demonstrated a strong identification with their roles. Distance was removed through a direct identification between actor and role. Some participants chose to tell humorous stories about positive experiences, thus providing themselves with a safe margin of distance. Others chose rather serious and negative experiences, told in some detail, thus underdistancing themselves. The director intervened rarely. His intervention would have been necessary had the imbalance of distancing been extreme. In that case, his intervention might have been through suggesting the use of either humor or seriousness, positive or negative emotion, past or present time orientation, observer or participant role, etc. During this part of the exercise, catharsis was evident through laughter, tears, shaking, and blushing, thus indicating a balance of distancing.

During the closure of the sociodrama, partners were asked to provide feedback to each other, out of role, and speak about the degree of their identification with the character portrayed by their partner. Too, individuals spoke of the degree of their identification with their own characters. Finally, the group ended with a more objective discussion about male and female roles within society.

Again, various degrees of distancing were evident in the closure. Some became aware of a strong identification with a character portrayed by their partner, by someone else in the group, or by themselves. Others expressed feelings of disconnection from the portrayals, but these individuals were in a distinct minority. The director helped these participants break through the overdistanced posture through focusing upon a single portrayal that was provocative and providing a double to help the person move closer to an expression of feeling toward that character portrayed. In the final discussion of male and female roles, the director brought the experience back to a more overdistanced, sociological perspective, but one based in a dramatic experience in which aesthetic distance was the main objective.

There are a wide variety of other drama therapy experiences that make use of aesthetic distancing principles. Generally speaking, any time the drama therapist makes a decision to work with a psychodramatic role (role of self) or a projected role (role of other), he is choosing an approach to distancing. His choice of technique, e.g. puppetry, mask, storytelling, caricature, also implies an approach to distancing. However, roles and techniques that appear to be skewed toward one pole or another can, as we have seen, be used for an opposite purpose. Projective techniques of overdistance can be used as means of underdistancing; psychodramatic techniques of underdistance can likewise be used as means of overdistancing, according to the nature and need of a specific client. The cognitive, conscious distancing of a client who, like the Brechtian actor, separates himself from empathetic relationships in order to take on a more rational viewpoint, is of quite a different order from the affective, unconscious distancing of a catatonic schizophrenic in a psychiatric hospital setting. Thus, the therapist must be fully aware of the client's style of distancing and clinical diagnosis, as well as the techniques appropriate to moving him toward a balance of attention.

Drama therapy techniques can be viewed, then, on a continuum from underdistanced to overdistanced with the understanding that, although any given technique might seem to be inherently over- or underdistancing, it can also be used, when appropriate, throughout the spectrum of distancing.

Drama therapy work, like drama/theatre enactment, in general, is representational in nature (Landy 1975, 1982b); that is, the participant represents a real or imagined experience, through action, within an environment that is removed from yet reflective of everyday life. If this is true, then there is a notion of two realities, that of the everyday and that of the dramatized. It is within the space between these two realities that the drama therapist best functions. His goal is to help the client better understand the everyday reality through working within the dramatic reality, like the classical psychoanalyst helps the client understand significant issues in his everyday life through exploring the transference occurring at the present moment in the relationship between client and therapist.

More precisely, the drama therapist works to help the client see the continuity of and interplay between the everyday and the dramatic, the imaginative, the intuitive, the expressive part of the client's psyche. To do this, the therapist needs to be skilled in balancing distance. As a concept, distancing in drama therapy does not make sense apart from the notion of representation. It is through the manipulation of the distance between the everyday and the dramatic and between the participant and the observer roles that the drama therapist attempts to create balance and equilibrium, a state of seeing as well as being, thinking as well as feeling.

The balance of attention is achieved, according to Scheff, through a process of catharsis. The result is a therapeutic one as the client is able to see his dilemma more clearly. In a fascinating critique of the classical notion of catharsis, the theatre artist, Augusto Boal, refers to Aristotle's conception as coercive and reactionary. Boal (1979) speaks of Aristotle's notion of catharsis as 'the purgation of all antisocial notions,' as a way of leading the spectator into a deadening of critical thinking and feeling, as an elimination of 'all that is not commonly accepted' (pp.46–47). Boal's poetics, like Brecht's, are revolutionary, viewing theatre as a means to encourage the spectator to act, to transform his society.

The notion of catharsis as put forth by such theorists as Scheff and Moreno leads toward a similar revolutionary, transformational goal. The change, however, is an intrapsychic and interpersonal one, political in the sense that personal and interpersonal transformation is a political and radical act. In the case of aesthetic distance leading to catharsis, the personal becomes the political; possibilities for new action are liberated through a process of balance. The actor and the spectator become one. Because one is not overflooded with feeling, one can think. Because one is not overly analytical and withdrawn, one can feel. Is this not a radical psychic posture?

The notion of balance does not negate the values of more extreme positions within the spectrum of distancing. There have been many theatrical, anthropological, and social-psychological studies of the extreme states of ecstasy, trance, and meditation, as they relate to both theatre aesthetics and healing (Sarbin 1962; Eliade 1972; Cole 1975; Schechner and Schuman 1976; Scheff 1979; Turner 1981). However, at the mean of aesthetic distance, the possibilities for insight and for psychic healing are very great indeed. If, as Scheff has conceptualized, the paradox of repressed emotion can be resolved in this state through the simultaneity of participant and observer role-playing, then the client will have the capacity to reexperience and see clearly that which was formerly repressed. This capacity to see is in itself a radical notion. If this process can occur through a balancing of distance, then the drama therapist must be adept at applying the techniques of distancing to the treatment of his clients.

# CHAPTER 3

# Conceptual and Methodological Issues of Research in Drama Therapy

As the field of drama therapy develops, more and more students ask for a clear conceptual and theoretical framework in which to understand its essential nature and therapeutic effects. During the past several years, such a framework has been slowly emerging. Early writing has been rather general and descriptive in nature. The kind of research that now appears in scholarly journals tends to address conceptual issues and looks toward ways of formulating a theoretical basis and a methodology for researching drama therapy.

In this chapter I will examine the research literature in drama therapy and related disciplines and discuss future directions of conceptual and methodological concern to researchers, students, and practitioners of drama therapy. Research has many and varied meanings. In the physical sciences, research is generally empirical, based upon observation, quantification, and generalization. Social scientists often model their research designs after those of their colleagues in the physical sciences. Many psychologists and sociologists, for example, are dependent upon empirical approaches, even though they are concerned, at times, with phenomena that are not directly visible and quantifiable, e.g. motivation, mind, and self. In that contemporary western institutions exist in a research climate of accountability through numbers and empirically verifiable fact, social scientists have devised methods to quantify not only observable behaviors, but also such unobservable constructs as cognition and affect.

In the arts, research is more difficult to define. Creative artists engaged in the process of making art can be seen as researchers. Their methods are aesthetic, often implying a search for the unique case, rather than the general condition. Researchers of the arts, engaged in a reflective, rather than an experiential process, often work through qualitative, historical, and aesthetic kinds of inquiry. Some borrow the quantitative methods of the physical sciences and carry out empirical studies of artistic processes.

If one is in a hybrid discipline, such as drama therapy, which is inherently both an art and a social science, the temptation to quantify in order to achieve academic respectability is unavoidable. However, in a discipline that is concerned primarily with nonobservable phenomena, e.g., insight, feeling, and creative processes, empirical behavioral research should be tempered with more qualitative approaches, more clinically and aesthetically verifiable methods.

However different the orientations and concerns of researchers in the social sciences and arts may be, there are certain commonalities that might help a fresh breed of researchers in drama therapy develop research that is more powerful than general descriptions of sessions, and more relevant than diminutive statistical analyses.

## Theoretical Models

One commonality shared by researchers in most disciplines is the grounding of their research in a theoretical and conceptual framework. As drama therapy has yet to develop such a framework, research in the field is problematic. However, researchers have freely borrowed from the related fields of psychoanalysis, sociology, educational drama and performance studies, among others, and are building an eclectic framework.

There are several theoretical orientations in the published drama therapy writings. David Johnson, who writes often from a developmental perspective, states:

> Whereas other paradigms suggest human dysfunction is due to something missing or out of balance, requiring things 'to be put right,' the developmental perspective sees human disorder as a blockage or halt in development... The overall goal of development...is... increasing the range of expression, so that the person has access to, and flexibility to move among, all developmental levels. (1982a, p.184)

Johnson's theoretical model comes from such developmental psychologists as Werner (1948), Erikson (1968), and Piaget (1971). Based on the developmental model, Johnson (1982a) posits a new concept, that of transformation, which he defines as: 'the flexible alteration of self in response to the ever-changing world about one.' This concept, which has been widely used in linguistics as well as humanistic and existential psychology, can prove quite useful to researchers, but it needs substantial refinement and a clearer relationship to existing theory.

Johnson also writes from a strong role-theory orientation. In a recent paper (1981), he posits a structural role model, characterizing improvisational role-playing by four conditions: impersonal, the relationship between two actors in their roles; intrapersonal, the relationship between an actor and his role; extrapersonal, the relationship between one actor out of role and another actor in role; and interpersonal, the relationship between two actors out of role. This model seems very useful in researching the effects of therapeutic role-playing on helping clients sort out their relationships to self, to others, and to their environment. In a related research article, Johnson and Quinlan (1980) examine differences between paranoid and non-paranoid schizophrenics by means of an improvisational role-playing task. The prime interest in this research was on intrapersonal and interpersonal role-playing.

Johnson's work in role-playing can be related to the theoretical framework of role theorists such as George Herbert Mead (1934), Theodore Sarbin (1954), Erving Goffman (1959), and Robert Selman (1971), who have worked primarily from a sociological perspective to define human behavior in terms of social interactions.

Eleanor Irwin and her collaborators generally favor a more psychoanalytically-based framework for their research in drama therapy, taking the position that repressed material can be enacted symbolically through such dramatic techniques as puppetry and storytelling. Much of Irwin's work focuses in play therapy, puppetry and related projective techniques that are essentially dramatic in nature. In examining the roots of play as therapy, she quotes Freud (1920) as saying:

> It is clear that in their play children repeat everything that has made a great impression on them in real life, and that in doing so they abreact the strength of the impression and...make themselves master of the situation. (p.17)

Irwin draws freely from the writings of those psychoanalysts whose interests include inquiry into the psychology of the child through playful means. These theorists include Anna Freud, Melanie Klein, Margaret Lowenfeld, and Erik Erikson, whose work has led Irwin (1983) to the conclusion that 'the child's spontaneous "acting out" of concerns in therapy is a kind of language to be examined and understood'. (p.149)

Like Johnson, Irwin also draws upon developmental psychological theory in examining the developmental roots of pretend play. She cites, for example, Piaget (1962), Singer (1966), and Sarnoff (1976) as important in providing research evidence for developmental processes in play.

Irwin frequently cites Margaret Lowenfeld's work in having children create dramas in the sand. Through their sandplay with specific toys and generalized objects and materials, children recreate 'the planet on which we live, with its mountains and lakes, its forests and deserts, its animals...people...their way of seeing and feeling...of loving and hating' (Lowenfeld 1970, p.xi).

This psychoanalytical perspective is reflected in an educational drama model, most clearly present in the work of Dorothy Heathcote and Gavin Bolton. The children and adults who work with Heathcote and Bolton also recreate a representational world and project onto it their ways of seeing and feeling, loving and hating: 'Bolton led the participants into building new sets of laws, governments, and systems of education and family life... In creating a new world the participants were, in fact, recreating the old one' (Landy 1982a, p.27).

As a theoretical model, educational drama is somewhat underdeveloped. Its relevance to learning and therapy is grounded more in practice than in theory. However, the writings of Gavin Bolton (1979) and Richard Courtney (1974, 1982), among others, provide a substantial body of theory.

I base much of my inquiry into drama therapy upon the drama education models mentioned above. Further, I adopt the developmental models of Piaget in cognition (1971), Selman in the development of role-taking competencies (1971), and Kohlberg (1976) in moral development. The psychoanalytical model is also relevant to my work, especially as it relates to the processes of projection, seeing the other as self, identification, seeing self as other, and transference, seeing the other in symbolic terms, as representing still another character.

A fourth theoretical model that informs my work is a sociological one, that of the symbolic interactionist perspective. This perspective is based in the notion that 'human beings interpret or "define" each other's actions... Thus human interaction is mediated by the use of symbols, by interpretation, or by ascertaining the meaning of one another's actions' (Blumer in Rose 1962, p.145). Human behavior, then, is not reactive, but interactive, interpretive and proactive. The implications of this idea for drama therapists can be seen most powerfully in the work of George Herbert Mead. Mead theorized that a person acts toward himself as others have acted toward him.

In Herbert Blumer's words, 'the human being can be the object of his own actions' (Blumer in Rose 1962, p.146). According to Mead (1925), the symbolic interactions occur through a process of role-taking. As a person takes on the roles and attitudes of others within his social environment, he is able to develop a conception of himself. He internalizes their roles and views himself as they have viewed him. Mead (1925) writes:

> It is only by taking the roles of others that we have been able to come back to ourselves... The self can exist for the individual only if he assumes the roles of the others... We appear as selves in our conduct insofar as we, ourselves take the attitude that others take toward us. (p.57)

Interestingly, Mead also speaks of play as essential in child development as the child becomes the endless imitator, taking on the roles of others within his social environment and acting toward himself as they act toward him.

Charles Cooley (1922) refers to the notion of the looking-glass self where the individual becomes a mirror for each person that he encounters. In other words, a person becomes himself to the extent that he has taken on the reflections of those within his social environment.

The body of symbolic interaction theory has provided a framework for much research in the social sciences and can provide a similar basis for research in drama therapy.

A fifth theoretical model is that offered by twentieth century theatre performance theorists, most notably Stanislavski and Brecht. Stanislavski's theoretical notions of psychophysical actions and emotion memory have deeply affected the practice of theatre. The Stanislavski method, as conceived by himself at the Moscow Art Theatre and scores of imitators throughout the world, is a psychological method, or a psychophysical method, where the actor's craft is not only about observable actions, but also about an understanding of motivations underlying actions, an accessibility to unconscious forces, and a connection to past affective experiences. Stanislavski (1936) wrote, '...periods of subconsciousness are scattered all through our lives. Our problem is to remove whatever interferes with them and to strengthen any elements that facilitate their functioning' (p.293).

With the pervasive application of the Freudian analytical model to almost every discipline after the 1930s, theatre, too, became an arena for psychologizing. As a reaction to the naturalistic, psychological model of theatre, Bertolt Brecht and other expressionists developed an alternative theoretical model – one based upon the notion of aesthetic distancing. Brecht's model of an epic theatre was one that demanded a separation from the primacy of affect and verisimilitude so that the spectator would not be hypnotized by the theatre and falsely led to mistake theatrical life for real life. In order to see clearly, Brecht speculated, one needs distance from the ordinary and the expected, reflexive responses to everyday life.

Both theatrical models are useful for generating research in drama therapy. For in drama therapy, the client sometimes needs a naturalistic, affectively-based mode of presentation, and sometimes a more stylized and distanced cognitively-based mode. The efficacy of either or both for clients of various clinical types has yet to be tested.

The primary concept that I have gleaned from a combination of twentieth century performance theory and social-psychological theory is that of distancing. As developed most recently by the sociologist, Thomas Scheff, the process of distancing in psychotherapeutic terms is about helping a client find a balanced psychic position between an overdistanced state of repression and an underdistanced state of emotional flooding, so that catharsis may occur, thus helping the individual restore psychic equilibrium and move toward an understanding of his therapeutic dilemma. Catharsis occurs, according to Scheff (1981), when the individual, in enacting a therapeutic drama, re-experiences emotions without becoming overwhelmed by them. There continues to be research in this area, most notably Scheff's own (1979). However, there has yet to be research in the area of drama therapy concerning the effects of distancing and the ensuing catharsis.

Although the theoretical positions mentioned above are taken from different disciplines, they are very much interrelated. Developmental theory, role theory, psychoanalytical theory, play theory, educational drama theory, sociological theory, and performance theory all view the human being as changeable, as capable of interpreting experience, and as developing toward healthy functioning through such dramatic processes as role-taking, pretend play, identification, imitation, affective memory, distancing, and catharsis. Even the most verbal and apparently nondramatic of the models mentioned thus far, that of psychoanalysis, views the relationship between human beings, in general, and the therapist and client, specifically, in terms of transference, which is a dramatic process in that one character represents another and the client acts toward the representational character 'as if' he were another.

## Research Questions

Given this body of theory, researchers in drama therapy can begin to draw out relevant research questions. Examples of questions already addressed include: Can the use of improvisational role-playing differentiate paranoid from non-paranoid schizophrenics (Johnson and Quinlan 1980)? Can the use of improvisational role-playing aid schizophrenic patients in seeing and experiencing a 'whole set of complex interrelationships' (Johnson 1981)? What effects do theatrical productions have on the lives of hospitalized psychiatric patients (Johnson 1980b)? Can the use of storytelling help hospitalized children cope with the stress of their hospitalization (Irwin and Kovacs 1979)? What is the value of play for learning-disabled children (Irwin and Frank 1977)? What is the relationship between art and drama as diagnostic tools in a child guidance center (Rubin and Irwin 1975)? Can a child's level of affective and interactional communication be positively modified as a result of repeated experiences in drama (Irwin, Levy, and Shapiro 1972)?

Some of these research questions have been grounded solidly by their authors in role theory, play theory and psychoanalytical theory. Others, such as the effects of theatrical performances on psychiatric patients, have not. It is most important that all further research in the field be clearly based on existing theory. That theory might be a single model or an eclectic one, consistent with the eclectic and interdisciplinary nature of drama therapy.

## Research Methodologies

Given a theoretical model and a group of research questions, the researcher then has to decide upon appropriate methodologies for research. This becomes problematic as drama therapy is both an art and social science, each area perhaps implying a different methodological approach. I use the word perhaps, because it is now commonplace to find researchers in the arts using quantitative methods, most often the domain of physical scientists and social scientists.

Social scientists, likewise, have used qualitative and impressionistic methods, more often associated with aesthetic inquiry.

Richard Courtney makes a distinction between experiential and reflective research. Experiential research concerns a subject having an experience. The experience itself is data for the subject. The subject is the object of his own research. He is the experimenter as well as the subject. When I compose music at the piano, for example, I am engaging in a search for the right sounds. When I repeat the process time and again, using a method of trial and error, building a melody inductively, note upon note, chord upon chord, I am engaging in a form of experiential research for the purpose of discovering the proper combinations of sounds that will become the finished song. Many theatre ensemble companies, such as the Open Theatre and the Living Theatre, engaged in a collective experiential research process in creating their pieces for the theatre.

Experiential research is the domain of the artist involved in the creative process. It is often existential and ahistorical. It draws heavily upon such nonobservable processes as intuition and sensation. It often proceeds inductively through a process of trial and error.

Reflective research is 'inquiry about enactment' (Courtney 1982). The researcher is no longer creating something himself, but distancing himself from a creative, psychological or social process in order to make sense of it. In drama therapy, there are several reflective methods that have been used. Many researchers take a descriptive approach. Through logs, journals, and the like, they tell about their experiences in the field with, for example, psychotic patients, the elderly, blind, deaf, incarcerated, among others. In the two volume anthology, *Drama in Therapy* (Schattner and Courtney 1981), examples of descriptive approaches include: Ramon Gordon's 'Humanizing Offenders through Acting Therapy' and Stuart Lawrence's 'Journal: Drama Therapy with Severely Disturbed Adults.' Although descriptive papers are valuable in informing the student of specific techniques applied to specific populations, these approaches are rarely couched in theory and tend to over-generalize.

A second primary method exemplified in published drama therapy research is that of the case study or field study. The writer will illustrate a conceptual position or elaborate upon the effects of a particular dramatic treatment strategy through examining an individual case, or a group of related cases. Examples include Eleanor Irwin and Marvin Shapiro's (1975) case examples in 'Puppetry as a Diagnostic and Therapeutic Technique;' David Johnson's (1981) case studies in 'Drama Therapy and the Schizophrenic Condition;' Elaine Portner's (1981) case study in 'Drama in Therapy: Experiences of a Ten Year Old.' When case studies are linked to theory, as these four authors have done, they provide an in-depth view of the effects of the drama therapy experience upon a limited sample. Whether the results are generalizable or not remains to be demonstrated.

A third method is empirical, quantitative research, in which the investigator will conceptualize his research questions in behavioral terms and choose an instrument, such as the Rorschach Index of Repressive Style (Irwin, Levy, and Shapiro 1972) or Fluid Boundary and Rigid Boundary Scales (Johnson and Quinlan 1980) to determine the effect of the dramatic experience upon a particular treatment group. The empirical researcher will generally compare the treatment group with a control group and proceed through a statistical analysis of a selected sample of subjects.

Empirical research is sometimes used in related areas of theatre arts, educational drama and theatre, and psychodrama. Quantitative studies in theatre published in the journal, *Empirical Research in the Theatre*, concern such subjects as dramatic involvement, counter attitudinal role-playing, and actor–character personality identification, among others. Much of the research is centered in the connections between theatrical and psychological processes and is thus relevant to research in drama therapy. Most notable is an article published in the first issue of *Empirical Research in the Theatre*, 'Psychology and Drama,' which examines many commonalities between the two disciplines and posits a useful instrument, Assessment of Dramatic Involvement Scale (Sutton-Smith and Lazier 1971).

The journal, *Children's Theatre Review*, also publishes empirical research and has devoted one of four issues published each year to research in the field of creative drama and children's theatre. Recent examples of empirical research studies include an exploration of improvisational dramatic activities as they effect self-worth and spontaneity (Huntsman 1982); and of creative drama as it effects comprehension skills in children (Furman 1981).

Although these empirical studies attempt to emulate their counterparts in the physical and social sciences, their research designs are often problematic. Further, researchers often run into problems in randomizing subjects, establishing validity and reliability, and finding appropriate instruments and statistical measures for analysis. The fault might lie in the training of the researchers or in the nature of the discipline researched or a combination of the two. Even with the most elegant research design and the most appropriate analytical tools, the questions remain: What is the value of measuring behaviors in an area where nonobservable processes are so crucial; and generalizing in an area where the individual case is so crucial and variation from one population to another, from one individual to another is so great?

Another methodological approach is a more qualitative one, that of the drama and puppetry interview devised by Eleanor Irwin (1975, 1976) and her colleagues. With this approach, the subject symbolically tells or enacts a story often in dialogue with the therapist. The therapist helps to elicit the story from the child. The child often projects the content of the story onto a puppet, who then becomes the storyteller. The content and form of the story will provide the basis for the therapist's diagnostic and treatment strategy. This approach can be seen as an adjunct to the clinical interview procedure often used by Piaget and his colleagues, where a subject engages in an open-ended dialogue with the researcher in order to uncover modes of thought, rather than specific behaviors. The method of the clinical interview was used successfully in related research in the field of children's theatre where the researchers, using a developmental scale to analyze data, looked at levels in which children of various ages identified with characters and interpreted scenes in a theatrical performance (Landy 1977). The drama and puppetry interview, like the clinical interview, is intended to look at modes of thought and affect, rather than at specific behaviors. It is an in-depth and qualitative method of inquiry.

A fifth approach to research in drama therapy is an analytical one involving the development of appropriate concepts for a theoretical base to drama therapy. Such concepts as distancing (Landy 1983) and transformation (Johnson 1982a) have been posited as basic to a theoretical structure. The work of researchers in building theory is still in its early stages and requires much collaborative effort among those in the drama therapy and related fields.

Neither historical nor aesthetic research has been used as a method of inquiry in drama therapy. In that the field is still in its infancy, any form of historical research would have to look at the disciplines, procedures, and concepts that are at the roots of drama therapy. Most obvious ones would include play therapy, psychodrama, and ritual, each of which has been researched quite thoroughly.

Aesthetic inquiry would examine drama therapy as a creative process, specifying which parts of the process to investigate, how the process works, and what effects that process has upon the functioning of subjects. As of yet, there is no significant published research in drama therapy that takes an aesthetic methodological approach.

## Analysis of the Data and Results

In analyzing the data that have been gathered through the above mentioned methods, drama therapy researchers have used several approaches to establish their results. In working with the puppet interview, Irwin and Shapiro (1975) analyze the stories presented by a child in terms of their form and content. Through case examples, the authors show how they proceed and what they discover. Their results are stated within the context of each case study. An example is of an eleven-year-old boy who is cured of chronic night terrors through play with puppets. In later work, they offer a more precise means of analyzing story content in terms of main character, theme, setting, affective tone, and ending (Irwin and Kovacs 1979).

Irwin and her colleagues have also used more quantitative means of analysis, such as rating scales (1979), judges (1979), and form analysis, including ratings from nine categories, e.g., organized/disorganized, clear/confused, and complete/incomplete (Rubin and Irwin 1975). In an ambitious study utilizing several instruments of analysis, the Rorschach Index of Repressive Style (RIRS), the verbal fluency test, the semantic differential, and the parent competency scale, to assess the effects of drama therapy in a child guidance setting with emotionally disturbed children, Irwin, Levy, and Shapiro (1972) found that those children with low RIRS scores were less repressed after the drama therapy experiences, and that their language became more personal and less stereotyped. Those in the drama group, as compared with two other control groups, demonstrated no significant changes in self-concept, as measured on the semantic differential, and no significant changes in the ways their parents viewed them, as measured in the parent competency scale.

In their research, Johnson and Quinlan (1980) used raters to assess fluid boundary and rigid boundary behaviors in their improvisational work with schizophrenic patients. Their findings were as predicted – the paranoid group scored lower than the nonparanoid group on the fluid boundary scale and higher on the rigid boundary scale. They concluded that rigid and fluid boundary behaviors can be reliably assessed by means of improvisation and that groups of paranoid and nonparanoid schizophrenics can be differentiated in terms of their approaches to dramatizing characters, objects and settings.

In a further study advancing their research on representational boundaries in schizophrenics Johnson and Quinlan (1982) used a highly promising analytical instrument, the diagnostic role-playing test, which Johnson (1980a) developed earlier to assess nine aspects of a client's role-playing: organization, action representation, integration of action, motivation, interaction, ending, accuracy, content, and movement.

In another study (Johnson 1980b) reporting the effects of a theatre experience upon a group of hospitalized psychiatric patients, Johnson used two scales: the social contact scale and the clinical state scale. Participants were rated by the nursing staff before, during, and after the presentation of two plays. Johnson discovered that, in comparison to a control group, patients in the first play had greater social contact and a healthier clinical state while in rehearsal. During a four-week period following the play, though, they became more withdrawn and clinically symptomatic. Noting this, Johnson worked on a second play and provided for weekly meetings following the performance to discuss problems and anxieties. In analyzing his data for the second play, Johnson found that, although social contact decreased in the days and weeks after performance, the clinical state of the patients did not worsen as it had in the first play.

Other means of gathering data that come more from the field of educational drama and theatre include the use of instruments developed by drama researchers. Of particular value to drama therapists might be Ann Shaw's (1968) taxonomy of educational objectives in creative dramatics. Based upon Benjamin Bloom, David Krathwohl, and Bernard Masia's (1956) taxonomies of educational objectives, Shaw's instrument translates artistic processes of child drama into observable behaviors and classifies these behaviors according to cognitive and affective processes specified in the model. The processes in the cognitive domain include: knowledge, comprehension, analysis, application, synthesis, and evaluation. Those in the affective domain include: receiving, responding, valuing, organization, and characterization.

Further research has evolved from Ann Shaw's work, most notably Linaya Leaf's (1980) doctoral dissertation in identifying and classifying educational objectives in creative drama as applied to handicapped individuals from five to eighteen years old. Leaf also used the Bloom *et al.* taxonomical model in analyzing her data, and extended Shaw's work with normal populations into the area of disabled populations.

A third drama-based instrument for gathering research data is Sutton-Smith and Lazier's (1971) Assessment of Dramatic Involvement Scale, mentioned briefly above, which looks at nine behaviors to be assessed through dramatic enactment. They include: focus, completion, use of imaginary objects, elaboration, use of space, facial expression, body movements, vocal expressions, and social relationships. A related instrument, developed a year later by Lazier and Karioth (1972), the Inventory of Dramatic Behavior, examines improvisational enactments by a single actor in terms of time, space traversed, number of stops, dramatic incidents, novel dramatic incidents, dramatic acts, repeated scenes, and characters created.

To summarize, thus far I have looked at existing research in drama therapy and related areas. I have delineated a number of theoretical frameworks that inform research in drama therapy. These models include: play theory, developmental theory, role theory and symbolic interaction, psychoanalytic theory, educational drama and performance theory. One unexpected omission is psychodramatic theory. Although most researchers in the field would, I think, affirm the value of that body of theory developed by Moreno and his followers, it does not appear much in the drama therapy literature as a conceptual model. That could be because drama therapists are attempting to establish an identity independent of psychodramatists, or it could be because the field of psychodrama has long had its own publication, *Group Psychotherapy and Psychodrama,* and research concerns. My sense is that psychodrama is both a theoretical root of drama therapy and a series of role-playing techniques that are subsumed under the larger umbrella of drama therapy practices.

After looking at theoretical frameworks, I looked at several research questions based at times in those frameworks. Next, I delineated kinds of research methodologies that have been used to examine the research questions. These included descriptive methods, case studies, empirical methods, clinical interviews, and theory building.

In looking at the analysis of data and results of selected research designs, I found researchers often borrowing instruments from the fields of psychology and education, depending often upon statistical, quantitative analyses, and discovering results that support the effectiveness of drama as a diagnostic and treatment strategy. The conclusion that researchers in drama therapy most often state is that such dramatic techniques as play, puppetry, improvisation, role-playing, and the like are powerful diagnostic and treatment tools that should be utilized more frequently as part of a team approach in hospitals, clinics, schools, and related settings.

## Future Directions

What form should future research in drama therapy take? Should it be empirical, conforming to the overwhelming trend in the behavioral and social sciences to quantify in behavioral terms? In his article supporting a scientifically-based, behavioral research in the theatre, Lazier (1976) begins:

> The principal dilemma of theatre research is that the essence of art is inexpressible. It is unquantifiable. It is beyond reason. It is the peak experience of Maslow, the sublime of Longinus, the goal of mysticism. It cannot be analyzed directly. (p.148)

Lazier solves the dilemma by arguing for meaningful empirical research based upon a systematic behavioral analysis of improvisation with children. His chosen method of inquiry is content analysis, used often in the social sciences and communications fields. Content analysis relates directly to western culture's obsession with computer technology and information processing. It is defined by Paisley (Paisley in Holsti, 1969) as 'a phase of information-processing in which communication content is transformed, through objective and systematic application of categorization rules, into data that can be summarized and compared' (p.3)

Yet neither the artistic experience nor the psychotherapeutic experience is, in essence, communication content transformed into data. And the technological metaphor, which can be stated as: creative states and feeling states to be experienced are like data and information to be processed, is not necessarily a rational argument for the primacy of scientific research into artistic and psychotherapeutic processes.

At the conclusion of his excellent article, Lazier questions the 'limits and pitfalls' of scientific research in theatre. He cites P.D. Ouspensky, a mathematician and philosopher, who was ever able to see a pure confluence of scientific and artistic thinking, and yet viewed the artistic process as a valid method of inquiry. Says Ouspensky (1971):

> Like science and philosophy, art is a definite way of knowledge... An art which does not reveal mysteries... does not yield new knowledge, is a parody of art, and still more often it is not even a parody, but simply a commerce or an industry. (p.33)

Art can be seen as a definite method of knowing. Further, when the therapeutic process is one based in an artistic, dramatic experience, then we need to look more closely at dramatic ways of knowing that reveal mysteries and yield new knowledge. In that many social scientists and philosophers have been using the dramatic metaphor for years, there is a clear relationship between the disciplines. Examples include Mead's (1934) sociological model of role-taking as a means of self-concept formation; Erving Goffman's (1959) analyses of social processes as dramas; Piaget's (1962) psychological notion of play as essential to cognitive development; Kenneth Burke's (1972) philosophical developmental model of dramatism.

Researchers in drama therapy borrow research methods freely from colleagues in the social sciences who have just as freely borrowed their theoretical metaphors and models from those in the field of theatre and therapy. But in the rush to do what they have done, that is, to specify human internal processes in behavioral terms and to measure them through quantitative means, drama therapy researchers have sometimes lost sight of Ouspensky's point of art as knowledge, of drama as a method of inquiry into essentially dramatic processes.

The task of the researcher in drama therapy is to examine those processes that are essentially dramatic and to look at how colleagues in the social sciences use those processes to talk about psychological or sociological processes that at least at first glance seem nondramatic in nature. David Johnson and Eleanor Irwin, to mention two, have made progress in that direction by looking at processes of role-playing and projection through puppetry, storytelling and play, processes that are essentially dramatic.

Further, researchers in drama therapy should not limit themselves to quantitative means of analysis. As the artistic experience of drama is not about thresholds and data processing and other mechanical images, but rather about thinking, feeling, moving and other humanistic images, then the means of uncovering the essence of a field based in an art should be more qualitatively-based. Researchers can move in that direction by means of more in-depth case studies, clinical interviews, and theory building conceived and written with a precision of thought and a foundation both in practice and in relevant interdisciplinary concepts.

The key word here is in-depth. As a teacher of the artistic discipline of playwriting, I instruct my students frequently to avoid philosophical writing about the great social and political ills of humanity. That is not to say that I don't want them to write about social and political issues. But the way to get there is through the personal, for at the heart of the single case, the minute and the small is a universe that is infinite and all pervasive.

A powerful image elucidating this thought can be seen in an extraordinary film about scientific research, Frederick Wiseman's *Primate*. In the film, a researcher who practices vivisection is interviewed as he casually decapitates a monkey, extracts the brain, slices the brain into smaller and smaller segments, until he has a tiny piece of tissue, which he slices even smaller. When he has extracted a single cell, he prepares a slide and feeds it into his microscope. All at once that miniature fragment of a once living being explodes in a universe of microscopic density. What was invisible to the naked eye becomes overwhelmingly gigantic through the eye of a powerful microscope.

In some ways, this scene in portraying a callous researcher who is not quite aware of the implications of his process points to the power of the artist. Wiseman, the filmmaker, shows that the camera is mightier than the microscope. The artist and the scientist see the same thing through the microscope, but the artist sees it with a different set of lenses and attaches a different set of meanings to it.

It would be difficult to discover or invent a scale or an analytical instrument that in itself is sufficient to take us as artfully as Wiseman's camera did into the large world of dramatized human experience. However, it is important to examine those scales and instruments that are dramatically-based and useful in analyzing specific dramatic processes. Also, there is a need to develop new means of evaluation that are qualitative and dramatic in nature. Johnson has begun to do this in his research with schizophrenics through developing rigid and fluid boundary scales and the diagnostic role-playing test.

Behavioral research in drama therapy is important but limiting. Researchers can well move beyond behavior toward the conceptualization and documentation of therapeutic performance. Therapeutic performance can be seen as enactment where the actor/client plays a psychodramatic role of himself or a projected role of another within a therapeutic context for the purpose of examining certain problematic areas of his existence. Therapeutic performance can be as simple as a creative dramatic exercise where, for example, one participant mirrors the movements of another, or as complicated as an autobiographical performance piece, where the participant recreates a piece of his life through dramatic means.

Therapeutic performance is not audience-centered. If an audience is present, it consists of those who are part of the therapy group. Therapeutic performance is about behavior, but it is also about thinking, feeling, intuiting, creating, wishing, fantasizing, dreaming – all processes very difficult to conceptualize behaviorally. Research based in therapeutic performance should account for the effect of the act of dramatic creation on the health of the client. Researchers can draw upon a number of theoretical models mentioned above, most notably performance theory. One method of investigation would be theory building, exploring such questions as: what are the essential concepts operative in the process of therapeutic performance? Therapeutic performance can also be researched through video-documentation. A substantial body of research in therapeutic uses of video has been developing that suggests a powerful technique and method of inquiry (Berger 1970; Fryrear and Fleshman 1981).

Finally, the therapeutic performance can be seen as a form of experiential research into the nature of performance as healing.

In his article, 'Research on the Arts and in Aesthetics: Some Pitfalls, Some Possibilities,' Morris Weitz (1976) states:

> ...if scientific research – theory-building and testing – is to be carried on in this area, we must begin not with testable theories about artistic creation but with the questions we need to ask and to answer. What are these questions about the role of research in the arts and, in particular, in artistic creation, that we want to ask and answer? (p.226)

A series of such questions about the role of research in drama therapy which might prove useful in guiding further research follows:

1. Who is best equipped to do research in drama therapy? What kind of background should the drama therapy researcher have?

2. Which populations should be researched? Should we use different approaches in researching different populations?

3. Should drama therapy be conceived primarily as a science? An art? A confluence of science and art? What are the methodological implications of these choices?

4. If we are indeed researching an artistic process through qualitative means, how do we talk about our findings in a precise way without falling into vagaries and generalities?

5. If drama therapy is based in the art of drama, are there dramatic methods of inquiry to guide our research? What are they?

6. What is it about the process of performance that lends itself to forms of psychological healing?

7. What issues in drama therapy should be researched through behavioral means? What are dramatic behaviors?

8. What kinds of quantitative methods are best suited for research in drama therapy?

9. What kinds of qualitative methods are best suited for research in drama therapy?

10. Is therapeutic performance a method of research in its own right?

11. How do we best analyze the information we gather through our research in drama therapy?

12. What kinds of dramatic 'information' are we looking for?

13. What kinds of outcomes do we expect through the process of drama therapy?

14. If drama therapy is not a primary means of therapy, and if clients also attend individual and group verbal psychotherapy sessions, how can we know what specific effects the drama therapy has upon the client?

15. How can those of us who practice or teach or study drama therapy best engage in conversation with our social science or performance colleagues and among ourselves to keep generating dialogue around issues of research in drama therapy?

# CHAPTER 4

# Puppets, Dolls, Objects, Masks, and Make-Up

In a recent article, Akhter Ahsen (1983) queries:

> But how is it that artists often have only resolved the contradictions of their lives in the parameters of their art; they do tend to suffer from neurotic symptoms. They have not made of their lives the art they have made in their imagination. (p.166)

If Ahsen is correct, then a possible solution to the dilemma of the creative artist, or others in non-creative, neurotic states, is to utilize the creative process, the imaginative act, as a means of restoring or revitalizing healthy functioning. In this chapter, I will look at several projective techniques gleaned from the dramatic arts and discuss how they can be used to restore or revitalize healthy functioning in everyday life. I will further relate Ahsen's (1983) notion of image as not only a link to memory, but also an instructional and transformational phenomenon related to the healing process of drama therapy.

Drama therapists use dramatic and theatrical processes to help clients develop a more satisfactory and functional existence. Unlike verbal psychotherapists, their methods are grounded in the aesthetic experience of making dramas, of dramatization. Like the director, the drama therapist helps clients discover appropriate imagery to guide them through the dramatization of their personal experience. That imagery, though based in memory, will serve a therapeutic end if it is both instructional and transformational in a present time frame. As Ahsen (1983) notes: 'The image fathoms life in a strong and total way and in this sense it embodies new understanding and enlightenment' (p.161).

Imagery generated in drama therapy has both external and internal sources. The external source is often embodied in a story or, as will be demonstrated later, in a projective device. The drama therapist might use, for example, a classical myth, fairy tale, fable, or parable, rich in relevant imagery, as a treatment strategy. The story becomes a representational environment upon which the client may project his fantasies, wishes, expectations, anxieties, or from which he may introject the same. The therapist will choose a story with imagery that is relevant to the client's search for clarity.

One example of externally generated imagery is in a story I heard at a workshop in 1976 told by the British educational drama expert, Gavin Bolton. I have used this story with several drama therapy groups where a prevalent issue was unresolved Oedipal conflicts. In the story, a young boy of 10 is very attached to his mother. So deep is their love that he is unable to establish friendships with his peers. As he reaches the age of 12, he befriends a peer and becomes very committed to his new relationship. The friend, jealous of the boy's love for his mother, demands that the boy choose between the mother and the friend. 'If you wish to retain my love,' the friend says to the boy, 'then you must kill your mother and bring me back her heart as proof.' The boy, although in profound turmoil, decides to obey his friend's wishes. He murders his mother, cuts out her heart, puts it in a sack, and travels through the forest to his friend's house. Along the way, the boy trips on a stone and falls. The sack also falls to the ground and the heart is revealed. The heart looks up to the boy and says: 'Are you hurt, my son?'

The image of the heart, for one, can serve as a focus for the therapeutic dramatization. In assuming the role of the heart or, as will be described below, the roles of the other characters or objects in the story, the client can explore his Oedipal relationships as well as other friendship and love relationships.

An internal source of imagery is that generated by the client from his unconscious. The drama therapist would provide a stimulus to tap the unconscious source. As an example, a therapist might help the client work into a relaxed body position, then with eyes closed, focus in on a sound created by the therapist. The therapist might, for example, drag a chair across the floor or pull a window shade up and down. As soon as the client has become aware of an image or series of images associated with the sound, he is ready to apply his imagery to a therapeutic dramatization.

## Therapeutic Dramatization

Therapeutic dramatization is the aesthetic method in which the client uses externally or internally generated imagery to enact a problematic aspect of his existence. The enacted image can take the form of a character or an object. The enactment can be in movement, sound, monologue, dialogue, or soliloquy; it can be a one-person performance, a dyadic or group performance. The enactment can be re-presentational, in the sense that an event that has already taken place is reenacted or reviewed in order to be better understood. The enactment can also be a pre-view of a future event. Or the enactment can have a present orientation that neither looks to the past nor the future. However, most therapeutic dramatizations will reflect the complex images of time where time present, time past and time future fold in on one another.

The experience of the enactment might in itself be healing. Many professional actors report therapeutic benefits from acting workshops and/or performance situations. One actor reported to me, for example, the effects of performing an improvised exercise concerning the opening of a letter, a prop which contained, in fact, a blank sheet of paper. His objective was to 'see' an actual message and to react. When he opened the letter, he immediately saw the text as a telegram announcing the suicide of a former student. He reacted by constricting his musculature, cutting off all feeling, then visualizing the student in a manic moment. Finally he took a chair and smashed it against the wall. The director simply said: 'Either repair or replace that chair, please.' Nothing further was ever said. The actor reported that he felt a sense of relief and clarity after the incident and that he was able to let go of an old feeling that he had in some way been responsible for the suicide. Although this was a therapeutic moment, it was not therapy *per se*. The implicit therapeutic function of acting becomes therapy when the director, trained in the arts of drama and psychotherapy, uses his training to reach explicit therapeutic goals.

In drama therapy, therapeutic dramatization might indeed be healing and require a minimum of reflection and verbalization. However, both therapist and client are engaged in a process to determine the therapeutic effectiveness of the dramatic experience. There is a time of readiness, a time to look at, to make sense of the dramatization or series of dramatizations created by the client. In the drama therapy process, action precedes (re)cognition, but does not necessarily preclude it. Sometimes, action is sufficient for 'new understanding and enlightenment' – two significant therapeutic goals. This certainly is true in the case of Hamlet, who reverses the therapeutic chronology in that for him, cognition precedes action. But his final action, though deadly, does bring about a new understanding and tragic re-cognition.

Ahsen (1983) relates action to imagination. He says:

> In the realm of the image the essence of knowledge is finally not conceptual but a flow of elusive action and activity; in the image, action becomes ethereal and meets imagination, and imagination, without becoming alienated, becomes action. (p.161)

It is Hamlet's act of imagination, the image of himself as an actor who can act, that leads to his ability to take the dark, tragic voyage toward enlightenment.

In drama therapy, action is often not sufficient for new understanding and enlightenment. There is a cognitive, reflective process that follows the action or at times is interwoven within the fabric of the action, that locates the imagination in reality, that bridges the gap between the neurosis of the artist in everyday life and the health of the artist in the spontaneity of the creative life.

It is this reflective period of talking about what has happened, of making reference to past and future, to self and others, that gives the aesthetic experience a further conscious healing function. Although the western drama therapist is like a traditional spiritual healer or shaman, his method is significantly different. He engages his clients in a reflective process outside of the therapeutic dramatization to interpret and help them see a context for their images and their actions.

## Distancing in Drama Therapy

In the drama therapy process, there is a distancing factor operative. There is a separation between action and reflection upon action. There is a separation between actor and role, even between actor and his own body.

Distancing is a concept that informs much of my work in drama therapy. Dolls, puppets, objects, masks, and make-up are all projective devices based in that concept. Though long used as an aesthetic concept (Bullough 1964; Willett 1964), distancing has in recent years been applied to sociological and psychotherapeutic contexts (Landy 1983; Scheff 1981). The theatre artist, Bertolt Brecht (1967), provided a model of distancing, the Verfremdungs-Effect, which viewed the actor as separated from his role, and the spectator as separated from his memory bank of conventional responses to dramatized human experiences. Brecht's model was an overdistanced one, based in a reaction against not only an aesthetic naturalism, but also a social-psychological emotionalism. For Brecht, the question was: how can theatre become a force for critical, dialectical thinking and for, in Ahsen's words, imaginative action? In his characters – the bourgeois thief, Macheath; the heroic anti-hero, Mother Courage; the sensual intellectual, Galileo; the whore with the heart of gold, Shen Te – and in his recurring images of justice–exploitation, sensuality–intellectuality, riches–poverty, Brecht explored this question over and over. Brecht's answer, though never fully realized, was in the alienation effect, in the overdistancing of actor from role, of spectator from expected response.

Perhaps Brecht failed in his aims because his means were imbalanced. The alienation effect implied too much overdistance. That is, in order for change to occur at both the socio-political and psychological levels, there must be a balancing of distance so that the emotional and rational parts are confluent, so that the person and persona, the individual and the institution, are interdependent.

This notion is explicated elegantly by the sociologist, Thomas Scheff (1979, 1981). Scheff claims that a balancing of distance occurs when an individual is able to play both the actor and observer roles simultaneously and re-experience a problem of his life without being overwhelmed by the conscious awareness of it. Scheff claims that a person in this balanced posture can experience catharsis. He sees catharsis as a state of aesthetic distance, when one experiences formerly repressed emotions without being overwhelmed by them. Catharsis is a discharge of these emotions through proper physiological means, that is, crying, laughing, shaking, blushing.

Aesthetic distance is a balance between the Brechtian notion of overdistancing and the early Stanislavskian (1936) notion of underdistancing, of fully identifying with a character through emotional recall.

## The Use of Projective Techniques in Drama Therapy

In drama therapy, the concept of distancing finds a natural focus in projective techniques. The client playing with a doll, puppet or object, wearing a mask or make-up, is first making a clear separation between self and non-self. However, the non-self has properties of self, and through the act of projection can easily be viewed as self. A projective technique provides a margin of safety. The client is no longer enacting his life, but the life of a puppet or a doll with another name and in another setting. The therapist's aim in using projective techniques is to bring the client to a properly balanced catharsis, a dialectical moment of thinking and feeling, of imaginative action and active reflection.

### Dolls, Puppets, and Objects

Dolls, puppets and objects are the most distanced of the projective devices, as they are most detached from the body. Generally, they are the basic elements used in play therapy situations (Schaefer and O'Connor 1983; Woltmann 1971). Eleanor Irwin, a prominent drama and play therapist, uses puppets for both diagnostic and therapeutic purposes (Irwin and Shapiro 1975). She and her colleagues have devised a technique of a puppetry interview where the child enacts or tells a symbolic story through the puppet (Irwin and Rubin 1976; Irwin and Shapiro 1975). This often occurs in dialogue with the drama/play therapist. In that the story is told through the puppet, the child has created a safe margin of distance. For diagnostic purposes, the therapist is able to analyze not only the form of the story, but also the content, including the images created by the child in the puppet role. These images can lead to further dramatization and analysis.

In play therapy, the puppets, dolls and objects should be carefully chosen to represent a variety of images. Images of aggression, passivity, neutrality, of positive, negative, and neutral moral states should be present. The aggressive puppets might be in the form of animals with prominent mouths. There might also be devil puppets and dolls and soft objects that can be used for hitting. The softness of a bat, for example, distances the aggressive object from causing any real harm and thus allows the child to safely discharge his aggressive energies. More positively charged projective devices might include soft, friendly animal dolls, teddy bears, and kindly animal puppets. Neutral devices might include rubber balls and other rubber objects, sock puppets with simple human features, etc. There might also be puppets and dolls with more defined human characteristics representing family members and certain moral figures such as policemen and firemen. These human figures, though inherently protectors, are less distanced than the animal figures and thus more apt to be positively or negatively charged by the children within a short period of time.

The therapist generally encourages the child to play with the various dolls, puppets, and objects, intervening sparingly. At times, he might ask the child to tell a story while engaged in the play or following the play. In noting the imagery created by the child, the therapist will have a means not only to enter into the child's unconscious experience, into the world of his imagination, but also to fashion a treatment strategy.

Many play/drama therapists will allow children to play out the same story repeatedly, until they reach a transformational moment in the play. That point might be reached when, for example, a negatively charged object becomes neutralized, when an image of aggression is transformed into a utilitarian image. This intuitive leap can happen through an imaginative act on the child's part. Like Odysseus outsmarting the negatively charged Cyclops through an act of imagination rather than aggression, a child can resolve his feelings of entrapment by a parent through a similar leap of imagination. If, for example, he is biting a parent doll with an animal puppet that has an extended mouth, the mouth might be transformed into a source of reason, of words, of the expression of direct feelings, rather than a well of aggressive biting and fearful engorging. Of course, this transformational process doesn't always occur spontaneously in drama therapy. Thus, the therapist needs to become more of a verbal guide or active player in the drama and help to bring the needed images of integration within the puppet and doll play.

In playing with puppets, dolls, and objects, the therapist is working through a subtle dialectic that informs all creative action in the theatre. The actor on stage is actual and fictional at the same time. He is person and persona. He exists in a space that is both a real room and a series of flats and two dimensional backdrops. He handles objects that appear real, but that are props, fakes. The notion that the puppet is real and fake at the same time is the distancing factor necessary for the therapeutic dramatization to occur. The therapist will help the child increase or decrease that distance in order to move toward catharsis and understanding.

## Masks

In working with masks, the same principles of distancing apply. However, masks are inherently less distancing than puppets, dolls, and objects since they are worn directly on the face and cannot be seen apart from the face. The therapist might begin drama therapy sessions with masks by prearranging a variety of masks that are essentially positively, negatively and neutrally charged. The client, engaging in free play by wearing the mask, can then enact a story or incident improvisationally, in words and/or movement. The story might be further developed in dialogue with the therapist. Over time, with the aid of the therapist, the client can discover the meaning of the imagery he has created in his mask dramas and move toward unmasking his resistances to healthy functioning.

As a second approach, the drama therapist can ask the client to construct his own masks, each of three representing a positive image, a negative and neutral image. The therapist can warm-up a group by having each member introduce his three masks, giving each a name. Then he can ask an individual to choose three people from the group, one to wear each mask. If the group trust level is high, then the therapist might ask the protagonist to explain why he has chosen each person to wear a particular mask. Next, the client can sculpt the group of three into a frozen tableau, carefully choosing the body positions, attitudes, and relationships among the three. Following the sculpting, the client is to give each masked figure a name, then name the group still life. Following the exercise, the client can be asked to reflect upon his sculpture and his relationship to each character in the still life. Then, he can engage in an exploration of his relationship to the characters in everyday life represented by the masked figures. As a variation on this exercise, the client can assume a role in the still life by taking on the mask of a particular character in the sculpture. At the discretion of either the therapist or the client, the still life can move, vocalize, or verbalize. In fact, almost any dramatic variation would be appropriate if the therapeutic goal is to balance the distance and bring the client closer to catharsis and understanding.

The transformational quality of therapeutic mask dramas is centered in the paradox of masking as a means of unmasking. Many clients report a perceptual heightening when wearing masks. They talk about seeing better, seeing clearer, feeling more at ease in movement, and ironically, seeing others in the group or in the world as appearing to be wearing masks. So then, in the dramas, one masks oneself and assumes a stylized identity in order to be able to achieve the proper distance necessary to see reality more clearly.

The image of the mask is an omnipresent anthropological and theatrical one (Sorell 1974). It re-occurs throughout cultures and throughout the history of dramatic literature. In the theatre, masks are used to elevate the human to the superhuman, the person to the type, the individual to the group, the profane to the sacred. Masked figures in Greek drama represent gods and powerful noblemen. Masked characters in Renaissance *commedia dell'arte* represent human types, that is, the wise fool, the miserly father, the cowardly commander (Duchartre 1966). Masked actors in modern Brechtian and expressionistic drama become moral and political symbols. Contemporary street theatres and experimental theatres frequently employ masks and puppets, transforming the actor into a creator of ritual, social, and political acts, rather than particularistic psychological actions.

By working through masks in therapy, then, the client enters a less psychological, less personal plane. In wearing the mask, he is transformed into Zeus, who represents great power and judgement, into Harlequin, manipulating those of high status through his foolish wisdom, into a concentration camp victim in a Grotowski (1968) experiment who embodies all human suffering. And from this distanced, elevated, aestheticized realm, assuming a role of a generalized other – the gods, the clowns, the victims – the client can begin to see the judgmental, the foolish, and the victimized parts of himself. Too, he can begin to explore how these images have shaped his conceptions of himself. The movement of therapeutic mask dramatizations, then, is from an overly distanced, aesthetic, socio-political realm to a properly distanced psychological one, where feeling and thinking are confluent, where the individual can be viewed in relationship to the group.

## Make-up

The least distanced of the projective devices referred to in this paper is that of make-up. It is less distanced than the mask, because it is applied directly on the face. It is, however, less strange as a therapeutic device in that many clients use it regularly in everyday life, and those who have acted on stage accept it as a proper theatrical convention. In working with make-up, drama therapists sometimes use a free play approach where the clients create their own imagery through the free application of make-up on their faces (Breitenbach 1979). As in the work with puppets and masks mentioned above, the free make-up play might be interspersed with appropriate therapeutic intervention and reflection upon the experience.

Another approach is to link the make-up experience to a series of externally generated images. An example is working with the story mentioned earlier concerning the matricide. After telling the story to a group, the therapist can ask each client to choose one character he most identified with. The characters can be human – the mother, boy, friend – or inanimate – the heart, stone, sack. Then, each client is asked to assume that role through the application of make-up. The process of applying the make-up can take on a highly ritual quality. First, it is helpful if small support groups are arranged so that each individual feels connected. All are instructed to sit with their groups and cleanse their faces before applying the new make-up. The make-up, which should contain both stylized clown-like rouges, sticks, and greasepaints, as well as more conventional eye make-up and bases, can be shared among the individuals in each group. Following application of the make-up, each group can dramatize the story in movement and sound, not necessarily in chronological order, but rather in a form that corresponds to their need to explore character relationships and feeling states. The groupings themselves will be random in terms of the character arrangement, that is, one group of four might have two mothers, one heart, and one stone. After the dramatization, each client can be asked to speak a soliloquy in role, telling the others who he is and how he feels in relation to the other characters. Finally, after the soliloquies, each client, out of role, can verbalize similarities and differences between himself and his character.

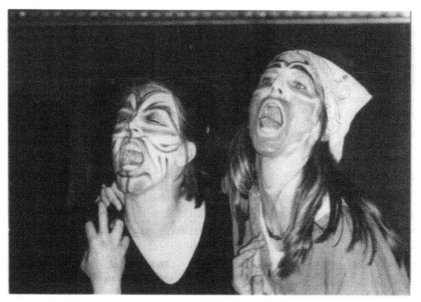

*Figure 4.1 Story dramatization through make-up*

This is a very powerful exercise that requires a substantial amount of time for closure. For one, the externally generated imagery is powerful in its violent resolution of the Oedipal complex by having the boy kill his mother in order to choose another love object. Too, the images might re-stimulate the Oedipal dilemmas of some of the group members. The use of stylized make-up and dramatization through movement and sound helps distance clients from possible overwhelming emotions. However, the soliloquies remove distance and bring clients closer to their personal experience as children who might have fantasized about killing a parent in order to live an independent existence; or parents who might have conflicting feelings about their ability to let go and allow their children the freedom to search for their own identity.

This experience can be further distanced by engaging the group in a ritual process of removing the make-up within their subgroups, of letting the role go as the make-up comes off.

The therapist, in using such powerful material, must be skilled in balancing the aesthetic distance. Again, a stylized, aesthetic, theatrical process leads to a psychological, therapeutic one. The creation or re-creation of the imagery through make-up, movement, sound, and soliloquy is necessary for therapy to occur. A further essential part of the process is a reflection upon the experience, a view of how the client is similar to and different from the role he has created. In the use of all of the projective devices, the therapist is a dialectical juggler. It is his task to help the client discover relationships and distinctions between self and role, between mask and face, between projecting the self and accepting the self. And it is his task to help the client discover the significant images essential in uncovering those relationships and distinctions.

## Conclusion

In the artistic process, the artist does not need to make conscious distinctions and see clear relationships between, for example, the notes in a musical phrase or the colors on a canvas or the actions in a play. The artistic process is not an analytical one. However, the artist both thinks and feels through the creation of imagery. The artist, in the act of exercising his creative imagination, is living through a dialectical moment of simultaneously thinking and feeling. It is a moment of balanced aesthetic distance, of simultaneously playing creator and observer roles. Repressed feelings are available but unformed, like clay yet to be molded. If this is true, then it is no wonder that, as Ahsen (1983) suggests, 'artists often have...resolved the contradictions of their lives in the parameters of their art' (p.166).

In moving toward resolving neurotic and psychotic personality disorders in everyday life, the unconscious artistic process can be consciously employed. If emotional disturbances are, in part, imbalanced feeling states and confusions in boundaries between self and role, one role and another role, then healthy emotional functioning can be restored through properly balancing emotional distance and helping the client see role/self distinctions.

The process of creative arts therapy implies not only aesthetic acts of the creative imagination, but also reflective acts of analysis in helping the client move toward a confluence of thought and feeling. There is much research to be done in uncovering the methods and effects of drama and other creative arts on restoring healthy functioning (Landy 1984). Given the practice and early conceptual speculation regarding the efficacy of such projective devices as dolls, puppets, objects, masks, and make-up, a powerful technique becomes available for fostering healing through action, imagination, and reflection.

CHAPTER 5

# The Image of the Mask
## Implications for Theatre and Therapy[1]

The image of the mask is ubiquitous throughout culture, history, stages of human development, and literature. As an object, the mask takes on human projections in play, ritual, magic and theatre. As a projection of the self, it can assume an infinite variety of forms – human, divine, animal, inanimate object. This chapter is a personal odyssey by means of the mask. During the journey, I will reflect upon my experience with masks in the theatre, in photography, and in drama therapy.

## The Mask in Theatre

As a young adult working as a theatre director, I became fascinated with the epic theatre style of Bertolt Brecht. It wasn't only the philosophical notions of the stage as a socio-political laboratory or the elegant poetic diction dripping with irony that converted me to the Brechtian world view; it was also the puppets, masks, and exaggerated objects that delightfully cluttered the set. This was truly an epic-scale theatre. The great events in human history and spiritual history would be enacted through actors in masks, through puppets, songs, and crankies, scroll-like contraptions that carried a story in funny pictures. The actors were often clowns, modeled after the great American comic, Charlie Chaplin. The epic theatre was in many ways a theatre for children who had no use for the well-made play or the realistic play, who had no need for a linear structure where beginning precedes middle. The epic theatre was truly a theatre about theatre. Speeches were made. Images were inflated. Ideas were debated. Songs were sung, stories were told, and characters would step out of role to explain the moral of the story.

---

1   This chapter was presented as a keynote lecture at the 8th Annual Conference of the International Imagery Association, New York City, 1984.

Given my childlike enthusiasm for epic theatre, I was eager to direct my first children's play, *Rags to Riches* by Aurand Harris, based upon the mythic characters in Horatio Alger novels. My first act as director was to reconceptualize Harris' melodrama as epic theatre.

Each character was to be a kind of figurative mask. Unlike the original melodramatic intent toward empathy and identification on the part of the audience, this epic theatre production aimed toward alienation, a separation of actor and role, role and audience. For in the separation, according to Brecht, one is free to think, to view the events objectively and consider alternative actions.

The masks of the actors were developed in their gestures, movements, facial expressions, and projections of character. They included the idealistic mask of Dick, the heroic personification of the rags to riches ethic; the demure mask of

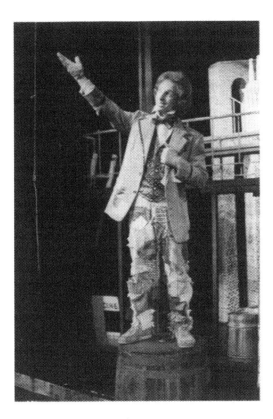

*Figure 5.1 Ragged Dick, from* Rags to Riches

Ida, the poor little rich girl; the grandiose mask of Mr. Greyson, the rich banker, exaggerated in costume by 12-inch elevated shoes; the clownlike mask of

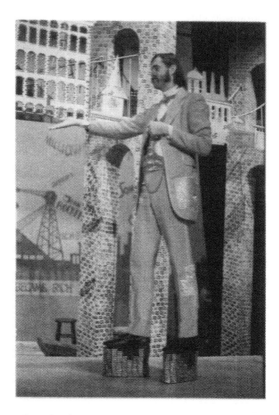

*Figure 5.2 The Rich Banker from* Rags to Riches

authority worn by the policeman; and the masks of destitution worn by the chorus of poor street children.

My dedication to this project was total and fiery. Most all of the actors were pulled into my magic circle of vision. But there was one malcontent cast in the role of a corpulent, callous, calculating businessman – a minor role. He would come late to rehearsals and speak disdainfully of the directorial concept. He had plans to be a successful commercial actor on television. One week before opening, he quit the cast and we needed a replacement desperately. Unable to find another able-bodied actor, we decided to replace the malcontent with a puppet, life-size, supported by a broomstick on top of which sat a grotesque mask in the style of George Grosz.

The puppet was a great success. Its commitment to the vision of the play was total. It never made a false move throughout the run of the play. It was, in fact, the consummate actor.

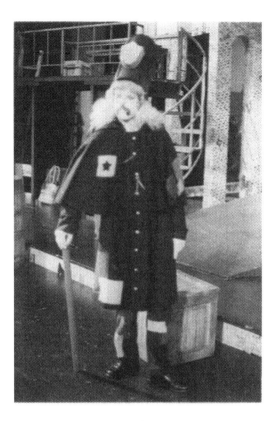

*Figure 5.3 The Policeman, from* Rags to Riches

The image of the mask has had a long and glorious history in the theatre (Smith 1984). In the ancient Greek amphitheater, the actor performed for a crowd of 30,000 viewers, and often portrayed a godlike of noble character. Thus, the human actor needed to be expanded in stature to reach the epic proportions of his role and to project outward into the crowd. Not only was he made taller by wearing coturnus, ten-inch platforms attached to his sandals, but he was also given an extension to his face, a mask that projected both the voice through a funnel-like opening in the mouth, and the spirit or emotional power of the character.

The mask continued to be a significant theatrical device throughout history and across many cultures. It appeared steadily in the European Renaissance *commedia dell'arte*, in the Peking opera, the Japanese Noh drama and the Indian Kathakali dance dramas, among many others.

In the early twentieth century, the British director and designer, Gordon Craig, editor of the magazine, *The Mask*, saw the puppet and mask as the supreme expressions of the dramatic arts. Craig (1919) wrote that the mask is 'that paramount means of dramatic expression without which acting was bound to degenerate' (p.118). For Craig, as for the Greeks, the mask transformed the human head into the godhead, the particular and mundane into the universal and sublime.

The contemporary alternative theatre, working within the tradition of Brecht, also frequently draws upon the mask as a powerful symbol. Perhaps the most outstanding example is in the work of Peter Schumann, founder of the Bread and Puppet Theatre. Schumann covers nearly all his actors with masks and has no place in his sacramental theatre for an actor with an ego to parade or a product to sell.

From my experience with *Rags to Riches* I understood the temptation to replace faces with masks, people with puppets. But as a director working with human actors, not yet convinced of the expendability of the human face and the tradition of naturalistic method acting, I engaged again in the human struggles. But I quickly tired of the endless clashes of ego and the moments of theatrical life that appeared and disappeared so quickly. There was too much motion for me. I needed more calm, more focus, less frenetic action.

After the thrilling experiments in theatre during the late 1960s and early 1970s, a long, tedious period set in. The Bread and Puppet Theatre was an oasis in a dry country of masked commercials, soap operas, Broadway musicals – pedestrian and sentimental.

The language of the theatre, which took a back seat to the Artaud (1958) and Grotowski (1968)-influenced spectacles of the 1960's, was revived in the plays of Tom Stoppard, Sam Shepard, and others. But it didn't ring true to me. Stoppard and Shepard were too fast, too facile, too far removed from the shamanic power of the mask.

## The Mask in Photography

In 1975, I borrowed a camera and started taking pictures. Now I had total control over my medium. People become objects for posing, among other objects. If I so chose, I could pose them in a mask and slow them down. In taking pictures, I experienced a whole new relationship between the two levels of reality – the everyday, which is imitated in art, and the dramatic, the magical, that which imitates. I took great pleasure in shooting everyday settings, always hopeful of revealing the magical.

One day, a student gave me a gift – a Pocahontas mask, fashioned after the famous early American Indian princess. In legend, Pocahontas saved the life of Captain John Smith, converted to Christianity, married an Englishman, and made peace between the Americans and the Indians.

Pocahontas means 'playful one,' and for me the mask signaled the beginning of a period of personal play. I put the mask on many friends and relatives, then photographed them. I had no idea why I was taking the mask pictures, but I couldn't stop.

Finally, I learned to make a mask of my own face, and I began to take self-portraits in mask. I felt powerful in the mask. I felt I could see the connection between my face and body in mask better than ever before. Looking at the finished images I saw myself transformed – not quite a god, but neither quite a mere mortal.

I needed more. I wanted to extend the role-taking theories of George Herbert Mead (1934) to photography, to explore the notion that one knows who he is by virtue of taking on the role of another, in this case through an aesthetic methodology, that of photography. To do that though, I needed the masks of all the significant others in my life. I could wear them, take my picture in their masks, and better learn the true nature of myself. But that was impractical. So I worked from the other way around. I put my mask on them and shot their pictures – an act of pure photographic projection. I put the mask on my parents, my sister, my wife and friends, on elders, children, couples – all in natural settings. I called these pictures 'Still Lives.'

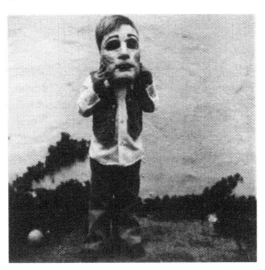

*Figure 5.4 Boy with mask, from* Still Lives

I contemplated the images for a long time, but didn't really understand them. The portraits were of me, but not of me. They were still, but not any more in my control. The particular person was transformed, but into an unknown entity. I didn't see an archetype or an image of great emotional power or a god. The pictures were too distanced for me. I experienced very little emotion in their

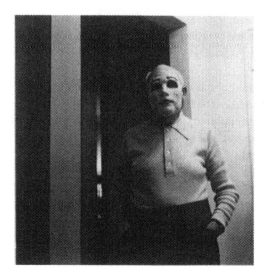

*Figure 5.5 E from* Still Lives

presence. They pleased me because they were strange and technically adept. But much of the mystery and power I imagined would be there was hidden from me.

### The Hunger Artist

At that time I became involved in a book project, illustrating Franz Kafka's story, 'The Hunger Artist,' through photographs. The story concerns a man whose art is fasting. While fasting is in vogue, he achieves quite a bit of acclaim for his excellent artistry. But when the public loses its interest in fasting, the hunger artist, although neglected, continues, breaking his own fasting records in obscurity. In the end, he sells himself to a circus, withers away in neglect, and is finally replaced by a panther. Before his death, he is asked why he didn't resume eating. He replies: 'Because I could never find the right food.'

In searching for the right images to illustrate the story, I came across a desolate structure on the waterfront of New Jersey and shot a series of rather desolate pictures of the mask of myself in a kind of suicidal pose. For the first time, I realized that these pictures of masks had something to do with dying, and that the dying was self-inflicted, about a vain search for the right sustenance. In many ways, this is the substance of dramatic tragedy, embodied in a protagonist who in his hubris acts out his art blindly, searching for the life-sustaining food that is always beyond his grasp. In the end, like the hunger artist, he brings upon his own death.

## Diane Arbus

Soon thereafter, I became aware of the charged world of Diane Arbus (1972), of her peculiar use of the literal and figurative mask, of her willingness to expose actors trapped in roles impossible to separate from. Arbus' photographs spoke to me directly. They were so painfully real, so full of feeling, yet so stark, stylized, and distant at the same time. The two levels of reality were suspended in a timeless tension. Hers were the images on Keats' Grecian urn, the foster children 'of silence and slow time.' Hers were Keats' gods bringing the message to us mortals that 'Beauty is truth, truth beauty.' But what a grotesque beauty – assorted giants, dwarves, transvestites, and disabled individuals. Their grotesqueness and strangeness was their mask, the part of the godhead under which was a human survivor. Arbus saw divinity in the persona, that elevated state of being that she could never find in her own masks or within herself and so, like the hunger artist, she stopped living.

## Ralph Eugene Meatyard

Soon after luxuriating in Diane Arbus' images, I was introduced to the equally extraordinary photographic work of Ralph Eugene Meatyard. Like Arbus, Meatyard was obsessed with the grotesque which means, literally, the painting of grottoes. His stated aim was to get people to read the image on the grotto as if it were a clear message. He wrote (1974): 'I want to get people to read stone, tree, so forth and so on through the construction of the picture' (p.82).

Many of Meatyard's pictures are of masks – adults and children in masks, masks in nature, people and natures as masks. All his subjects become endowed with an extraordinary power. Gene Meatyard must have seen them that way – nature and people as gods, demons, heroes, spirits. Unlike Arbus' stillness, Meatyard's pictures move. A recurring motif is an out-of-focus image, caused by the deliberate or random movements of head or body or wind in the branches of a tree. The distortions and the shadowy substance leads us further into the spirit world, the Mount Olympus of Lexington, Kentucky, where Meatyard shot most of his pictures.

As we look at Meatyard's images, we become immediately alienated from the conventional world that we know best. Through Meatyard, we come to see feelingly, as Gloucester does in Shakespeare's *King Lear* once he is blinded, to see beyond the veil or reality.

Meatyard's most ambitious work is *The Family Album of Lucybelle Crater*. The name is taken from a short story by Flannery O'Connor whose characters are Lucynelle Crater and her daughter, Lucynelle Crater. In Meatyard's work, which took the form of a one-man show and later, a book, we see two masks – one an overstated rubber fright mask of a woman; the other, a more realistic plastic mask of an old man. He photographed residents of Lexington, Kentucky in the masks, two in each picture. One of the two is his wife, Madelyn, wearing the female mask. In the final image, however, she appears wearing the male mask, dressed in Meatyard's clothes. He appears in the female mask dressed in Madelyn's clothes. The title of the picture is 'Lucybelle Crater and her 46-year old husband Lucybelle Crater.'

*Lucynelle Crater* is called a family album. All the conventional family roles are there – mothers and fathers, children and elders, brothers and sisters – but they are all one (or all two). Is the family one person, a woman and her double, repeated infinitely? And is this one person pure persona, a reflection of the godhead that is infinitely (pro)creative? Do the shadows, the blurriness, the distortions of the face suggest that the family and the community also have doubles, created spirit-like in the mind of the artist and the viewer who, willing to look, see the unseen?

As one pages through this bizarre family album, one becomes aware that the two masks change constantly according to different wearers. Then is Lucynelle Crater one person/persona or many? She changes yet remains the same. Says Catullus (Catullus in Meatyard 1974): 'Everything is water/if you look long enough' (p.83).

## A.D. 1952

Around the time I became interested in Meatyard's photographs, I embarked upon my most ambitious project – photographing my hometown, Hoboken, New Jersey, in terms of a mask, a rather human-like representation of Captain Kirk, the role created by William Shatner for *Star Trek*. Unlike Meatyard, I wanted my vision of Hoboken to be crystal clear – no movement, no heavy shadows, no distortions. I didn't quite understand my attraction to the mask except that it seemed to stretch the boundaries between life and death. That is, it appeared both alive and dead at once: alive in its representational quality, dead in its fixed expression, suggesting a cadaver after embalming or a death mask.

While photographing the mask in a vacant lot, alone, a man appeared, dressed conservatively in suit and tie, staring at me from a safe distance. He appeared frightened seeing the mask suspended from a wire on a brick wall. I assured him that the mask was, in fact, an object made of rubber. He responded by telling me the story of a murderer he had read about in the local paper who decapitated his victims. To ease his mind and to slow down my rapid heartbeat, I retrieved the mask and brought it to him, crumpling it up in my hands to demonstrate its inanimate quality. But he became more frightened by this demonstration and ran away. For him, I was, indeed, one who decapitates, a murderer of sorts.

I reflected upon the primitive warriors who demonstrated their victories by decapitating their enemies and shrinking their heads. How curious it is that the contemporary western healer, the psychotherapist, is referred to, ironically, as a 'head-shrinker.' Is it the mind of the neurotic that needs shrinking? Is his head too large, his ego too inflated?

Captain Kirk was just the right size for a head. But in the pictures he assumed many sizes and poses. He was malleable – at times appearing quite alive, other times, quite dead. I put together an exhibition entitled 'A.D. 1952' after a wall I discovered near the waterfront with that particular inscription. In the title photograph, the mask was centered on the wall.

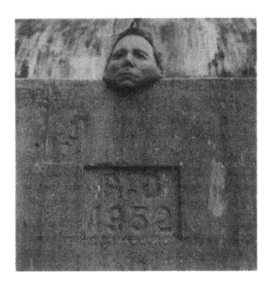

*Figure 5.6 A.D. 1952*

As before, I didn't understand quite what I had done. The pictures were technically the best work I had made. Hoboken was visible in quite a beautiful way. The seediness of junkyards and wire fences took on an elegance. And the presence of Captain Kirk was strong, rich, changeable, alive as a spirit presence.

When I named the show 'A.D. 1952' I had no understanding of why. In a recent therapy session, six years after the show, my therapist asked me if I could remember a time when I was really happy. I told her that when I was a child in Hoboken, living in a rich mix of cultures and classes, I was very happy. When I left to move to the suburbs at age eight, my unhappiness and sense of alienation set in. There, I was with others like me – all similar in religion, socio-economic status, race. We all looked alike, all Captain Kirks with fixed expressions, changing only in subtle ways with each new picture in our family albums. The year I moved was 1952.

Ralph Eugene Meatyard lived in Lexington, Kentucky for the last 22 years of his life. He saw his town clearly yet photographed it, as through a glass, darkly. Virtually all his pictures are of Lexington. I've lived in and out of Hoboken, never staying very long, always moving on. My vision of my

hometown is tinged with nostalgia, sentiment, memory. Because I could not
see it clearly in my mind, I tried to see it clearly in my art. The focus was always
as clear as I could make it. In 1952, I experienced a profound death – the loss
of my childhood. Captain Kirk sits upon the tombstone/wall, near the waterfront, commemorating that death. He is a vulture without eyes.

## The Mask in Therapy

For the past six years, I have been working toward the development of the
profession of drama therapy. Although there is a long history of psychodrama
and theatre performance by and for disabled and disturbed populations, the
profession of drama therapy, combining the several areas of psychotherapy,
improvisation, and performance, is new. Being new, there are few models of
theory and practice. Still resonant with the mysteries of masks, I began
experimenting with masked forms of dramatic projection – puppets, masks,
make-up and dreams, among others.

The image of the mask as death did not hold in my work in drama therapy.
Ralph Meatyard (1974) once queried: 'Am I looking at a mask or am I the mask
being looked at?' (p.83). The mask is alive, a persona that can see and hear. In
therapy, the mask is not the Greek actor assuming the role of Oedipus to be
projected to 30,000 viewers. In therapy, the mask is not the godhead reaching
toward Mount Olympus. In therapy, the mask is an image of the self. The
external focus of theatre and photography take a turn inward in therapy. The
godlike, emblematic, universal quality of the mask points not to the head and
the heavens, but to the heart.

I make a distinction in drama therapy between psychodramatic techniques
and projective techniques. The former refer to the enactment of the self,
unmediated. The latter refer to the enactment of the self as it is projected
outward upon a character, mask, doll, puppet, or other object. Each projective
object implies a certain level of distance from the subject. The less distanced
objects are those, like dolls, that are separate from the body. The mask, although
not attached to the face, is an object of minimal distance, because when worn
it becomes part of the face. It is, however, more distancing than make-up as it
can be removed easily and referred to as a separate entity in the therapy session.

In therapeutic mask work, then, the mask is used as a projective technique
to separate one part of the self from another. The masked part, the persona,
being stylized and dramatic, provides a measure of distance from the person.
Through the work with the persona, the person comes to see his dilemma more
clearly. The therapeutic masquerade aims to unmask the self through masking
a part of the self that has been repressed or seen dimly by the client.

Akhter Ahsen's (1972) work in eidetic psychotherapy often begins with an
image of the parents in the house where the client has grown up. The therapy
proceeds through a visualization of the images of parents and self, then through

a monologue or dialogue based in the visualization. In individual or group drama therapy work, the images are given a tangible form. A powerful container for that form is the mask.

Starting from the point of visualization, the client then builds masks of the characters imagined, most often mother, father, and self. The mask-making process itself is a ceremonial act of creation as the client reconstructs the image of his face three times. An additional fourth mask can be added to incorporate the image of a sibling. This fourth image would be consistent with Ahsen's (1984) notion of the primacy of the sibling relationship as described in *Rhea Complex*.

In building the masks on the face with gauze impregnated with plaster of paris, an exact imprint of one's facial features is fixed. Working to design the mother, father, and sibling masks, then, one begins with the image of self. The self mask becomes mother, father, and sibling as it is decorated with paint and material. Even those who are without siblings would work with the image of an imagined sibling. In superimposing the images of mother, father, and sibling upon the mask of self, those images become projections of the self.

The process of building the family masks is similar to the process of photographing significant others in the mask of self. The difference is that as the drama therapy proceeds, clients will wear all the masks themselves. In the photographs, 'Still Lives,' the face/mask remained the same while the bodies changed. In the drama therapy work, the body remains the same while the face/mask changes.

When the masks have been constructed, the client begins to reconstruct the world of his childhood with available objects in the room. His world is represented by the house he grew up in, including the rooms where he visualized his family and himself. Like the theatrical set designer, the client symbolically re-presents a piece of reality through objects and props.

Then, the client places the masks in the house, exactly in the proper places. With the therapist's help, as needed, the client interviews the masks, assuming the role of interviewer and all the roles of interviewee – mother, father, sibling, and self, in turn. Should the verbal interview prove too over- or underdistancing for the client, he can be asked to warm-up through a movement exercise. Taking the masks one by one, he can assume each of the four roles, finding the appropriate posture, gait, and emotional tone for each character as he moves through space.

Following the verbal and/or movement warm-up, the client is brought back to the house of masks. The drama can proceed in several ways. For one, the client can simply play with the masks, enacting a spontaneous scenario through a manipulation of the masks. The mask thus becomes a kind of puppet that is animated by the client in taking on the various roles.

Following the play, the client can be brought to reflect upon his drama in discussion with the therapist or in creating a narrative based upon the content of the drama. If the story is distanced by reference to the characters in third person and by a 'once upon a time' frame, the client can safely re-present his family drama. In working with the overdistanced client, the therapist might ask him to assume the point of view of one of the masks/family members and re-tell the story in first person.

A second approach is for the client to work in mask, assuming the roles of the family characters. This can occur spontaneously, as the client chooses masks at will, engaging in dialogue with the other characters. Or, the therapist might be more directive, encouraging the client to assume the point of view of one character at a time and to interact with the others in movement and/or monologue.

A third approach is a more psychodramatic one where the therapist or other group members play auxiliary ego roles, assuming the masks of mother, father, sibling, or self in relation to the client, also in mask. Through movement and/or dialogue the dilemma of the client can be brought into focus through a confrontation with the auxiliary ego.

Again, each enactment is followed by a period of closure or reflection upon the action. The closure can be a rather conventional discussion about what has happened or a more expressive, symbolic mode of storytelling or movement.

During the closure, the client is presumably unmasked. But is he really? Is there actually a part of a person that is separate from a persona? Is the reflective/analytical mode an unmasked mode? It seems to me that the image of the thinker is no less a mask than that of the actor. The backstage, at ease, relaxed behavior of a person is also a persona which can be as spontaneous and/or rigid as on-stage, performed behaviors.

The closure, then, is not an un-masking, but a shift from one reality to another, from that of drama/representation/fiction to that of the actual. Both realities have their masks. In the former, one consciously fashions his masks and wears them, knowing well that they can be discarded at any given moment. In the latter, one often unknowingly fashions his masks and wears them as if they did not exist. In the mode of fiction, one is free to come and go in and out of character at will. In the mode of actuality, one must work hard to achieve that level of liberation.

Beyond the persona is the person. Beyond the mask is the face. Beyond the face is the skull. And the skull is a ubiquitous image stamped on masks throughout history and culture. The skull is death, or life in death, or life remembered, or life re-lived. When Hamlet approaches the cemetery in Act Five of Shakespeare's play he discovers several skulls and speculates upon their origins as politicians, courtiers, businessmen, lawyers, even as the first murderer, Cain. Then he comes to the skull of Yorick, his father's jester. Yorick, the 'fellow of infinite jest,' wore a mask, a painted face. He was a player and a companion of Hamlet. He made the troubled Hamlet laugh. The troubled adult was once a joyful child in the presence of the masked Yorick. The jester that is left is a skull without a chin, a mask twice removed. That skull, universal emblem of the mask, leads Hamlet to muse upon the absurd cycle of life from flesh to earth. He recites:

> Imperious Caesar, dead and turned to clay,
> Might stop a hole to keep the wind away.
> O, that that earth which kept the world in awe
> Should patch a wall t'expel the winter's flaw! (v, i, 205–8)

The final image of the mask, that of the skull, is the great equalizer, the mask of Everyman, of Lucybelle Crater, of lawyer and courtier, of Caesar and Alexander and Cain. In drama therapy, as in verbal and visual imagery work, the mask reflects the universal. But, unlike the photographic and dramatic arts, it proceeds through an inward journey toward self. Paradoxically, that self is a reflection of the outside – of the family, the society, the culture that stamps its masks on the skulls of us all.

## The Significance of the Mask in Theatre and Therapy

The notion of drama as representation is central to psychotherapy. The mask is a link between western psychotherapy and universal cross-cultural ritual, magic, and healing. Freud recognized the power of the dramatic in his notions of transference and countertransference, a making present of the past through endowing the other in the therapist/client relationship with a new role. In psychoanalysis the crucial moments occur when the client is able to move from the narrative mode, the telling about what has happened, to the dramatic mode, the re-living of the past, transformed through present experiencing.

The mask of the classical analyst, like the classical Greek actor, is a distanced, neutral one. The analyst is Everyman, Willy Loman, Father, Mother. The analysand is the director of his own drama of transference, type-casting the analyst in his autobiographical script. Likewise, the analyst casts a mask upon the client, transforming him into the ingenue, the romantic lead, the heavy, the earth goddess – images of desire, fantasy, repulsion within his life scenario.

Jung was the first to overtly recognize the power of the creative arts in healing. Developing the notion of active imagination, Jung expanded upon dream images through creative expression in movement, drawing, drama. Studying the rituals, ceremonies, and healing rites of many non-western cultures, Jung incorporated a deep understanding of the mask into his analytic psychotherapy. His notion of mask took the form of the archetype, the substance of the collective unconscious. The archetypal images of the demonic, the godlike, the parental, the bisexual, were ubiquitous – in dreams, memories, fantasies, reflections. In order to move toward individuation, a sense of integration and wholeness, the client in Jungian analysis needed to wear his archetypal masks without guilt or fear of being taken for an imposter.

Other psychotherapists have incorporated images of the drama and of the mask in their work – the mask of play in the studies of Melanie Klein (1932), Margaret Lowenfeld (1967), and Erik Erickson (1952); the mask of the double and the auxiliary ego in the work of J.L. Moreno (1946); the mask of the top dog and underdog in the work of Fritz Perls (1947). Those therapists and counselors who deny the mask are left with only one mode of reality to work through – that of the actual. The behaviorist works best in the actual mode, focusing upon visible, tangible manifestations of personality. But without a notion of the other reality, that of the imagination, the mask, the double, an all too finite part of the human being is being addressed.

For centuries, healing and dramatic activity were enacted by masked practitioners – shamen, priests, mummers, *commedia* actors. They all recognized that the power of the mask lay in its power to link the two realities of the actual and the imaginative, the natural and the supernatural. They knew that the life of a human being was not only about visible behavior, but also about magical thought, irrational feeling, spiritual transcendence. To let go of the mask, which points to the notion of two realities, is to let go of a profound conception of mankind. To deny the connection between psychotherapy and drama, one that is clearly manifest in magic and ritual, is to settle for a method of psychological healing that is superficial, skin-deep.

In 1912, Gordon Craig warned that the theatre would degenerate if the mask were removed. In most arenas, the mask has been removed – in Broadway, in London's West End, and in countless third world countries that import the latest New York/London smash hit. Plays are packaged and sold by virtue of the drawing power of the leading performer. The personality of Dustin Hoffman, for example, has sold the 1984 production of Arthur Miller's *Death of a Salesman* to the public. The Broadway audiences come to see Hoffman perform, rather than to see the life of Willy Loman unfold. Hoffman's make-up notwithstanding, the actor is unmasked. The personality is the event, rather than the persona.

When the actor and the audience conspire to bury the mask, they enter into a narcissistic relationship, seeing each other naked, a reflection of a reflection; the former needing to maintain a star status in the eyes of the public; the latter wishing to be as important and as celebrated as the star. Such a relationship severely demeans the value of theatre.

The alternative theatre that still breathes in the forms of ritual drama, dance/movement, storytelling, song, and puppetry is a theatre of mask. It is a popular theatre in a way inconceivable to the press agents of Broadway. It is a theatre that evokes gods, demons, heroes and fools, that addresses issues of life and death, war and peace, change and revolution through archetypal figures. The audience's critical faculties are not dulled by an easy identification with the suffering of a single personality. Rather, they are brought to an awareness of the way things are and the way things can be though remaining at aesthetic distance from the actual events dramatized. The dramatic illusion is based in their knowledge that the mask is both a god, unlike them, and a person, like them. In the conventional theatre, the public sees the actor as a god and the issues presented as masks. The dramatic illusion is based in a consciousness that does not necessarily aspire to critical thinking or insight, but rather to the narcissistic celebrity of the star.

The mask in theatre and therapy is a projective device. It is an image of the transcendent part of the human being, that which strives toward a more perfect existence and battles with deep-rooted fears. It points outward toward the heavens and hells of myths, beliefs, and cultural practices, and inward toward the gods and demons of the unconscious mind. It hides and obscures the individual in order to reveal the universal. Its superficial and frozen appearance masks the profound and dynamic nature of the human mind. The mask is pure paradox – a mediator between the two realities of the actual and the imaginative, a link between ancient religious practices and modern psychotherapeutic and aesthetic ones, a midpoint between life and death.

In his book on Liberian masks, George Harley (1950) writes: 'The thesis that God made man in His own image is reversed when man makes a human image and endows it with godlike attributes' (p.3). With such a powerful object as a mask, both therapist and director can transform their art beyond the superficial, beyond the cult of the personality. In restoring the mask to its proper place in theatre and therapy, the director, actor, therapist and client can play, like Ralph Eugene Meatyard, among the stones and trees, learning how to read stone and tree, how to see the family and the self again.

Theatre comes from the Greek *theatron*, a place for seeing. Both the theatre and therapy session can become that place if all players agree to reveal that which needs to be seen, the actual, through participation in the masked world of the imagination.

# CHAPTER 6

# Reflections Upon Training
## The Making of a Drama Therapist

I have been a trainer of drama therapists and a writer and researcher in the field of drama therapy since 1980. In that time, I have come up with a list of competencies that I thought should be mastered by all of my drama therapy students (Landy 1986). My assumption has been that if one masters the several skills of acting, directing, counseling, conceptualizing, and developing a 'therapeutic personality,' one will become a competent therapist; if not, one won't. I also assumed that I had mastered all these competencies, and that I was to be the model for my students, at least at the level of knowledge and skills.

During the past few years, as students have graduated from the New York University Drama Therapy Program and become professional drama therapists, with varying degrees of mastery of the above competencies intact, I have noticed the surfacing of a quiet but persistent insecurity. It goes to the core of the person's professional identity and raises some very basic questions: Do I really have the competencies necessary to help people get better? How can I survive in an environment where I feel so alone and often unacknowledged? How do I know that drama therapy really works? Outside of my graduate school program, does anybody really care about drama therapy and, consequently, about what I can do? Did I become a drama therapist because I have failed as a theatre artist or because I didn't have the right stuff to succeed as a legitimate psychotherapist? Am I, in fact, a legitimate professional at all, or simply a pretender, a mere player?

Assuming the professional, nurturing role, I've often responded to these questions in a positive way. 'Be patient,' I've told my students, 'you are knowledgeable and well-trained. Affirm your choice of a new profession. Accept the reality that new professions threaten old, established professionals. Take on the pioneering spirit, as lonely as it is, and forge ahead. Trust yourself. Trust your training. Trust your teachers. Healer, heal thyself!'

Returning from a recent sabbatical, marked by visits to other drama therapy training programs and to faraway spiritual sites, I experienced a certain professional identity crisis. I could still go through the motions of teaching and training drama therapists, but I couldn't silence the kinds of questions mentioned above, this time turned back on myself. I suddenly felt that the little niche of drama therapy that I had carved out for myself wasn't enough. Several students were abandoning the program or the field, some transferring to social work schools, where, they reasoned, their professional identity and job prospects would be assured. Others were jumping ship in joining forces with the psychodrama community which they perceived as more organized and validated. Still others were applying to clinical psychology programs and Jungian institutes. I wondered if I, as teacher, should follow the lead of my students?

Lost as to my next step, I turned, as I had done many times before, to the classical forms. In this instance, the most classical form of all seemed to be psychoanalysis. I reasoned that if I became an analyst, trained in the classical Freudian orthodoxy, I would at last achieve legitimacy, if not intellectual clarity. Then I could return to drama therapy and really know what I was doing. Wasn't it, in fact, time to stop playing games and start doing some really serious work?

At the heart of my questioning were the same insecurities I had heard expressed by my students. The years had passed, but the world was still not safe for drama therapy. There were finally jobs available, but they were primarily with severe and difficult populations – psychotic in-patients, homeless mentally ill, disoriented, frail elderly – those who often frustrated more established mental health professionals. There were local, national, and international organizations hard at work, but I still felt isolated and disconnected from a professional community. If only I had gone to medical school. If only I had entered a conventional clinical psychology program. If only I had the proper credential or the appropriate training. If only I had a mentor and a safe collective that desired me. If only I were different from what I was.

The more I raised these kinds of issues, the more attractive psychoanalytical training appeared. I was invited to participate in a symposium on play therapy at New York University, centered around a paper, 'The Myth of Play Therapy,' delivered by Martin Silverman, a child psychiatrist. Dr. Silverman and all the other presenters were psychoanalytically trained. The thesis of the paper was that play therapy is a myth, a fiction, as children are not healed through mere playing. It is the verbal expression of feelings and its analysis that leads to the therapeutic results, the play being a device the helps facilitate the verbal, analytical process.

My voice was the only dissenting one. Play can be seen as a valid therapy in its own right, I said. It could well be that the healing comes through the playing rather than the talking. Myth is not, I continued, a misrepresentation of some objective truth, but rather a set of subjective assumptions we trust in to explain a piece of reality. Thus, the myth of play therapy is as subjectively true as the myth of psychoanalysis. My critique wasn't very forcefully delivered. I didn't want to offend potential colleagues in psychoanalysis, whose club appeared very attractive to me.

After the symposium, we all shook hands amicably, and I went home to fill out my application for the psychoanalytical training institute, feeling somewhat ambivalent and isolated. Dr. Silverman presented a dramatic case in his paper of a seven-year-old emotionally disturbed boy named Billy, who took excessive responsibility caring for his mother, a depressed emotionally immature woman who was only content when pregnant. Throughout Billy's young life, she was pregnant most of the time and had suffered three miscarriages.

Billy liked to build model airplanes, one of which remained unfinished and became an object of conflict between his therapist (Dr. Silverman) and himself. Billy demanded that Dr. Silverman help him complete the model. Dr. Silverman informed Billy that he would only when Billy agreed to speak about why the model was so important to him. Billy was initially incapable of articulating this thought. Through a difficult verbal, analytical process, Billy was finally led to realize that he had been suffering terribly because of his inability to understand and control his mother's pregnancies and pain. The therapeutic breakthrough (catharsis? insight? behavioral change?) came when Billy was able to release his pain through sobbing and verbalize the connection between model and mommy. Yet, I felt that what really lead to the therapeutic change within the boy was not the talking and the analyzing, but rather the authentic moments of spontaneous drama, most noticeable in the peak moment when Dr. Silverman (Silverman 1987) physically stopped the boy from smashing the model airplane, and: 'he collapsed backward against the wall and sobbed bitterly: "I want a new model! I want a new model! I want a new molly! I want a new mommy!"' (p.15).

It was summertime. The psychoanalytic training in the fall would include my own analysis, five times a week. To resolve whether or not I should enter therapy five times a week, I began therapy once a week with a rather unconventional man, a classically trained clinical psychologist, who proceeded to violate all the classical rules: He talked 50 per cent of the time; he allowed sessions to exceed the sacred 45 minute rule; he offered me food and drink (juice) and prepared tuna fish sandwiches in the kitchen adjacent to the consultation room when he got hungry; he answered his telephone during sessions; he told corny jokes while in session.

As a client in therapy, I again realized the power of the therapist as model. He became a point of identification, a touchstone. I found myself at first critical and angry in the face of his flagrant disregard of therapeutic protocol. I reflected back on my early days as a drama teacher of severely emotionally disturbed adolescents. Whenever one of my students regressed or acted out in a manic fit of destructive behavior, I would be held accountable by the equally unstable headmaster and branded with the term 'unprofessional.' And I was an easy target, because I often felt unprofessional, insecure and tentative in my early application of dramatic techniques to behavior well beyond my understanding. The epithet 'unprofessional,' however, became a wall, a defense against the headmaster's own inability to resolve apparently unresolvable behavior. But in my mind, I retained the sense that a 'real professional' knew the curative methods, the answers to the mysterious questions raised by the reality of mental illness.

At first, I judged my therapist to be unprofessional. Then, as the therapeutic bond developed and the judge retreated, that label melted away. Couldn't I, too, be 'unprofessional' and still be knowledgeable and effective? I realized certain confusions I had among the terms unprofessional, uncertain, and unconventional. To clarify these confusions I turned each word around: professional therapists were those who had mastered a body of knowledge and skills which they applied to help foster the psychological growth of a client. A code of ethical principles also accompany the knowledge and skills. Harder to define than the more external skills, ethical principles refer to the relationship of the therapist and client in terms of power, confidentiality, and behavior in role.

Unprofessional therapists were, first, inadequately trained and acquired their knowledge by minimal exposure to the field – through workshops, readings, occasional coursework, and unsupervised fieldwork. I reflected upon the first course I taught in drama therapy. Although I felt somewhat prepared academically (it was 1980 and there was little available literature), I certainly felt unprepared as to the actual function and clinical purpose of the drama therapist. This first course was a pure improvisation. I hoped the students would be sophisticated enough to validate my vaguely formed thoughts. On the last day of class, one of my least knowledgeable students informed me that she and her husband were moving to the country and asked if I thought it was alright for her to begin a drama therapy practice – based only on the experience of this one course. Unprofessional! I said, both to my student and myself.

Further, unprofessional therapists, no matter how well trained, subscribe to a dubious ethical system. Such a system is not necessarily dependent upon whether they offer food or answer telephone calls during therapy (although for some clients and therapists this might be a real professional issue), but rather upon their ability or inability to maintain a respectful, tolerant, non-judgmental, non-coercive relationship with a client, to examine their own countertransferential issues in supervision, and to assure confidentiality. I certainly had no intention of being unprofessional according to these criteria.

The next term, uncertain, seemed to me more comfortable and more clearly self-descriptive. Turning the word around, 'certain' therapists were ones who had not only mastered a certain technique or approach, but believed that it was certain to work most of the time. Certainty applied to those psychiatrists, for example, who treated a symptom rather than a person, prescribing medication to quell the hyperactive and stimulate the depressive, those whose treatment was based upon achieving predictable behavioral results.

Uncertain therapists were ones who acknowledged the mysteries and complexities of behavior, thought, feeling, intuition. Uncertain therapists worked with individuals who appeared catatonic, ignorant, senile, rigid, self-destructive, totally lost within themselves, and first dared to acknowledge the limits of their techniques and understandings. Then, engaging their professional skills, they devised strategies, uncertain as to the outcomes.

I find myself praising uncertainty too much here and echoing the notion of Bertolt Brecht that of all things certain, the most certain of all is doubt (see Brecht 1977). Uncertainty need not be a therapeutic ideology, but rather a way of validating the complexities of the human condition. Certain of their skills and orientations, of their careful readings of the research literature, certain, too, of the limitations of the same, therapists enter into the uncertainties of new therapeutic relationships. I wanted to be both certain and uncertain – a professional certain of his knowledge and skills, yet open to the uncertainties of the therapeutic process.

The third term, unconventional, proved the most difficult of the three to specify and understand. The field of drama therapy, with a short history, had not yet established an image of the conventional drama therapist. The conventional psychoanalyst, in the image of Freud, is wise yet distant, unseen, unheard; the conventional Jungian analyst, in the image of Jung, is intellectual, mystical, and creative; even the conventional psychodramatist had a model, that of Moreno, the magician, the powerful, often manipulative director who creates emotionally charged, cathartic moments. For me, conventional therapists adhered to the principles and techniques of their mentors. If they deviated from the hard line, their deviations were minor, later to be confessed to an orthodox supervisor.

With no hard line established in my field, and with the burden of becoming simultaneously unconventional, in the sense of breaking with classical models of psychotherapy; and conventional, in the sense of having established one of two extant drama therapy training programs in the United States and becoming a model for my students, I became uncertain and fearful of underlying unprofessional tendencies.

In the summer of 1987, I withdrew my application from the psychoanalytical training institute and began to re-build my professional self-image and reaffirm my primary commitment to the healing inherent in the art of drama/theatre. I turned back to an earlier paper I had written (Landy 1982b) setting forth a four-part model for training drama therapists. The four areas of training were, as follows:

1.  The self, involving the development of personal creativity and psychological awareness;

2.  The client, involving an understanding of various disabled groups;

3.  The techniques, involving a range of interdisciplinary practices;

4.  The theory, involving interdisciplinary principles and philosophical considerations.

I needed to review my own recent development in these areas and, more generally, to reevaluate the efficacy of the model. The most problematic area for me was that of the self in terms of creative and psychological development. For the past several years, I had very much focused my attention on theoretical and analytical matters, researching and developing theory and searching for ways to reconcile both psychoanalysis and analytic psychology with drama therapy. I had moved far away from the theatre. My former creative work as performer, director, and writer halted. I even had difficulty sitting through a play, feeling an odd mixture of boredom, repulsion, and jealousy toward the actors, director and writer.

The one medium I still embraced as a means of personal creativity was music. I had a long history of playing various instruments, of improvising and composing music. In my recent study of composition, I struggled against the demand from my teacher to be concrete and wedded to specific feelings and a coherent narrative. When connected to my feelings, I was able to find the tonalities that expressed the sense of isolation and loss I experienced in my early 40s. But all too soon, following the return from my sabbatical, the music stopped. For unknown reasons, I had difficulty hearing and composing music. Without theatre and music, my major means of aesthetic expression were silent.

At the same time, I had discontinued both psychotherapy and an ongoing process of transcribing and analyzing my dreams. I was no longer a client and a maker/consumer of art.

In my separation from the role of creative artist, I began to question the primacy of art as the base of the drama therapy experience. Around this time, my graduate school was also going through a kind of identity crisis, looking to reorganize and streamline its various offerings in education, health, communications, therapy, and the arts. I wrestled for long hours with the question: 'Should I support the move of drama therapy from a theatre department to a counseling/psychology department?' At first, I supported that move, a decision I saw as congruent with my desire for personal training in psychoanalysis. But then, I recognized how I was projecting my own sense of artistic alienation upon the discipline. I finally returned to the argument that the creative arts therapies are distinct from other forms of psychotherapy primarily by virtue of being based in the various art forms.

The picture of the self broadened further when I realized that my criteria for self-development were limited. Although I was not in the midst of an artistic project or a self-analysis, I was deeply involved in other equally creative acts: a kind of spiritual journey far away from home through ancient cultures and religions; and a love relationship, back at home. The twists and turns of these non-analytical acts demanded an intensity of synthesis and presence. Confronted in middle age so directly by God and Lover, the solid ground of Self became shaky. Being in relationship to forces outside myself, my very core trembled.

Extending this thought, I began to question the very existence of the self. An individual's role repertoire seemed to be ever expanding with each move into and away from the world. I know a role, new or old, by virtue of taking it on then moving, speaking, feeling, and sensing through it. And when a particularly compelling role sits on my shoulders, forcing me very much into the present, the sense of a core, a self, becomes lost. The social-psychologist, Sarbin (1954) wrote: 'The self is what a person "is," the role is what a person "does"' (p.244). But in an intense role, my actions and my being are one. I am, at the moment of role enactment, fully an intimate lover or a spiritual searcher. That is not, of course, all that I am. But is the 'all' something called self or simply more roles?

With this question in mind, I began to re-think the first area of training. Related questions surfaced: What is the self? What is its relationship to role? What is its place within a theory of drama therapy? In developing aspects of the self, shouldn't trainers know what aspects they are training?

In my case, I had to leave behind the roles of client, self-analysand, and creative artist in order to allow new roles to enter. In doing so, my professional identity became shaky, requiring support. I needed to renovate myself (my self) – break down walls and provide more space in my internal house for new roles. Nearing completion of this round of renovations, I found that the old roles of educator, scholar, and solitary thinker returned, somewhat transformed. In training the drama therapist on a personal level, there should be, I thought, plenty of room for expansion as the person discovers new personae.

The second area of training, that of understanding the client, appeared less problematic to me. In the several years that drama therapists have received formal training, with master's degrees in hand, the availability of jobs has dictated the realities of the client populations. The three most prominent client groups, at least in the New York metropolitan area, continued to be children situated primarily in a child life program of a medical hospital, some of whom were there for minor surgery, others who have been abused or in treatment for life-threatening diseases; elderly people situated in nursing homes, senior centers, and hospitals, some of whom were self-sufficient, others who were frail and/or disoriented; and short-term adult psychiatric patients, many of whom were diagnosed schizophrenic and/or substance abusers.

As a practitioner of drama therapy, my experience had been primarily with emotionally disturbed children and adolescents and neurotic adults. I did not feel prepared within myself to work with the client populations with whom my students interned and practiced. To remedy this situation, I spent many hours in the playroom of a large hospital in New York City. I was there in the role of internship supervisor, impressed with the skill of my students. Much of the time I felt like an imposter, for I was actually the student, learning how those academic matters I had taught actually translated into practice with children. Following a session in play therapy, I would resume my critical supervisor role and serve up a critique, usually still in awe of the work observed while in a student role.

I also observed work with the elderly, both in improvisational drama and the creation of theatre based in shared cultural experiences. While marveling at the patience, care, and skills of my students and of professionals, I clearly kept my distance from the group members. I began to recognize that my resistance to working with a frail elderly population was based in unresolved family issues. I feared the dependency, the infantilizing, the many losses of control of mind and body. I came from a family that regarded elders as either an extreme blessing or a hellish curse. On the one hand, a son was supposed to worship his aging parents; on the other, be dutiful and self-sacrificing, even as he secretly wished to escape the torrent of complaints and demands. Of all the groups available for drama therapy intervention, this was the one I avoided most in my professional career. Could I still encourage and supervise others in their work with the elderly while harboring these feelings within myself? I remained the distanced observer while I wrestled with this question.

But the observer role felt too distanced, too clean. Having just completed a textbook on drama therapy, I was able to assuage my fears and resume my professorial role, within which I felt rather safe. But it was time to work directly with a group again. I choose a large city hospital and a group of short-term psychiatric patients.

I was to be a volunteer in a large city hospital and like all volunteers, I was subject to the bureaucratic paperwork, interviews, and physical examinations. It took several days of endurance to pass through the often humiliating initiation rituals of the hospital.

Walking into my first group in a locked ward, with two supervisors present, a flood of regressive feelings overcame me. During the session, one supervisor intervened in the midst of a role-playing sequence with one man. Later she explained: 'He had gone too far. He got lost in the role. I had to bring him back. That's the point of our creative arts groups – to keep them in reality. After all, their illness is about delusion and flight from reality. You have no right to support their delusions. Stay away from fantasy!'

Lesson number one. So I was really back in school, and after I had written the textbook! How far should I go? I asked myself. If drama therapy was about working through a projective fiction in order to explore a deeper level of truth, then how could I manage to 'keep them in reality' without denying the essence of the dramatic experience?

There was an underlying message given by the supervisor, a trained creative arts therapist herself, that I heard over and over again from many supervisors in many activity therapy departments: 'This is what schizophrenic patients need – a large dose of reality, comparable to that doled out in their daily medication. The arts are great. They love plays, but be careful of encouraging unstructured role-playing – they get lost, excited; and stay away from masks and puppets – too stimulating. Why don't you give them plays to read?'

The double message – to do drama but not to do drama, or rather, to do theatre and not drama therapy – was a weight on my shoulders each day I led groups at the hospital.

As I began to become familiar with several of the patients, I relaxed into my role of drama therapist. I resisted the proddings of some of the staff to bring scripted plays to the group, and instead continued to explore fantasy work with puppets, masks, and stories. But it seemed that each time I gained a small victory, another roadblock would surface. For example, I wanted to know more about those few clients who faithfully returned to the group each week. At first I wasn't permitted to read the charts. Then one day, without notice, I was escorted into the chart room, with permission to read the documentation of my clients under the watchful eye of a supervisor. Shortly thereafter, I was reprimanded by another supervisor – volunteers were officially forbidden to read the patients' charts, she said, officiously.

Over several months, the group would change quite frequently. At times, I would appear at the scheduled hour to discover the group had been cancelled for one reason or another. The trips to the hospital became more tedious. The actual patient contact was becoming a smaller and smaller part of the experience. Like the clients, I, too, became a short-term person, defeated by a large city institution that denied me access to communications I needed, not only as information, but also as a lifeline from the community of human beings in the hospital environment to myself. And as a short-term person, the long waits for the elevators, the long wasted hours of bureaucratic indignity, the transience of the population, and endless frustration and weariness of the legitimate staff finally got to me.

Despite the personal frustrations, I left the hospital with not only a greater knowledge of adult schizophrenics, but also with a sense, however tentative, that projective techniques were effective in their treatment. There were actually strong moments in the group work when Ann was able to distinguish between characteristics of herself and those of her role; when Bea was able to reclaim her mother role through building a puppet; when Carl was able to move out of his chronic catatonic state for a short time and relate to another client through rhythm and movement. Even so, I was still left with the feeling of being a short-term therapist working with a short-term population with no means of follow-up. As such, I felt unable to claim any lasting therapeutic gains. Nor did I realize that such work could be valuable in and of itself. In the field of drama therapy, in 1987, there was no valuative instrument available.

In my role of volunteer/non-professional, in part self-chosen, in part imposed by the institution, I often felt powerless and isolated. Thinking about the four-part training model, I realized that a knowledge of the client population was insufficient in itself. The client group needed to be viewed in the context of an institution or community. As an uncertain therapist in an unconventional field I needed to be knowledgeable of the conventional psychiatric wisdom, but I also needed to trust that my unique approach might make a real difference in the lives of institutionalized clients. That trust was difficult to maintain when the institutional environment is harsh and indifferent, when supervisors are distracted, suspicious, or disinterested, when small clinical victories could not be shared, and when self-doubts crept in with regularity.

Further, I needed to develop an understanding of the limits of working with a short-term population, one that was fast becoming the norm in hospitals. Because the group was constantly in flux, the creative arts therapist had an ethical responsibility to shun depth therapy. Goals with short-term clients needed to be formulated to support defenses and contain excessive feeling, even while the process moved clients in and out of states of imagination and reality. With a group of hospitalized schizophrenics, many of whom are medicated, some of whom may be actively delusional, that process might involve taking on and playing out relevant roles, culminating in a single but significant realization of ways that they are the same as and different from their fictional personae. The naming of a role that is both me and not-me is ultimately a support of a client's need for reality testing. Through drama therapy, the knowing of reality occurs through the knowing of fiction and through the ability to distinguish one state of being from the other.

I had intended to explore these notions further in my work at the hospital. Through puppetry and mask work, especially, I wanted to validate the application of distancing theory in drama therapy to the healing of schizophrenic adults (Landy 1983, 1986). But with too much theory in hand, I ran my head against the hard reality of institutional life.

The third part of the training model concerns a mastery of drama therapy and related techniques. During the past twenty years, with a wide training and experience in theatre, in Gestalt therapy, psychodrama, group psychotherapy, and the like, I gathered a seemingly endless array of games, exercises, and toys. During the past three years, I have begun to realize a more difficult goal – that of letting them go. In the past, I had led most of my groups, whether therapy, education, or training, by preparing a particular exercise/technique, which provided a structure for the experience. The technique might be story dramatization, based upon a story I had chosen for the group. Or the technique might be one of many I was particularly fond of, most notably projective work through masks, puppets, and play objects. Many of my groups became workshops in the sense of providing a highly structured, short-term experience in drama therapy. The common denominator seemed to be control. If I controlled the means of working/playing, I thought, then the ends would be fairly well predictable.

Immersed in a theory of distancing which aimed toward a balanced emotional state and shunned both excessive emotional outbursts and hostile withdrawn behavior, I set out to work all too rationally. A series of early successes as a group leader, using highly motivating and creative techniques, filled me with confidence bordering on smugness.

During one year-long therapy group, which I co-led with a creative arts therapist who taught me the importance of letting go of plans and controls, my sense of technical competence was strongly challenged. While wielding my distancing techniques whenever the opportunities arose, an angry woman, Doris, less than dazzled by the magic, began: 'Speak to me directly. You are cold and distant. You keep hiding behind your techniques, which are fake.'

As a therapist with certainty, I interpreted her several outbursts as examples of transference and tried, through dramatic means, to get her to see whom I represented. But Doris resisted my attempts and remained in her angry role, railing against my refusal to see that she was angry at me, not at a symbolic counterpart.

After some months of this repeated behavior, coupled with many long talks with my co-therapist, I began to doubt my sacred techniques. For Doris, the dramatic experience of playing and reversing roles, of disguising some essential personal qualities in order to uncover a deeper sense of truthfulness, was artificial, false, and cold.

Doris and I did not get too far beyond our mutual barriers. There was, however, a mild reconciliation at the end of the group, when she agreed to reverse roles with me, and we were both able to enact a rather open and touching portrayal of each other. I remained convinced that my failure with Doris was based, in part, in her inability to creatively work through the transfer ence. I further thought that it was based in my inability to help her work through her resistance, as well as my own countertransferential issues of insecurity when confronted by an aggressive woman. My hunch was that Doris' sense of frustration remained based in a mistrust of the drama techniques and the drama therapist, both of whom she continued to see as too indirect, removed, and inaccessible to her needs. Maybe I should have been willing to meet her needs more directly. But I was so invested in the dramatic approach that I was unable to let go.

The work with Doris led me to question the limitations of dramatic techniques and structures. As exciting and motivating as they have been for many, the drama techniques were certainly not universally valid. Some, such as Doris, might need more direct contact with the therapist and to her everyday life experiences, feeling threatened by having to project parts of herself onto artificial roles. I learned that for those unwilling to engage in the artifice of drama, another approach to treatment seemed more appropriate.

Doris' resistance to the drama therapy approach was also a valid critique both of my dependence upon excessive structure and technique and my concurrent difficulty to be fully present. As I have been able to trust my technical knowledge and let go more of the need to control and prove, I found myself becoming a more competent therapist. In giving up a bit of the magician, who can dramatically transform one state of being to another, I became more the human being, able to be there and allow the dramatic and commonplace moments to unfold naturally. Sometimes that natural process is inhibited and individuals need the specific structures and techniques. A large issue in my self-training concerned developing the ability to know when to be more the model, the teacher, the leader, providing the structures, and when to be more the facilitator, the follower, drawing upon those structures provided by the client.

Doris also posed a challenge to my theoretical thinking. She was often too angry and confrontational, unwilling to project that anger onto a role. According to the distancing model, she was unable to release her anger, experience catharsis and thus, balance. During the past several years, I have employed the model to explain a range of emotional states, measured against a midpoint of balance and equilibrium. I defined balance as a healthy state, one rich in potential creativity, insight, spontaneity. At balance or aesthetic distance (see Scheff 1981), the individual is capable of feeling, without being flooded by excessive anger or shame; and thinking, without becoming overly intellectual.

I used the distancing model to assess clients, students, myself. I used it as a means of choosing techniques for treatment and education: if the client was too overdistanced, too removed from her feelings, I would choose a more reality-based psychodramatic technique; if the client was too underdistanced, too close to feeling out of control, I would choose a more fantasy-based projective technique. Further, I used the distancing model as a means of evaluating a drama therapy session or, more generally, a treatment over time. The measure of a client's health was determined by her ability to reach a balanced state and thus, to become more playful and spontaneous. If that state could be sustained over time, and if the client was able to bring herself there, unaided by the therapist, the therapeutic work was to be terminated.

The model became my oracle. It took on not only an analytical, rational power, but also a predictive, magical one. It was my rock, my article of faith. Even as my students pointed out inconsistencies in the model, I had answers. But as I began to listen to my answers, I became less certain. I couldn't help Doris by means of either over- or underdistanced techniques. I couldn't even decide if she was over- or underdistanced in her behavior. Her expressions of anger were sometimes loud and 'dramatic,' but they were coupled with a reflective quality not usually associated with underdistanced behavior. She wasn't only trying to express her feelings, but also to reflect upon them, to understand her position in the group.

I also noticed that some rather withdrawn, overdistanced schizophrenics reacted well to the distanced projective techniques of mask and puppetry. Others acted in ways more consistent with the model. The questions kept coming. One student asked: 'You say that depression is an overdistanced emotion, yet when I get depressed I sometimes lose control and cry for days. Explain that.'

I tried, but my attempt was feeble. The distancing model had become too heavy, and I grew weary trying to carry it around. As an article of faith, it lapsed.

I was slipping. I was so in need of answers, and it wasn't Freud or Jung or Perls or Moreno or Brecht or Stanislavski who had the answers. It wasn't the unconventional therapist who fed me tuna fish sandwiches, or the Jungian analyst who read my astrological chart, or the Pakistani guru who straightened out my misplaced mental images. It wasn't even theory that embodied the answer anymore.

What was the question? Was it the one I had raised so many times in my classes to those very practical souls resisting the study of theory: 'Why is it important to understand psychoanalytical theory, performance theory, any relevant theory? How will this understanding enhance your practice of drama therapy?' And always the eager hands shot up: 'To give us a way to make sense of our experience.' Yes. But I didn't encourage the discussion to go much further than that. What happens when the sense breaks down, when the balance is not restored as promised in the distancing model, when, in Yeat's words, 'Things fall apart; the centre cannot hold.' And what if there is no center at all? Maybe that was the question that I needed to ask myself in order to proceed with an understanding not only of drama therapy, but also of the general task of helping others seek their own paths.

I came to the conclusion that even in the face of breakdown, chaos, and irrationality, a central framework is necessary. That framework is provided by theory which can be conceived of as a map, a point of balance, a golden mean, a symmetry, at least a dialectic. Even in recent postmodern attempts to deconstruct art and language, a point of departure is established and identified as a model with an intact structure. Heiner Müller and Robert Wilson's play, *Hamletmachine*, deconstructs the solid text, *Hamlet*; in his non-book book, *Glas*, Jacques Derrida deconstructs the writings of Jean Genet.

The drama therapist also needs a point of reference, a framework, as a way to make sense of conventional life experience which is routinely deconstructed as clients take on and play out refracted views of reality. But given the complexities of human experience and a mind reflecting upon that experience, the single point of reference is often not enough. A text deconstructed is infinitely less complex than a mind deconstructing. If this is so, could it be that a single theory applied to the process of uncovering and reclaiming the self (if there is a self) is inadequate?

Several years ago, I discovered a theory, based in a philosophy of art (Bullough 1964, Scheff 1981, Willett 1964) that helped to explain, in part, the psychological and aesthetic phenomena embodied in drama therapy. But in the enthusiasm of discovery, I applied the theory of distancing too broadly, viewing it as the way to understand the substance and form of drama therapy. Distancing theory has been valuable. I trust it will continue to be so, but only if I can let go of it somewhat and stop squeezing it for more answers than it can yield.

As a trainer of drama therapists and as a practitioner of drama therapy, I feel I must continue to wrestle with issues of theory, practice, and personal growth. There will be regressive periods, when I abandon the struggle to renew and grow. And there will be times that I withdraw, retreat, and follow the path of the alienated Beckett characters who seem to only have enough energy to wait. There will be times of self-pity and jealousy, of chastising myself for all the missed opportunities in my life. At those times, I will try to remind myself why I have chosen drama therapy as a profession. It is a home that well contains my personality, with all its often contradictory pushes and pulls toward expression. It is a single thing, a framework, that contains a multitude. It is a domain for the parts of me that are foolish and heroic, powerless and powerful. It holds together my deepest interests in life – to act and to reflect, to live through the body and through the mind. It is a path to do good deeds while in the presence of demons. It is a way to stay very much alive in the world which, when it sings, is so very much like a stage. Through drama therapy I can be artist, healer, and celebrant – all at once. It is truly the house in which I live and even when I run away from home, it is one place to which I can always return.

# CHAPTER 7

# One-on-One

## The Role of the Drama Therapist
## Working with Individuals

## Introduction

Basketball is one of the most popular team sports in the United States. It is highly competitive and dependent upon physical, strategic, and creative group work. The team coach is a crucial figure, as he is responsible for shaping the group dynamics – the team spirit and strategy – that will prove effective in defeating a common enemy. Although basketball teams have star players, their effectiveness and health are dependent upon an integrated group of five men or women, all having a sense of their roles in relation to those of others on the team.

A more intensified form of basketball is called 'one-on-one'. In this version of the sport, one player competes against another. The group is that of two individuals, each assuming a similar role. That role, however, is complex. The one person embodies the five players on a team. S/he plays all positions and must perform all the actions ordinarily divided among five specialists. Furthermore, the two players must constantly reverse roles with one another. When Player A has the ball, Player B must take a defensive role and vice-versa. Each exchange of the ball implies a change of role from offensive to defensive and back.

One-on-one can be played in other sports and games, but the larger the arena and cast of players, the more difficult it is to collapse the many into one. Much of psychotherapy, as practiced worldwide according to the classical psychoanalytic model, is a game of one-on-one. However, according to the dictates of Freud and his orthodox followers, the roles of the two players tend to remain fairly stable. For the orthodox practitioner, psychoanalysis is not a sport or an art, but a science, practiced with fairly stable rules that govern the role relationship between the two participants. It is predicated upon reaching a given goal, the resolution of the transference neurosis, and aims toward the capacity to generalize – if it works for one, it should work for all who meet similar criteria for being suitable analysands.

In both Britain and the United States, an alternative psychotherapy tradition has developed, one that is based more in flux, ambiguity, intuition, play, doubt, and shifting role definitions. Less overtly scientific and encased in stable principles, it has evolved from many diverse sources: the transpersonal and imagery-based work of Jung (1968); the creative action approaches of Moreno (1946, 1959) and Perls (1969); the creative play approaches of Lowenfeld (1939) and Axline (1947); the humanistic approaches of Rogers (1961) and Maslow (1971); the existential approaches of May (1969) and Laing (1967); and the object-relations and transitional phenomena approach of Winnicott (1971). The alternative tradition has spawned many non-directive, imagery-based, and humanistic approaches. Most recently, this tradition has been exemplified in the work of the many creative arts therapists working through the media of art, dance, drama, music, and literature.

In the United States, a plethora of university-based training programs has developed respectively in art, dance, and music therapy. One, the Expressive Therapies Program, based in Lesley College, is eclectic, training students concurrently in art, music, movement, and psychodrama to become creative arts therapists. Several private institutes have also developed to train creative arts therapists; yet in the United States, they do not have the resources or credibility of the university programs. Drama therapy is a relatively new field. Unlike psychodrama, which has been practiced in the United States since the 1930s, it has found a safe haven in American universities. Several colleges and universities offer undergraduate and graduate courses in drama therapy and two offer fully blown graduate degrees in drama therapy, one at New York University, and one at California Institute for Integral Studies in San Francisco. The kinds of jobs that are available in the United States include those in psychiatric and medical hospitals, out-patient clinics, nursing homes and senior centers, facilities for substance abusers and developmentally disabled individuals, and hospices and treatment centers for those with terminal illnesses and AIDS. The majority of jobs tends to be in and around large cities, especially New York and San Francisco, where the two training programs are located.

## The Role of the Drama Therapist in Group Treatment

Drama therapy, like psychodrama, has tended to be a group therapy. Much of the focus in a drama therapy group has been upon group dynamics, role and communication structures. As such, drama therapy has remained true to its natural connection to the theatre and the theatrical event. Embodied in the theatrical event is the notion of enactment in role, in a particular space, with others who sometimes participate overtly, as fellow actors, or more covertly, as observers. In group drama therapy, the role of the therapist is similar to that of the theatrical director. S/he holds a vision of the whole, a concept of order, a beautiful form, often in the face of those resistances, struggles, and ambiguities essential to the creative process. It is this vision which provides the structure in which the participants can work creatively to discover, uncover, or recover the meanings of their enactments in role. The vision is not necessarily fixed, but shifting, consonant with the alignments and realignments of the group.

Like the basketball coach, the drama therapist helps the group develop strategies to defeat a common enemy. The locus of that enemy, however, tends to be within the individuals in the group. That internal enemy tends to take on demonic shapes as fears and insecurities are projected and transferred onto individuals in the group. A drama therapy group experience can be quite dizzying as projected roles dart about, bat-like. And like that of the basketball coach, the role of the drama therapist is a strategic one – helping to shape a group strategy that will lead individuals to a knowing of what their social roles are and what they can become in relation to others in a group.

## The Role of the Drama Therapist in Individual Treatment

The role of the drama therapist changes in a one-on-one situation; or, rather, it expands. The drama therapist remains essentially a creative, strategic thinker. S/he continues to hold a vision of the whole. But that vision is often less clear, less based upon a model of how things should be, for in the game of one-on-one, therapists are more visible, as they comprise 50 per cent of the group. The vision of the whole, then, is based upon the therapist as much as the client. The dynamics are intensified and in the interplay of the two actors on the therapeutic stage, many roles, often contradictory, ambiguous, ill-formed, will be called out. Also, as therapists become more active players, their ability to see themselves more objectively becomes impaired. In the heat of the drama, the player risks the possibility of identifying too deeply with the character.

I have used a model of aesthetic distancing in earlier writings (Landy 1983, 1986) to characterize the relationship between individuals in a group drama therapy situation and the intrapsychic relationships among internalized roles. I would now like to apply that model to the relationship between client and drama therapist in a one-on-one situation.

The model is based upon aesthetic principles represented most directly in the twentieth century by Edward Bullough (1912) and Bertolt Brecht (see Willett 1964). Developed by the sociologist, Scheff (1979), the distancing model speaks of human relationships in terms of degrees of closeness and separation. Intrapsychically, overdistanced people are those who are very removed, cut off from their feelings, highly self-protected. In psychoanalytic terms, they are under the control of their superegos. They tend to be overly intellectual, rational, and compulsive.

Underdistanced people tend to be too manic and excitable, too vulnerable, too close to the bone. Controlled primarily by the id, they appear to be overly emotional and impulsive, at times irrational.

The ideal state of aesthetic distance is one where the emotional and rational parts of the self are in balance. At aesthetic distance, the individual is capable of feeling, without fear of being overwhelmed by the emotion, and thinking, without fear of losing the ability to respond passionately. In the language of Witkin (1974), the state of aesthetic distance is one of an intelligence of feeling. According to Scheff (1979), the person at balance is able to respond to the paradox: how can I allow myself to recall repressed feelings, if the reason I repressed them in the first place was because they were too painful? The answer is that in the balanced state, the person is simultaneously playing actor and observer roles, a paradoxical situation that provides an emotional safety net. If, as I vent my rage, I can see myself – that is, if I can separate out the observer part that watches the actor part of myself enact a drama of rage – then I will be safe to release that emotion and perhaps, to reflect upon it. The enraged, murderous actor does not actually kill; the client acts the role of one who feels like killing.

Hamlet, as presented by Shakespeare, is not a balanced character. He is either overdistanced, 'sicklied o'er with the pale cast of thought,' (III, i, 93) or underdistanced, when he actually resorts to the violence that is ultimately homicidal and suicidal. In drama therapy, Hamlet might choose to conjure up the ghost of his father in the person of the therapist, or act out sexual and aggressive fantasies on dolls; but then the Shakespearian play would disappear. A balanced Hamlet, or any character purely acting at aesthetic distance, tends not to be theatrical, as the balanced state is one of resolution, rather than one of conflict. However, in classical theatre as well as drama therapy, aesthetic distance is the aim, the point of insight, catharsis, resolution. The means to that end is through the enactment of the more enhanced states of over- and underdistance. Thus, in moving toward resolution, the actor/client works through the spectrum of distance, playing with moments of rage, moments of depression and withdrawal, until a point of balance, of thoughtful feeling or sensitive reflection, can be discovered.

In applying the distancing model to the one-on-one drama therapy situation, let us look at the client/therapist relationship. According to the classical psychoanalytical model, the analyst remains overdistanced in relation to the patient. S/he is a physician – cool, analytical, in control. Even when analysts are not in control, they remain rational, holding in check their subversive tendencies toward countertransference. In a current British study of the psychotherapeutic process, Casement (1985) refers to the need for therapists to develop an internal supervisor, an observer role that will monitor their countertransferential reactions during a session. The implication here, I think, is to at all times get hold of oneself, to hold or contain oneself, as one holds or contains one's client. Most drama therapists might well argue that they need ultimately to assume a balanced role *vis-à-vis* their clients, checking themselves for moments of excess merging or separation. It seems to me, however, that the overdistanced role of the therapist is useful in drama as in other therapies, at least in the sense of providing boundaries and separation from their clients. Unlike more verbal, classical analysts, drama therapists have rather 'dramatic' ways of demonstrating separation and boundary setting. Their primary media are the stage, the story and the role.

One example of the stage, which becomes a separation of the reality of the imagination from that of everyday life, is in sandplay, enacted in a box with definite borders. These borders contain the imaginative enactment built in the sandbox by the client. According to Margaret Lowenfeld (1939), clients build miniature worlds in the sandbox, and through their 'world technique' external-ize their inner lives.

The story creates distance by framing experience in another time and another place: 'Once upon a time there was a little girl who grew up in a town far, far away...' Through the fiction of the story, the client tells the truth about her present circumstances.

Role, the most distinguishing feature of drama therapy, provides a further means of separation. In role, a person is reduced to personae as he unconsciously or consciously separates out discrete, coherent aspects of his personality. Roles are based in such categories as occupation, socioeconomic status, cognitive and affective state, and developmental or family position. In psychoanalysis, the role structure is covert; in drama therapy it is overt. A central rule of the game is that the client and often the therapist will play roles. The roles that each chooses to play create a boundary from the other. If he, as client, is in role of Mouse, and she, as therapist, is in role of Elephant, then a dramatic separation has been made.

By virtue of consciously working in role, the drama therapist differs radically from the overdistanced stance of many of her colleagues. The drama therapist does not, and cannot, remain permanently overdistanced if she is to effectively enter into the one-on-one drama. In working through a relationship where differing levels of power are delineated, i.e. elephant and mouse, mother/father and daughter/son, therapist and client, the drama therapist must be able to shift not only from one role to another, but from one level of distance to another. Thus, the safety of remaining in control and super-rational becomes difficult to sustain.

At times, the therapist needs to act underdistanced in order to evoke a response from an overdistanced client. For example, the client in the role of the mouse, makes himself very small. His movements are tight, tiny. His voice is barely audible. He avoids any contact with the therapist in role of elephant. The therapist fills herself up with her role. As the mouse shrinks, she expands. The smaller he becomes, the larger the therapist becomes. She trumpets, flailing her trunk; she swaggers around the room, knocking things off the table, threatening to crush the mouse under her big, round, wrinkled foot. In her fullness, being most threatening, challenging, clumsy, provocative, the therapist/elephant acts at being underdistanced.

Psychodynamically, this underdistanced enactment might very well be indicated to help the client/mouse experience, then become aware of his predicament when confronted with a large, clumsy, powerful authority figure. However, intrapsychically, the therapist might not feel underdistanced; that is, she might actually be balanced, having consciously or intuitively chosen a series of actions that might well provoke the kind of response she feels is necessary.

Ideally, the therapist, even in the heat of a dramatic enactment, remains balanced. She is, in fact, the consummate actor. Her moments are like those in a theatrical performance where the actor as Ophelia, on the brink of suicide, utterly despondent, is capable of releasing the imbalanced pain of Ophelia while simultaneously containing or retaining her own balanced sense of herself as intact performer.

In this balanced state, the therapist does not become so identified with the elephant that her own clumsy, elephantine power is on display. There needs to be an actorly reserve in her therapeutic performance and a repertory of roles easily accessible. For at any moment, she might ask the client to reverse roles with her, to take on the behavior and feeling of the elephant as she mirrors the diminutive mouse. And to the extent that the client is unable to take on the powerful role, the therapist must be able to meet that resistance within her new role, conjuring, seducing, provoking a willingness on the part of the client to pour life into the elephant shell.

Further, the therapist can move beyond the mirroring of the client's mouse. Drawing upon fable and myth, the therapist can present a mighty mouse or a clever mouse, who can run circles around the elephant, move elegantly, think and speak wittily.

The drama therapist, then, in a one-on-one situation, strives to find a balance between the part of herself that *is* actor, capable of conjuring up an excellent performance, and the part of herself that is therapist, audience, observing the effects of the drama and determining when and how to move it to another level of role-enactment and distance. She is in many ways both elephant and mouse: on the one hand, large and imposing, slow, clumsy, frightening; and on the other hand, small and sleek, quick and elegant, witty and frightened. In fact, she needs to be stereotype, prototype, no type at all, and even iconoclast. She is more than Hamlet and Ophelia; she is the entire *dramatis personae*, as well as stage manager and director. She is the consummate repertory player, a juggler of roles, a one-person masquerade.

## The Role of the Client in Individual Drama Therapy

Does the same burden fall upon the client in the dramatic game of one-on-one therapy? Must he, too, embody the many in one, and enter into drama therapy with an impressive theatrical resume? No…and yes. For the game of one-on-one to be truly a balanced one, both players must be relatively equal; that is to say, capable of surprising the other, capable of rising above one's apparent abilities or disabilities. It is the surprise element, the connection to even greater levels of excellence in performance that makes sports, arts, and therapy most vital.

The client surprises as the therapist surprises, through a kind of dramatic transcendence – unrehearsed, unconscious. This occurs when the client transcends his everyday role of mouse and accepts the challenge of the therapeutic stage – the permission to play. To play what? The many complexities of mousedom; and the many complexities of an expansive, inner repertory of roles. Each part or role of one's inner life, and each object or image in one's external world is a potential skin to be entered. These skins or masks are entered for a time, played through, then shed. And like the snake, a growing takes place when the skin is shed. A new creature appears, both different from and the same as the original – slippery and vulnerable, but ready to move on.

So the client must do what the drama therapist does – identify roles, take them on, and play them out. But there is a significant difference between the two players. The therapist's repertory of roles is larger than the client's – at least by one. And that one is the director role as well as what I referred to above as the consummate actor role – the part that calls for a consciousness of the movements into and out of the looking-glass. It is the consciousness of the process of role enactment, the deliberateness of the moves and plays, and the ability to manipulate roles that distinguishes the therapist from the client. The therapist attempts to remain at balance much of the time. As the balanced anchor, she helps the client sway between states of over- and underdistance, encouraging him to rock the boat, to journey out into stormy seas, Odysseus-like, until he can safely steer to the calmer waters of aesthetic distance, Ithaka, and home.

The ultimate role of the client in the one-on-one is, I think, a murderous one. In order to claim that one extra role formally belonging only to the therapist, he symbolically kills the therapist. Then, upon internalizing the therapist role, he becomes his own healer. The violent image of the murderer might not be appropriate in relation to those clients tending toward psychopathic or sociopathic behavior, as it might trigger further violent fantasies, leading them away from the possibilities of closure. Yet for some, locked into an Oedipal struggle with the family, unable to separate from mother or father and take on another intimate adult relationship, the image of murderer might well be an apt one.

From a drama therapy point of view, regardless of the pathology or problem of the client, the process is complete, the resolution is successful, when the client has recognized the existence and significance of the healing part of himself and begins to act toward himself as the therapist has acted toward him.

The client who, through the therapeutic process, has discovered a way to become familiar with his own internal cast of characters and to acknowledge its presences, demons and gods alike, is now the consummate actor. A complete, available repertory is the goal. A working through of each role in thought and action is the method by which one achieves the goal and through which one continues to expand one's skills as a future performer in everyday life.

## Transference in Drama Therapy

As in psychoanalysis, the drama therapist needs to be concerned with moments of transference and deal with them through the drama. In many ways, transference is a dramatic concept as 'an individual transforms an actual role of another into a symbolic one,' and 're-creates reality according to one's subjective world view' (Landy 1986, p.95. See also Jennings 1987). Both players in the one-on-one cast the other in various roles and act toward the other as if he or she were in role.

The focus of much of classical psychoanalytical work is in establishing the transference neurosis and resolving it. As the rule of the game is to talk through a process of free association, the transference occurs covertly, without the patient's knowledge (see Eliaz 1988).

In drama therapy, the primary rule of the game is to play, to enter into an 'as if' context where I am both who I am and who I am not. In other words, in drama therapy, transference is overt. Both client and therapist, by definition, cast each other into alternative roles. It is a healthy act, rather than a neurotic one. However, within the imaginative act of transference, an unconscious component might arise as, for instance, the client attributes an excessive amount of energy to a role enacted by the therapist. The elephant role, for example, might become overly threatening, provoking extreme anger or extreme with-drawal reactions from the client. In such an instance, the therapist uses her role of elephant to help the client work through the spectrum of distance and toward a point of balance.

That moment of reaching the point of aesthetic distance is a cathartic one, at times characterized by an overt discharge of emotion. Within the distancing model, catharsis implies a balance between the two roles of actor and observer, and an ability to feel and reflect simultaneously. The cathartic moment can thus be a subtle, gentle one, difficult to observe from the outside.

Dramatic transference becomes most pronounced when the client (or the therapist, in the sense of countertransference) chronically casts the other in the same role. That is, the client might always see the role of the therapist as elephant-like, even if she is, in fact, playing a relatively neutral role. In exploring this repeated pattern, the therapist again works through the spectrum of distance, weaving in and out of role, leading the client to do the same, then reflect upon his enactment.

A prolonged transference necessitates a prolonged treatment in role. But unlike her counterpart in psychoanalysis, the drama therapist does not remain in a neutral, overdistanced role. She works both from within and without the drama. Following each enactment in role, during the closure period, she asks the client to consciously distinguish between the two realities, that of the imagination, the state of being en-roled, and the everyday, the state of being out of role or de-roled. Theoretically, the transference can be resolved to the extent that the client can distinguish between the two realities and see how the dramatic impinges upon the everyday. In that understanding, the persona of the therapist can be seen for what it is – a mask of the father, mother, etc. – and can thus be lifted. In working through the transference, the therapist takes on the masks handed to her by the client who, when ready, unmasks the therapist to discover a person there.

## Role Seduction and Countertransference

Throughout the centuries, a certain seductive quality has subsisted in theatre. Actors have not only been seductive to audience members, who might tend to view the actor and character as one, but have also tricked themselves into believing the same myth of the persona. I would state that myth as follows: in enacting the role, I believe my own act, and thus, become the role. In many ways, this is similar to the myth of Narcissus, who is seduced by his own reflection in the water. The actor's reflection, or mask of himself, is indeed seductive. One can easily be taken in by one's own act.

One of the most memorable pantomime performances I have seen was that of Marcel Marceau's Mask-maker, in which the maker of masks mimes the putting on of a series of emotionally-laden faces. When he puts on the happy face, he discovers that it is stuck to his actual face. He tries in vain to take it off. He frantically tears at it. He is frustrated and his body reacts in panic. The power of the piece is in the extreme tension between the agonized body and the happy face.

For the drama therapist, countertransference, the imposing of her issues upon the client, is one danger. The greater one, I think, is self-seduction, the danger of being trapped in a large mask stuck to the flesh. If there is no way for the drama therapist to de-role herself, to let go, to restore the balance between mask and face, body and mind, her value as a dramatic healer will be negated. The drama therapist stuck in a single persona will not be a poseur but an imposter, a fake.

Countertransference can, I think, be handled within the movements from one role to another, from in and out of the therapist and player roles. But this assumes that the therapist has the ability to be aware that countertransference is occurring, catching herself, then making the appropriate role adjustment so that she is safe to carry on.

As an example, I was working with a client who was a gifted singer. As a young girl, she had been sexually abused. At one point, she had unconsciously cast me in the role of an abusive male. With very little provocation on my part, she began to verbally attack me. Neither of us was in a dramatic role at the time. I felt on very shaky ground, and although I didn't know who she was becoming for me, I did know that I was frightened by her power. To ease my counter-transferential fears, I channelled my feelings into a musical competition. We assumed the roles of opera singers and began to vocalize at one another. The vocalizations became aggressive and intense, building to a kind of vocal catharsis. In de-roling, we were able to speak about our perceptions of the other for the first time. Later, in my own therapy, I was able to explore the shrike-like image I had imposed upon my client. But in using the safe distance of the role, I was able to discharge my own anxiety in a way that was also appropriate for the client.

I find it more difficult to counteract the moments of self-seduction. I find that I often need more recovery time after I have endowed a role with a bit too much feeling. In a one-on-one session with a client who works professionally with schizophrenic adults, some of whom live in the streets of New York, I took on the role of a lost, destitute woman, begging in the streets. I knew that my client had made a strong identification with this role, and I was attempting to uncover her feelings toward the character. As I become more involved in my role-playing, I experienced not only a deep sadness, but also a certain sense of dignity in suffering. The role was getting larger and I felt trapped. The bag lady was taking over. I became Mother Courage, Charlie Chaplin, my great-grand-mother from Poland. The images were intense. It was difficult to find my balance and allow my client equal time. I was up-staging her. It was my game.

The session felt very powerful to me, but upon examining it in retrospect, I realized that I had been unwittingly seduced by my role. The seduction was so complete, that I couldn't really re-focus upon my client. The session felt good, because I was working in role on my issues, using the client as a foil. I was Iago; she, my Othello. In actuality, the session might have been good theatre, but ultimately, poor therapy.

Perhaps what I have described as self-seduction, an underdistanced role-en-actment on the part of the drama therapist, is simply another form of counter-transference. As such, the therapist uses the role to entertain her own issues. This occurs unconsciously and needs to be monitored by the drama therapist in her supervision and/or in her ability to develop an internal supervisor, an observer part of herself that stands by in the wings during each moment of role-enactment (see Jennings 1990). To the extent that the drama therapist can work toward a balance of self and role, she will be most effective in working through a process of dramatic role-playing.

## The Drama Therapist as Follower and Witness

The drama therapist in a one-on-one situation does not always work in role. At times, she may take on a more distanced stance, encouraging the client to work on his own. (See Jennings 1990 for description of four internal states of the drama therapist.) The effectiveness of the drama therapist in this more distanced role is measured by her skill in providing a playful stage for the client to enact his own issues in role, and then move toward integration.

Let me illustrate with an example. An institutionalized schizophrenic woman, Susan, had been capable of working at a very basic level for some weeks. She was part of a drama therapy group and would appear in a disheveled, almost catatonic state. She would only stay for a short time, with minimal, if any, participation in the movement and improvisational activities. During her eight weeks in and out of the group, she was non-verbal. I began to work with her in a one-on-one situation, and she showed an interest in building puppets and masks. I remained in a neutral but supportive role, encouraging her projective play.

One day, she constructed a female puppet and for the first time, agreed to speak. I encouraged her to take on the role of the puppet, and when she did, she began to direct her dialogue toward another small object in the room. When I asked her who she was, she replied: 'The babysitter.' When I asked whom she was talking to, she replied: 'To Susan's daughter.' She had a daughter, and for the first time in months, she was able to verbalize that she missed her daughter and wanted to leave the hospital.

In remaining apart from Susan's drama, the therapist was able to follow Susan's lead to the projective objects, recognizing that Susan could express her feelings only through the safety of the puppets. Susan was now ready to integrate a split-off role – that of the caretaker of the baby. The taking-on and recognition of the babysitter role helped Susan move toward an acceptance of her mother role and eventually, a return back home.

This example illustrates another role of the drama therapist in a one-on-one – that of the follower, a less active, more patient, less controlling and manipulative role. For many, drama therapy suggests overt activity, action, movement. Certainly drama therapy is about these physical acts. But it is also about subtle activity, action, and movement. It occurs in the making of a puppet, the animation of the puppet, the putting on and naming of a mask. It occurs as a disabled child, paralyzed and permanently confined to a wheelchair, spots an airplane on a shelf in the room and begins to 'take off' in flights of fancy. It occurs as an angry, abused ten-year-old builds a chaotic scene in a sandbox, with small objects, and names it, 'My House.' It occurs as a frail three-year-old, dying of AIDS, bound to an intravenous tube, carefully picks up a stethoscope and listens to the heartbeat of a doll.

In these examples, the therapist needs to stand back, to let go of the role of equal player, provocateur, trickster. In taking on the role of follower, she needs to accept the ability of confused, unhappy, unwanted, ill, and disabled individuals to express their needs symbolically, and ultimately, to heal themselves through acts of the imagination.

She becomes not only the follower, but also the witness, one who is there to see and affirm. At best, she is a brave and compassionate witness who can remain intact yet caring as demonstrations of darkness are re-enacted.

## Provocateurs, Evocateurs and Invokers

Working one-on-one is fairly new for me. Much of my past clinical experience has been with groups of emotionally disturbed children and psychotic adults. My clients now tend to be neurotic individuals who wish to look at their lives and their work though a more creative means. I sometimes take an active role in this work, enjoying a vigorous game of one-on-one. But I most prefer a quieter, more covertly active role, at times steering people into sandboxes and masks when they seem to be driving in those directions. At other times I ask clients to translate their personal stories into mythic ones, taking on fictional roles in order to reenact dreams, fantasies, past realities. I am comfortable with the distance that these forms of projective techniques provide both of us. In order to do my best work, I need to feel safe: not complacent, not overdistanced and overly-intellectual, judgmental, or analytical, not cold and separated from my own feelings or those of my clients – but safe enough to be authentic, to let something dramatic happen, to allow myself to witness it, contain it, and use it as a point of reference in the context of the ongoing therapy.

Working as I do sometimes takes a bit longer to help a client zero in on a particular issue. A more active drama therapist, more in the role of the provocateur, might move more quickly toward an issue. Such a model is quite prevalent in gestalt and psychodrama, especially when the therapists are working along the lines of Perls and Moreno, two highly provocative individuals. The provocateur role is one where the therapist becomes an active role-player, often taking on an antagonistic stance that frustrates the client just enough to lead him often to the point of active catharsis.

The advantage of taking on the provocateur role is that one moves quickly and, when skilful, the therapist is able to help the client pinpoint an issue. This approach tends to be most helpful with overdistanced people who have great trouble expressing emotion. The disadvantage is that in working quickly, the subtleties of the dramatic form are often compromised. If Hamlet were to quickly resolve his indecision and murder his uncle at the beginning of the play, a rich, complex character would be lost to us. So, too, might a client, who after one long weekend of treatment discovers that in symbolically killing his step-father he has resolved his primary Oedipal issues.

The more gentle, covertly active role can be seen as that of the evocateur, one who evokes, facilitates, actively follows. The advantage to this role is that the therapist becomes less obtrusive, less the object of judgement and permission. The provocation must come from within the client. The disadvantage is that the evocateur can become too passive and miss opportunities to heighten the drama of the therapy.

The ideal drama therapist would need to present qualities of both the provocateur and evocateur, but these qualities are not sufficient in themselves. Another *vox* is necessary; that is, another voice, another calling. That voice can be characterized as an invocation, a call for inspiration. The classical poets would invoke the muse. The drama therapist invokes the imagination, the source of creative and healing energy. As such, she takes on a religious or ceremonial role – she is a priestess who will remind the celebrant/client that the source of healing is within the person.

The drama therapist, then, provokes, evokes, invokes. She plays many roles in the game of one-on-one: director, coach, consummate actor, object of transference, provocateur, evocateur, invoker, leader and follower, witness, masker and unmasker, persona and person. Unlike the client, the drama therapist needs to be conscious of the effects of her role-playing before she begins to practice. She further needs to allow her repertory of roles to change and expand with each new client and with each new movement of old clients. And as she changes, she needs to retain a self-critical stance, an internal supervisor that can help catch the moments of self-seduction and countertransference, and later, work them through.

## The Roles Less Traveled

If we were to accept the ideal of the drama therapist as consummate role-player, then it would seem there are few inessential roles for her to play. I would argue that in the practice of drama therapy, some roles are less equal than others. The one most easy to abuse is that of the analyst/interpreter.

The aim of drama, whether in play, performance, education, recreation, or therapy, is to have an experience in an imaginary realm, one that mirrors the reality of one's everyday life, and to undergo some sort of transformation as a result. The dramatic experience is essentially subjective, even though certain role types and certain archetypal scenes embody universal qualities. The actor in any dramatic mode has the responsibility of making sense of his own dramatic experience. Should a therapist presume to know the meaning of a client's drama, she moves into an analytical model that diminishes both the aesthetic and healing nature of the experience.

I do not mean to imply an anti-intellectual stance on the part of the drama therapist; like other therapists, she needs to develop a fine critical ability in order to make sense of the client's material. But the way she makes sense of the material is not simply cognitive; it is qualitatively different from that of her colleagues in analytical therapies. She sees with the eye of a witness to a dramatic event, whether director, audience member, or fellow performer. She looks at forms, roles, rhythms, images, tensions, ironies, masks, and other aspects of the dramatic experience. She is a skilled reader of text and subtext. With a keen knowledge of the vicissitudes of role-taking and role-playing, she understands the paradoxical and delicate balance between actor and role, person and persona. She attempts to make sense of the dramas from inside the creative process. Thus, she becomes a creative collaborator, who might well be critical, but also humble in her inability to enter the experience of another and respectful of the other's creative process.

A role less traveled in therapy is that of the critical, challenging co-creator who is neither analyst nor interpreter, but rather looks for meaning in the role enactment and helps the client to do the same.

There are occasions when the drama therapist needs to assume the role of teacher. For example, in working with severely regressed emotionally disturbed children who have never learned how to play, the drama therapist might gradually begin to model play behaviors, teaching ways to use dolls and toys. But as a rule, I think it wise to avoid a didactic approach. Like didactic theatre, didactic drama therapy easily falls into prescription and cliché, often depriving clients of the dignity to formulate approaches to solving their own problems. A positive conception of the drama therapist as teacher would be one who encourages others to learn how to learn through a dramatic process. In teaching the skills of play, the drama therapist presents a method of creating external forms that contain the repressed cries and whispers it is essential to express if one is to move toward healthy functioning.

A third role model that is often problematic when taken on by the drama therapist is that of the guru. Just across the line from the mentor, the guru tends to be more needy than her client. Often charismatic and narcissistic, the guru encourages a worshipful attitude on the part of the client, transforming the purpose of the relationship from therapy to religion. As I have mentioned elsewhere:

> The more the leader encourages a cult of personality, the more obscure any other purposes… become… If psychotherapy is about aiding individuals in developing the ability to solve their own problems, then charismatic leaders must work against their own and others' needs to transform them into oracles. The leader's charisma in the service of the participant's ego can truly help foster a therapeutic purpose. But when the charisma attaches itself to the superego needs of the participants,

then the form of the workshop becomes more about obedience and guilt, more truly about religion than about therapy (Landy 1987 p. 280).

The role less traveled would be that of the drama therapist as mentor, one who provides a model of dramatic learning and healing, one who can let go of her own power needs and pass on 'the mantle of the expert' (see Wagner 1976 on Heathcote).

## Supervision and Re-Creation

Many argue that the drama therapist, or any therapist for that matter, needs to engage in supervision throughout her professional life. The reasoning is to monitor and work through those moments of countertransference and narcissism that impede the therapeutic process. Further, a clinically sophisticated supervisor also provides information as to diagnostic, treatment, and valuative issues. I would argue that supervision is indeed helpful, and that the process of supervision mirrors the process of therapy in that the goal is to ultimately 'do in' the supervisor/therapist and internalize his image.

But I would add another aspect to the professional ongoing needs of the drama therapist – the need to play with peers. One-on-one drama therapy work can be quite intense. It implies a playing in the service of another's development. The extra need, then, is for replenishment and re-creation. This can be met through a peer group, playing through improvisatory means, or through a more conventional theatrical experience of rehearsal and performance.

## Conclusion

At the heart of the drama therapy experience is the art form, the act of creation through a process of impersonation. The essential role of the drama therapist is to embody the creative principle and, mirror-like, to turn it back on the client. That principle implies that through the act of creation, new lives and worlds can be born and developed, and old ones can be shed. That principle implies that the creative act is a revolutionary act, a healing act.

The dramatic healer, as we have seen, is multi-faced. In the one-on-one, many of those faces are required, and face-to-face, the two players mask and unmask. As the ball passes from one to the other, the defensive and offensive roles shift. At the end of the game, the fakery is exhausted. Each player removes his make-up, costume, role.

At the end of the classical story, the Wizard of Oz becomes a simple, vulnerable man again, his machinery exposed. But even so, he gives gifts, and all return home, in their everyday roles. Such is the wizardry of the drama therapist. After all the play and drama, the one-on-one ends, as one-and-one, two people, complex and intact, say goodbye.

# CHAPTER 8

# The Concept of Role in Drama Therapy

In the beginning of the drama therapy experience, only two media are essential – the role and the story. This is because they are the essential means of conveying messages from client to therapist. All communication that occurs in drama therapy, both intrapsychically and interpersonally, at least from the point of view of the client, proceeds through these media. They can be called primary media in that many of the specific mediated forms of expression, such as puppets and masks, video and story dramatization, spring from the source of role and story. The specific forms, then, become secondary media, which embody the projections a client makes while in role and while telling a story.

Dramatic media are mediated forms as they stand between two levels of reality, that of the everyday and that of the fictional. In playing a role and telling a story, the client in drama therapy enters the imaginative, fictional reality for the purpose of commenting or reflecting upon the everyday reality. Secondary media are effective means of treating clients to the extent that they can illuminate the nature of clients' roles and stories. It is incumbent upon the drama therapist to help clients find the appropriate roles to play and stories to tell, those that will provide a mirror reflective of their lives.

In the beginning is also the creative act, the source from which media spring. The creative act is the *illud tempus*, the time of origins, the spontaneous moment of verbal, tonal, or gestural enactment. The client in drama therapy is charged with a kind of birthing, a calling into existence of the parts of the self and the world, an arranging of his creation.

This chapter is an attempt to examine story and role not only as practical media, 'the tools of the trade,' but also as theoretical concepts, important in constructing drama therapy theory. The two concepts are interrelated as clients give voice to their role enactments through story. By story, I do not only mean a conventional, spoken narrative with a beginning, middle, and end. Story is the utterance, the gesture, the sound, that informs the therapist or group therapy members as to the nature of the client's role. If in role of the fictional character, Rumpelstiltskin, I depart considerably from the classic fairy tale, starting at the end and beating my leg angrily against the floor, uttering obscenities at the therapist and accusing him of abandoning me, I am indeed telling my story. The fact that I have broken with the chronology or narrative line of the fairy tale is less significant than the fact that I have found a way to express a role, the Rumpelstiltskin part of myself, that feels deceived and angry.

Role, then, becomes the container of those qualities of the individual that need to be enacted in drama therapy. Story is the verbal or gestural text, most often improvised, that expresses the role, naming the container. The client as creator, invents stories, some based upon published literature or popular secondary media, some springing entirely from the unconscious, as a means of revealing role. At the end of one's story, sometimes unfolded through months or years of therapy, one should be able to answer the question, Who am I? And the answer involves both an identification of individual roles I play and an integration among my many roles. Throughout this paper, role, a term derived from theatre, rather than self, a term derived from literary, philosophical, theological, and social-psychological sources, will be seen as the concept most responsive to the identity question. In the following pages I will argue that it is time to move from the myth of the self to the myth of the role and story in order to frame one's personal fiction.

Social-psychological interest in role dates back to the 1930s in the United States with the early work of G. H. Mead (1934), Charles Cooley (1922) and Ralph Linton (1936). All three were looking at the dimensions of the self from a social point of view. It was Mead who first used the term, role-taking, to conceptualize the development of the self through the internalization of significant roles in one's social environment. Cooley's sociological notion of the looking glass self echoes Shakespeare's poetic metaphor of holding a mirror up to nature. For Cooley, each person in one's social environment becomes a symbolic mirror, reflecting back images of oneself. Thus, I come to know myself through internalizing images of the other.

The anthropologist, Ralph Linton (1936), further defined role in terms of status, which he saw as a socially-defined collection of rights and duties. Role became the dynamic aspect of status, the fuel that mobilizes the status, transforming it into action. Further, Linton saw two kinds of roles: one, a collection of specific roles based in one's various socially defined rights and duties; the other a general role, representing the totality of all specific roles and determining one's relationship to his society.

These two notions of role are similar to the 'I' and 'me' of William James (1948) and G.H. Mead (1934), the former being the self as object, the more general, primary, core characteristics or central intelligence; the latter being the self as subject, the specific roles that one plays in relation to special social circumstances.

The work of Mead and his colleagues clearly presents the origin of role in society. Yet role is not a significant concept in its own right, but is rather subsidiary to the more general concept, self, which, in turn, is dependent upon the related concepts of mind and society. The 'I' and the 'me' are parts of the self. The role is a process of action that gives direction to one's status and provides the social substance to be internalized by a person so as to become a self in his own right. Role, then, was a convenient metaphor, borrowed from theatre, but unacknowledged as to its dramatic roots.

Moreno (see Fox 1987) attempted to restore the metaphor to its proper source. Criticizing Mead and Linton for limiting their conception of role to its sociological origin and function, he expanded the notion of role to include three dimensions: the social, the psychosomatic, and the psychodramatic. The psychosomatic dimension of role represented the biological aspects of the person; and the psychodramatic dimension represented the psychological aspects. For Moreno, the psychodramatic and psychosomatic aspects of role precede, in a developmental sense, the social aspects of role.

Yet Moreno's conception of role, like much of his theoretical writing, remains incomplete and inconsistent. On the one hand, he critiques Mead and Linton for being two narrow in their understanding of role; on the other he uses their sociological orientation with some frequency (Fox 1987):

> The form (of role) is created by past experiences and the cultural patterns of the society in which the individual lives...(p.62)

> The function of the role is to enter the unconscious from the social world and bring shape and order to it. (p.63)

Further, Moreno offers a dual conception of role not unlike that of the general and specific role or the 'I' and the 'me.' In his words (Fox 1987):

> Every role is a fusion of private and collective elements. Every role has two sides, a private and a collective side. (p.62)

The most significant contribution of Moreno to the dramatic conceptualization of role is his notion of a human being as a role-player. For Mead and many of his colleagues, in contrast, the human being is primarily a cognitive creature, developing a self with and through the mind, in relation to significant others in the society. Man is, thus, essentially a role-taker, rather than a role-player. This distinction, though apparently subtle, is of great importance. Mead's conception is primarily a cognitive one: I become a self to the extent that I can internalize the roles of others and see myself as they have seen me. Moreno's conception is a more active, dramatic one: I become a person to the extent that I can play out the many roles of myself and also play out the roles of others through the process of role-reversal. Unlike Mead, Moreno did not rely upon a notion of self in which to contain role. For Moreno (1953), role becomes the predominant concept. The ego, personality or self become too abstract and 'wrapped in metapsychosocial mystery' (p.75).

This dramatic conception helps re-focus our discussion on the theatrical origin of role, the source of the metaphor used so frequently by social psychologists. According to Moreno (Fox 1987, p.61), in antiquity, the word role referred to a round piece of wood upon which sheets of parchment were fastened. The role would facilitate the reading of a document, whose text would appear as the wood was turned. In the classical theatre of Greece and Rome, actors' parts were written on the roles, then read to them by prompters. The actors would memorize their parts based upon this process. Later, in the Elizabethan theatre, a character's dialogue would be written out on paper. This text, the character's role, then came to be associated with the substance of the actor's part in the play.

Thus established, Moreno developed a whole system of therapy, social analysis and education, which he named psychodrama and sociodrama, based in a dramatic notion of role. Yet Moreno's break with the conserves of dramatic literature and social-psychological thinking in relation to role theory was a partial one. He, too, was grounded in a social theory, where healing occurs in a group and where taking on and playing out the role of the other, role-reversal, becomes a predominant aspect of the theory and practice of psycho-and sociodrama. He, too, was trying to fashion his epistomological narrative, his myth of the creation of life – biological, psychological, social, but essentially, dramatic.

The two most prominent contemporary social-psychologists who have advanced the notion of life as drama are Theodore Sarbin and Erving Goffman. In Goffman's now classic study, *The Presentation of Self in Everyday Life*, we find an analysis of social life filtered through the lens of the dramatic metaphor. Goffman begins his book by offering a definition of role, not unlike that of Linton. It is: 'the enactment of rights and duties attached to a given status' (p.16). Nevertheless, he breaks significantly from his earlier colleagues by offering a global analysis of social life as role enactment. Finally, he concludes that the self is not a cognitive construct, but a staged artifact, a 'dramatic effect':

> The self, then, as a performed character, is not an organic thing that has a specific location, whose fundamental fate is to be born, to mature, and to die; it is a dramatic effect arising diffusely from a scene that is presented…(pp.252–253).

Goffman does not specify the distinctions between self and role. His language tends to equate the two. He does make a distinction, however, between the terms, character and performer, reminiscent of Mead's 'I' and 'me.' For Goffman, the character is the more stable part of the person, the object, the 'I', the ego. The performer, like the 'me,' is more subjective and flexible, the person as persona, the face as mask.

Goffman begins his book with the premise that: 'All the world is not, of course, a stage, but the crucial ways in which it isn't are not easy to specify' (p.72). Yet he ends by unmasking the *theatricum mundi* metaphor:

> And so here the language and mask of the stage will be dropped. Scaffolds, after all, are to build other things with, and should be erected with an eye to taking them down (p.254).

It was for others, like the novelist, Philip Roth, an astute observer of human social behavior, to reinforce that scaffold, and to retain the essential dramatic quality of his character as performance, of his self as role, of Roth as the fictional double, Zuckerman, the protagonist of his last five novels. Roth's play with role goes far beyond Goffman's. In creating a fictional alter-ego who has appeared every two years in each of five novels, Roth is able to dispose of the self, leaving intact two media, the role and the story, in one act, that of the imagination. Through his creation of a 'healing fiction' (see Hillman 1983), Roth is able to work through many of his persistent social-psychological concerns with gender, sexuality, nationality, religion and guilt. His tools of work are the role played and the story told. At the end of *The Counterlife* (1986), Roth, in the guise of Zuckerman, writes:

> Being Zuckerman is one long performance and the very opposite of what is thought of as being oneself. In fact, those who most seem to be themselves appear to me people impersonating what they think they might like to be... If there even is a natural being, an irreducible self, it is rather small, I think, and may even be the root of all impersonation – the natural being may be the skill itself, the innate capacity to impersonate... It's all impersonation – in the absence of a self, one impersonates selves... All I can tell you with certainty is that I, for one, have no self, and that I am unwilling or unable to perpetuate upon myself the joke of a self... What I have instead is a variety of impersonations I can do, and not only of myself – a troupe of players that I have internalized, a permanent company of actors that I can call upon when a self is required... I am a theatre and nothing more than a theatre...(pp.319–321)

The idea of the self as performed role is a powerful one that pervades all aspects of social, psychological, and even political life. The recent book, *Landslide, the Unmasking of the President, 1984–1988* (Mayer and McManus 1988), focuses on the role of president as movie star. The thesis of the book is that Ronald Reagan has performed the role of President as he has performed other dramatic roles in film and television. The authors' pejorative tone tends to imply their dismay at this revelation. But why should Reagan have been expected to be any different in this particular role? He has always been known as a mediocre actor who has tackled new parts with an equal lack of imagination. It could be that he has just been a consistent performer, whose roles have tended to be indistinguishable from one other. According to the role theory implicit in Roth's work, Reagan's repertory of roles is very limited indeed. It is not surprising, then, that Reagan, the actor, would perform the role of President of the United States. All individuals elected President do that. What is surprising is the quality of the performance, the inability to shift from the role of Hollywood actor, so dependent upon scripts and directors and make-up artists, to that of President of the United States, a role that, when enacted by more substantive performers, fills up with complexity, spontaneity, and vision, incorporating both the comic and tragic masks. From the distance of history, President Reagan will undoubtedly be pictured as the man in the comic mask, the family man, the man of banal wisdom, who ended each presidential narrative with the credo: 'And they lived happily ever after.'

During political campaigns we listen to the candidates' stories and try to make sense of their performances in debates and speeches and commercials. How do we know who they are and what they might really do if they are president? In answering these questions, we need to look at their potential roles as elected officials, which we base on their performances not only in the current role of candidate, but also in the past roles of political officials.

To assess their past, present and future competency as presidential role-players, let us turn to a model offered by Sarbin. Sarbin, like Goffman and earlier social-psychologists, sees role as a social artifact based in a dramatic metaphor. He uses the term, role enactment, as the basic focus of behavior in role. Sarbin and Allen (1968) specify three aspects or dimensions of role enactment: number of roles, organismic involvement, and preemptiveness or time.

The first dimension, number of roles, refers to the person's role repertory. The more roles one is able to play, the better he should be able to deal with a variety of social circumstances. This notion is similar to the goals set by several drama therapists (Emunah 1983, Landy 1986) who see their task, in part, as expanding one's role repertory.

The second dimension, that of organismic involvement, refers to the degree of intensity or to the degree of distance (see Landy 1983) manifest in one's role-playing. Distance has been conceptualized in drama therapy as a measure of a client's affective/cognitive involvement in a task. The point of optimal involvement is referred to as aesthetic distance, a balance of affect and cognition. Two points of imbalance are identified as overdistance, a compulsive state, manifested by an excess of thought, and underdistance, an impulsive state, manifested by an excess of feeling.

The degrees of organismic involvement vary from a low end of noninvolvement (similar to overdistance; Landy 1983), to casual role enactment, ritual acting, engrossed acting (similar to balance of distance; Landy 1986), classical hypnotic role taking, histrionic neurosis (similar to underdistance; Landy 1983), ecstasy, and finally to the state of sorcery and witchcraft at the upper end. At the lower ends of the scale, leaning toward overdistance, there is minimal affective or cognitive involvement, little effort, and role and self are fully differentiated. Toward the upper ends of the scale, leaning toward underdistance, role and self are undifferentiated and the person demonstrates maximal involvement and much effort.

The third dimension of Sarbin's model represents the amount of time one spends enacting a single role in relation to the time spent in other roles.

In making determinations about our candidates, we can apply Sarbin's model. Which one is the more balanced, incisive role-player? Which one seems to be able to play more roles effectively, including those of spouse, parent, negotiator, compassionate patriot, disciplinarian, balancer of budgets, and other roles that the voter deems essential? Which one is able to best move among the levels of organismic involvement, finding appropriate moments to be more or less distanced, without indulging in the extremes of noninvolvement, typical of puppet heads of state, or ecstasy and sorcery, typical of leaders of ecstatic cults or charismatic movements?

And finally, which one is best able to take the time to enact the role of negotiator or peace-maker or communicator, without becoming so over-whelmed in the role that the rest of his personality collapses under its weight? Jimmy Carter at Camp David successfully balanced these several presidential roles, using his time carefully to persuade Anwar Sadat and Menachem Begin to sign the historic peace treaty between Egypt and Israel (see Hare 1985).

In answering these questions, one might know, at least in part, for whom to vote. But one must also listen to the stories of the candidates, their visions of America, spoken in the language of myth – the political order as conservative or liberal, reactionary or progressive, threatening or peaceful.

In Sarbin's recent work (1986), he shifts metaphors from role to story. Human beings are not only role players, but also storytellers, who make sense of their lives through taking on the dual roles of storyteller and protagonist within their own stories, another variation on the theme of the 'I' and the 'me.' The metaphor of life as story has proven so appealing to Sarbin and his colleagues that they have postulated a new field of study, that of narrative psychology, which Sarbin (1986) subtitles 'the storied nature of human con-duct.'

In building a model of role for drama therapy, let us turn away temporarily from the social-psychologists, psychodramatists, novelists and politicians, and look at the primary source of the role metaphor, that of theatre.

In its early usage, as we have seen above, role was a theatrical term. Throughout much of theatre history, role indicated a character as type, rather than as psychologically complex human being. The person, who was the actor, was amply hidden beneath a mask or make-up or costume or exaggerated gestural and vocal apparatus, in order to present the persona, the universal character type embodied in the dramatic narrative.

The role of the actor in classical Greek drama was very much determined by his mask, which became the essence of his character, the link between the religious nature of the drama and the dramatic form (Harrop and Epstein 1982).

Each role, therefore, became a kind of archetype, larger than life, fixed by the nature of the mask, and projected outward to an audience of many thousands. The role was not necessarily unidimensional, as Oedipus and Antigone, for example, are richly drawn characters, capable of a wide emotional range. Yet, by virtue of conceiving the role as a mask, the Greek dramatist highlighted and objectified a particular behavioral or psychic quality: the suffering of Antigone, the treachery of Clytemnestra, the wit and wisdom of Lysistrata, for example.

Throughout most of theatre history, the actual or figurative mask continued to determine character roles. During the Renaissance in Italy, we find a stunning use of types in the *commedia dell'arte*. The actors, also in mask, assumed typified roles, such as: Pantaloon, the old, miserly merchant, the Doctor, whose favorite medicine was gold, the Captain, whose feats of bravery rival the Cowardly Lion in *The Wizard of Oz*, the much too romantic lovers, and Harlequin, the enigmatic trickster character, perhaps the most complex role-player of all.

During the English Renaissance we also find an array of character roles, including many of the *commedia* types. Shakespeare's Puck, Fool, Feste, and Falstaff can all be seen as examples of Harlequin characters.

From the seventeenth century through much of the nineteenth century, theatrical roles continued to be highly stylized. The actor took on the role as a social mask, again highlighting a prominent feature of a person rather than the person as a whole. The actor's costume, make-up, and gesture clearly delineated that feature, as did his name, such as Horner, Petulant, Teazle, Prism, and Malaprop.

And into the twentieth century, with the notable and nagging prominence of psychological realism, the role again surfaced as mask, prompting actors to again exaggerate gestures, stylize language, and assume such roles as Hamm and Clov in Beckett's *Endgame*, or Mother Courage and Swiss Cheese in Brecht's *Mother Courage*.

Even in the most psychologically complex characters, steeped in the modern tradition of psychological realism, from the early Ibsen portraits of Hedda Gabler and Nora Helmer, through O'Neill's Jamie Tyrone, William's Blanche DuBois, Miller's Willy Loman, and the contemporary losers and searchers in the plays of Lanford Wilson, David Mamet, and Sam Sheppard, even they become types of a sort. Although not in the tradition of *commedia* or drawing room comedy, these realistic characters, played often by actors trained in psychologically-based techniques, are nonetheless dramatic roles. And each dramatic role exists in a somewhat determined universe, limited by such factors as genre of play, concept and style of production, and predetermined dialogue, movement, and stage business.

Stanislavski (1961), as theorist and teacher, attempted to delineate the several factors or planes of a role in his book, *Creating a Role*. He mentions the external plane of facts and events; the social plane including class, nationality, and historical setting; the literary and aesthetic planes, dealing with ideas, style and scenery; the psychological plane, concerning feelings, inner action and characterization; the physical plane, centered in physical action and external characterization; and the plane of personal creative feelings, focused on the actor as person (p.11).

The role, then, at least from Stanislavski's point of view, is determined by social, psychological, physical and behavioral factors, as well as historical and aesthetic ones. This point of view is not too far removed from that of Moreno who conceived of the role as based in the three planes of social, biological, and psychological experience.

Twentieth-century performance theorists have added further planes criss-crossing the universe of roles. Gordon Craig (1919) conceptualized the actor as giant puppet, an uebermarrionette. Brecht (Willett 1964) conceived of the actor as narrator, storyteller, demonstrator, and social catalyst. For Artaud (1958), the role of performance became that of the plague, a cleansing through self-immolation. David Cole (1975) saw the performer as shaman, and Robert Wilson and Heiner Müller, saw the role of performer as sign, as another piece of the deconstructed text.

With the notable exception of Stanislavski and his able cadre of followers who have expanded his notions of the psychological creation of a role, much of theatre, past and present, is based in a typology of roles, a sense of the role as mask and type, a sense of the actor as god, shaman, symbol, and sign pointing to the audience, indicating ways that they have played their own everyday roles and told their own everyday stories.

Being one of two primary media in drama therapy, the role must be taken on, assumed. Without its assumption, drama therapy ceases to exist. When one assumes a role in drama therapy, one limits one's complex humanity to a particular type, a single status, a single 'me,' a single time and place, a single symbol or image, one mask, one name, one discreet series of actions. The role is a container of this oneness. The more finite and particular the role is drawn, the more the client can be able to explore its infinite dimensions, including its archetypal qualities and its relationship to one's total role system. For the role in theatre and in therapy contains a central paradox: by reducing a role to its essential actions and feelings, the actor/client opens up a universe of possibility. This paradox, like Blake's notion of seeing the world reflected in a grain of sand, finds the universal, the general, embedded in small, specific human actions.

In building a model of role in drama therapy, we work from the roots upward. In the beginning is the role and the role begins in theatre, and theatre begins with an imaginative act of telling a story in role. In keeping with its theatrical roots, role is mask and type, a particular form of action and charac-terization that embodies a universal conception.

The role is primary in drama therapy because clients are in search of those roles, either split off or buried, that will enable them to balance out their internal cast of characters. As in the most richly constructed dramatic scripts, they need to discover those parts of themselves that are hero and villain, lover and hater, deceiver and deceived, fool and wise person, tragic journeyer and comic homesteader, romantic dreamer and farcical buffoon. In the practice of drama therapy, the client engages in a particular form of action and characterization, through such secondary media as mask and story dramatization, in order to discover the nature of these types.

Applying Stanislavski's several planes of role, we can see how a client working through the role of Rumpelstiltskin, for example, moves toward such a discovery. The classical story, as collected by the brothers Grimm, concerns a girl of humble origins who is handed over by her father to the king, in hopes of marriage. The king sets extraordinary tasks before her: if she can spin his straw into gold, then she will be his bride. Feeling hopeless, a dwarf named Rumpelstiltskin appears before her and strikes a bargain. He will perform the task if she agrees to give him in return her first born son. She agrees, the task is completed, and the girl gives birth. A short time later, the dwarf appears and asks for his son. The princess pleads with him to allow the son to stay with her. Rumpelstiltskin agrees on one condition – that she guesses his name within three days. He then retreats to the forest. The princess sends her men after him who overhear him repeating his name. When he reappears at the palace, she guesses his name and in a rage, he stamps his foot so hard on the floor that it caves in and he disappears in the earth.

The following is a hypothetical example of work with the fairy tale. It is based upon several actual drama therapy group experiences led by the author. The session begins as all agree to work with the fairy tale. On the external plane, the story is told by the therapist or a client, and the characters and objects in the story are delineated: father and daughter, king and the dwarf, Rumpel-stiltskin, the eventual child of the daughter and king, and such objects as flax and gold.

One man, having identified with the Rumpelstiltskin character, begins to develop a particular characterization. On the social plane, he invents a social context for Rumpelstiltskin as an honest laborer, favored by the spirits with magical powers to do good, who, through a repeated series of rejections from his colleagues, has been forced to wander the countryside in search of others worthy of his offerings. The social plane intersects with the literary as he builds a rich story around his conception of the character. On the aesthetic plane, he fashions a mask of Rumpelstiltskin, decorating it with an earring and hat, and painting it in earth tones.

In developing the psychological plane, the client, in role, speaks of his feelings as an isolate, one whose simple life has been devoted to others, with few favors returned.He begins to create an inner life of the little man through his soliloquies and dialogues with the daughter, whom he helps to spin flax into gold and finally, to become princess. He further engages in dialogue with the baby, the child of the king and princess. He speaks of the significance of his name, Rumpelstiltskin, and his wish to remain nameless in order to claim fatherhood. And finally, he speaks of his rage and his need to disappear rather than to claim that which was his by contractual agreement.

On the physical plane, the client examines his masked image in a mirror, then lets it suggest various movements. As he feels his isolation and smallness, he projects these qualities in his gait, taking short, quick steps, often moving in patterns suggesting a caged animal.

At the conclusion of the drama therapy session, the therapist helps the client de-role and leads a closing discussion, focused upon the feelings of the actor as person, the plane of personal creative feelings. During the closure, the client, out of role, is able to identify the part of himself that is like the Rumpelstiltskin character. In naming that part 'The Little Man,' he is able to see how often he has felt enraged and exploited, and what part he has played in allowing that to happen – by not collecting the debts he is owed by others and by needing to hide his identity in order to claim what is rightfully his.

Thus, through particularizing the role-playing, according to the several planes of the Stanislavski model, the client is able to enact the Rumpelstiltskin type and discover a personal role, which he called 'The Little Man,' bearing much resemblance to the role model. In further drama therapy work, that client would be encouraged to see how 'The Little Man' works together with the many other roles in his internalized repertory.

Moving back to the social-psychological model, role is not only mask and type, but is also a cognitive and social construct. In keeping with this point of view, the drama therapist might well help the client in the above example to conceptualize his role of 'The Little Man' through an understanding of the identifications he has made and the significant role-models he has internalized. In viewing his father, for example, as a Rumpelstiltskin-type character, the client might be asked to take on his father's role in order to discover the origins of the view of himself as 'The Little Man.' Further, he might be asked to examine the social status of 'The Little Man' from the more distanced perspective of Rumpelstiltskin or the less distanced perspective of the father.

Throughout this chapter one point remains puzzling – that of the relationship between role and self. In an earlier publication (1986), I had written:

> Self is one's uniqueness, distinguishing a person from all other people... As a mediator between self and other, self and social world, role embodies qualities of thought, feeling, and behavior taken on from another and represented in a way prescribed by social convention. (p.92)

Thus conceived, self appears to be larger than role. Again quoting my earlier writings: 'The self has the capacity to take on a myriad of roles' (p.93). Yet now the concept of self, in the light of a more dramatic conception of role, seems misplaced and unnecessary. If the dramatic vision is one of flux, of movement in and out of role, and if drama therapy is concerned with helping people achieve a fluidity, a capacity for excellence in playing a single role complexly and integrating that role within a well-developed repertory of roles, why, then, impose upon it a non-dramatic, 'metapsychosocial,' overly-used concept implying stasis?

The myth of the self as prime mover has been exhausted. Narcissus drowned in it, Freud broke it up into three pieces, and Jung further decimated it into all the archetypes of the unconscious. Sarbin abandoned it in favor of role and story. Political actions of genocide and psychological actions of suicide, neglect, and abuse have hastened its demise. In the absence of the self, there still exists a primary dramatic process of identity. To Philip Roth, it is 'the innate capacity to impersonate.' And that capacity is expressed through role, the taking on and the playing out of heroes and demons, fools and wise people, lovers and sons and daughters and parents. Roles are the containers of all the thoughts and feelings we have about ourselves and others in our social and imaginary worlds. When those thoughts and feelings are given a dramatic form and safely played out, one has the potential of seeing oneself clearly, but not as a self, not as an 'I.' It is in the doing and seeing and accepting and integrating of all the roles, the 'me' parts, that the person emerges intact. 'I am a theatre and nothing more than a theatre,' says Nathan Zuckerman, one fictional storyteller taking on one role of Philip Roth. And drama therapists, too, looking for a way to conceive of their own roles and a theory in which to fashion their techniques and therapeutic objectives, might well look to the theatre that is their source and the role and story that are their primary media. For it is there that our work begins: in role, in story, in imaginary action.

# CHAPTER 9

# A Taxonomy of Roles
## A Blueprint for the Possibilities of Being

This chapter is an extension of two previous papers (Landy 1990, 1991) where I argued for a role theory based firmly in the aesthetic discipline of drama/theatre. I defined role as 'the container of all the thoughts and feelings we have about ourselves and others in our social and imaginary worlds' (1990, p.110), and I noted that an apparent source for those thoughts and feelings is to be found in the role types that reoccur in the history of world theatre. Many of these types (e.g. hero and villain, victor and victim) are repeated within the structure of drama therapy, and I offered several examples of how one works with such types clinically (1991).

Finally, I proposed a dramatic role model (1991) that looks at the following aspects of role: role type, quality, function, and style, attempting to bridge the gap between theatre and therapy in order to provide an effective means of clinical treatment. In concluding my thoughts concerning the dramatic basis of role theory, I offered the following:

> Further investigation might well reveal a full-blown typology of roles, a kind of theatrical archetype system... If such a system is valid, it may further guide the drama therapist in practical matters of assessment, treatment, and evaluation, as well as matters of research. (1991, p.41)

In this chapter, I will introduce the beginnings of a typology or taxonomy of role as a move toward a theatrical archetype system. Further, I will show how such a system guides treatment by presenting a case example and a description of the role method in drama therapy.

## The Case of Michael

Michael is a 28-year-old man from Chicago who wanted to become an actor. As he worked through various classes and showcase productions, he supported himself through temporary jobs. He committed himself to an extensive process of drama therapy in order to ameliorate certain feelings of isolation, depression, and rage. In our two years of drama therapy, he worked on many roles, including: gay man, fearful child, victim, moral person within an amoral universe, and son to an abusive father. The son role was quite prominent and demanded considerable attention. As Michael was a highly imaginative story-teller, I encouraged him to make up stories based on his present feelings. The following is an example told about one year into our work together:

### The Wooden Clogs and the Rubber Boots

There is a little boy who sings and goes with girls and stares at the ocean. His father is a fisherman. He smells of fish. He has shining eyes. The boy wears clogs. The father wears rubber boots. The boy walks down the cobblestone street toward the father, but the father thinks it's a girl.

'When are you going to become a man and wear rubber boots?'

'I like my clogs.'

'Women wear clogs.'

The boy is in the shower, his clogs on the floor. The father comes in and sees the clogs and is angry. He chops them up with an ax. The boy comes out and sees his father laughing.

'I've made you a man. I've cut up your clogs.'

'They were mine!'

The boy is furious.

'If you want to be a woman I will chop off your penis with my ax.'

The boy runs to his mother.

'Daddy's trying to make me into a woman!'

'He's just kidding. It's all right, son.'

The father buys a pair of rubber boots for his son. They fit well. He gives his son a big hug and tells him he loves him.

'Go away, I hate you!'

Everyone who sees the boy tells him how well he looks and that now he is a man. But the boy goes to the sea and throws away the boots and forever after he walks around barefoot.

The moral of the story is: no one can tell you who you are by the shoes you wear on your feet.

This tale, dealing with the relationship of son and father, is charged with much passion, fear, guilt and ultimately, confusion. The sexual masculine role is very much tied up with the father in this story. The father's threat is that if the son does not take on his role as man, then he, the father, will castrate him, transforming him into a woman. The father's function in the story is to leave his son a legacy of masculinity, even if he has to force it on him.

The role of the son is ambiguous. Although he is angered by his father's attempt to change him, he is ultimately unable to walk in his own shoes, that is, to choose his own sexual and developmental identity. In the story, the boy's function is to resist the demands of his father and to identify strongly with the child and with the female. At the end of the story, however, he becomes a sexual outcast, neither adult nor child, male nor female. The barefoot boy is a kind of eunuch, a castrated, lost soul. This role is self-inflicted because he is unable or incapable of resolving his ambiguities and choosing his developmental/sexual role.

The role of the mother is somewhat veiled, but present in its inability or refusal to protect the son from the terrible threats of the father. Unlike the archetypal mothering qualities of nurturance and protection, this mother is impotent, ineffectual. Her function is to deny the threat and to refuse to protect the son.

The final human role is that of a kind of Chorus, the townspeople who assert the voice of convention, urging the boy to take on his father's legacy, the boots, the trappings of manhood. The moral of the story is an ironic one in that the Chorus can tell the identity of the boy by his shoes. He, too, knows himself by his shoes. A more truthful version would be: everyone knows who you are by the shoes you wear on your feet, especially yourself.

Michael, at the time of the story, is attempting to find his way through a morass of ambiguities. He wants to know how to be a son to his father and to his mother, an intimate and lover to his mates. He wants to know how to be a gay man openly, how to allow the feminine and masculine parts of himself to be fully acknowledged and seen. He wants to know how to let go more and more of his many pariah roles and stop allowing the voice of the people to control his thoughts.

It has been through my work with Michael during the past two years that I began to develop the role method of treatment. Michael's ease in jumping in and out of roles, of inventing stories and making connections between one role and another was a constant inspiration. The harder part was facing up to my own father–son issues and recognizing the burden of assuming the transferential father role at a time when my immediate needs for fathering had barely begun to subside.

Early in our work, Michael told a story about a criminal lawyer who was protecting a homeless black man falsely accused of a crime. The lawyer role was invoked when I asked Michael to find an image that embodied his ideal lover/mate. His lawyer was an adult – mature, responsible, protective, conventional in taste and demeanor. Michael saw himself, in large part, as the black man in search of the lawyer, as the victim in search of a protector. The black man, however, was proud, suspicious of help offered by the conventional helpers. The lawyer/victim roles would play a large part in Michael's therapy.

I remained distant from Michael, rarely taking on an active role myself in his dramas. I remained witness, guide, supporter, scribe, questioner, sometimes teacher, sometimes interpreter. In the midst of our working together, I became a father to a daughter. The months following were difficult. I felt him withdrawing, finding more sustenance in the theatre than in the drama therapy session. He was rehearsing an adaptation of Harper Lee's *To Kill a Mockingbird* and was cast as the idealistic son of Atticus, a criminal lawyer who is defending a black man falsely accused of a crime.

All my father needs were met in relation to my daughter. So we danced around each other for a while. Then something shifted. For one, I was enjoying my father role tremendously and it began to spill over. Further, I saw a documentary film about Robert Bly and his devotion to working with men in search of their father and their masculinity. There was a moment when Bly asked all the men present who were over 50 to come forward. I remember that the younger men watched as if a magical rite were taking place and there was hope for them to be rescued in some way. I found myself choking back tears. The next day I had an appointment with Michael. I was almost twenty years his senior and I felt a responsibility beyond that of therapist to client. I was an older man and it was my place in the community of men to father Michael. I wasn't sure what that meant, but I knew that it must be done.

For Michael, the shift came when he was suddenly without a theatrical role and soon to be without a therapist for three months, as I was about to leave for Europe on sabbatical. His drama therapy work became focused as never before; he began dredging up roles and stories that helped both of us see more clearly into the nature of his dilemmas. One was Patty, an abused child, blind and deaf. During the session he was able to symbolically cradle her in his arms, offering protection and nurturance to that part of himself that was most hopeless and needy. As we parted, we both seemed truly sad.

While away on sabbatical, I voraciously read plays, mostly classics. I began to think of Michael's roles as just that – roles, parts in a play. So many of his roles were repeated – the innocent young boy, the angry young man, the enraged one, the lawyer and judge, and, especially, the victim.

As I plowed through the repertory of world drama, I saw the same – a multitude of characters, many of whom appeared and reappeared throughout time and throughout culture. My need to create a typology of roles was further inspired by reading Stephen Jay Gould's book, *Wonderful Life* (1989), which is based on a revision of a discovery of extraordinary fossil creatures at the Burgess Shale Quarry in Canada. These creatures were so unusual and distinct from any other life forms that they tended to defy conventional understanding of evolution. Because of this threat, the man who discovered the creatures, James Walcott, a most conservative scientist, attempted to fit these specimens neatly within the given biological categories of phyla and species, thus preserving the thrust of Darwin's argument that evolution proceeds in a linear and ordered pattern from simple to complex.

Rather than promoting the popular version of evolution, Gould theorized that these creatures challenge the Darwinian assumptions and actually offer an alternative theory that early life was indeed glorious and complex, that survival of and evolution from any one species was accidental, and that a truer evolutionary perspective should be envisioned as cyclical rather than linear.

All these extraordinary ideas came about because of the existence of the Linnean taxonomy of classifying animal and plant life. Gould argued that the new discoveries do not invalidate the old system of classification, but rather point to the need of such a system to be flexible and responsive to new discoveries, one that can potentially yield several theories about the nature of the things taxonomized.

Is it possible or even desirable to taxonomize roles? Why classify behaviors as if they were so many animals swimming on the ocean floor? Why take theatre and anatomize it, breaking it up into bits and risking the loss of its integrity?

I think such a system is desirable for several reasons: for one, it provides a kind of theatrical archetype system that responds to the universal quality of the theatrical experience. At a time when, generally, theatre forms and purposes are being questioned in terms of their relationship to commercial entertainment, education, therapy, spiritual values, and the like, such a system might provide coherence, or, at least, a point of departure. Specifically, a theatrical archetype system might well apply to the relatively new field of drama therapy, providing a tangible framework in which to formulate diagnostic, treatment and valuative strategies, and against which to evaluate new role phenomena. If I can know my actual and fictional role models, then I can have a good idea what I value and who I am. It could well be that through roles people create meaning in their lives.

Further, the theoretical implications of such a system are wide-ranging. Such a system might further advocate the notion that the era of the primacy of the Self as core object is dead and that we are now truly living within the era of the role. Role is a container of properties – somatic, cognitive, affective, social/cultural, spiritual and aesthetic – that define us as human beings, giving meaning to our behavior. To see a role is not to see a whole person, but a part. Role is only fully meaningful as it relates to its intrapsychic and interpersonal counterparts (i.e. my family role of father relates to my age role of adult and cognitive role of knowledgeable one); it also relates interpersonally to my daughter's family role of daughter and her age role of child.

We live in a culture of things, of stuff, of pieces and parts. We come to know ourselves by first naming the things that are meaningful to us and then claiming them as our own. We say: my mother, my father, my friend, my lover and later, if we establish effective relationships, we get to see ourselves as both worthy of parents, friends and lovers and capable of parenting, offering friendship and love to ourselves and to others.

If one needs a concept of centrality or core, I would like to offer that of impersonation. At the center of the person is the ability, the potential to take on other persona. This ability to impersonate, very different from imitation, which is essentially an external act, is a creative act in that a new part is generated, a new mask is fashioned, a new persona enters into the person's dramatic repertory.

The role concept, unlike the self-concept, which tends to be one thing – self as spiritual or self as conceptual or self as social – is inclusive and ecumenical. There exist roles for most all forms of human activity. The role is like the cell or the atom. It is a primary building block, diminutive at first glance yet expansive in terms of its own substance and function, as well as its powerful effects on the system as a whole. Speed up the atom or modify the cell and a radical, irrevocable force may be unleashed. Alter the role and a psychological counterpart to the physical and biological may also burst forth.

In order to fully grasp the role concept and its endless variations, we need a system that lays bare its infrastructure. The following is an attempt to provide such a system based in the original source of role – that of theatre.

## The Taxonomy of Roles – A Theatrical Archetype System

The taxonomy consists of the following nine parts:

1.  The Domains – the largest general category of role, responding to a holistic notion of human existence. Moreno (1960) offered three domains: the psychosomatic, pertaining to such basic body functions as eating and sleeping; the psychodramatic, pertaining to fantasy and inner psychological processes; and the social, pertaining to relationships in the social world. I offer six, as seen below.

2.  The Classifications within the domains – a sub-division of domain into kinds of roles germane to a particular domain.

3.  The Role Type – similar to Jung's notion of archetype (1964), a universal role form whose substance provides a meaningful constellation of related qualities.

4.  The Sub-type – a further sub-division of role type, useful when there are several related qualities of role, each of which imply somewhat different aspects of the role type.

5.  The Quality – descriptors of the primary role type, including physical, moral, emotional, cognitive, social, and spiritual aspects of the role.

6.  Alternative Quality – descriptors of the same sort applicable to a different set of role attributes, often contradicting the original set.

7. Examples, when relevant, from three different periods/genres in theatre history, e.g. classical Greek and Roman, Renaissance, and modern. This point substantiates, in part, the universal nature of the role types.

8. The Function – addresses the purpose of a particular role/persona for a particular character/person, the way that role serves the character as he or she plays it out.

9. The Style – the form in which the role is enacted, whether representational, presentational, or somewhere in-between. Representational style is that which is reality-based and drawn on a human scale. Presentational style tends to be more abstract and universal in nature, the mask rather than the face. Each style implies a specified degree of affect and cognition. The former implies a greater degree of emotion; the latter a greater degree of cognition.

The following presentation of the taxonomy, as I mentioned above, is incomplete at this time. Each role type is not fully developed as to sub-type, quality, alternative quality, theatrical example, function, and style. Further, certain role types need to be cross-referenced as they may apply to more than one domain or classification. Within the fully developed taxonomy to come, these issues will be addressed. Given the current development of the taxonomy, I will now offer one fully developed type per classification. All others will simply be listed.

## I. Domain: Somatic

*Classification: Age*

1. **Role Type: The Child**

   Quality:     playful, fun-loving, egocentric and guileless, young in years or childlike in attitude.

   Example:     Edward III (*Edward II* by C. Marlowe)
   The Child (*Woyzeck* by G. Buchner)
   Hedwig (*The Wild Duck* by H. Ibsen)
   Little Eva (*Uncle Tom's Cabin* by George L. Aiken)
   Tyltyl and Mytil (*The Blue Bird* by M. Maeterlinck)
   Hannele (*Hannele* by G. Hauptmann)
   Trouble (*Madame Butterfly* by D. Belasco)
   Peter Pan (*Peter Pan* by J.M. Barrie).

   Function:    to assert the playful spirit, innocence and wonder of childhood.

   Style:       presentational.

2. **Role Type: The Adolescent**

3.    **Role Type: The Adult**

4.    **Role Type: The Elder** (see Grandparent, 49)


*Classification: Sexual Orientation*

5.    **Role Type: The Eunuch**
       Quality:        castrated and impotent; sexually androgenous and
                       ambiguous; paradoxical in that s/he is both threatening
                       and trusted by those who are sexually insecure; often
                       witty and comical.
       Example:        Lucrezia (*Mandragola* by N. Machiavelli)
                       The Eunuch (*Volpone* by B. Jonson)
                       Two Eunuchs (*The* Visit by F. Durrenmatt)
                       Pothinus (*Caesar and Cleopatra* by G.B. Shaw)
                       Lauffer (*The Tutor* adaptation of J. Lenz novel by B.
                       Brecht)
                       Brick (*Cat on a Hot Tin Roof* by T. Williams).
       Function:       to stimulate sexual ambivalence and allow comic catharsis
                       through laughter; to perform the paradoxical function of
                       threatening and mollifying the threats to sexually
                       insecure men and/or women.
       Style:          presentational.
       Alternative Quality:   pretending to be sexually impotent; lecherous,
                       deceptive and scheming, ironic.
       Example:        Chaerea (*The Eunuch* by Terence)
                       Jack Horner (*The Country Wife* by W. Wycherley).
       Function:       to approach the object of lust under false pretenses; to use
                       impotence as a ruse for sexual conquest.
       Style:          presentational.

6.    **Role Type: The Homosexual**

7.    **Role Type: The Transvestite**

7.1   Sub-type:   The Queen


*Classification: Appearance*

8.    **Role Type: The Beauty** (see Innocent, 20 and Immoralist, 24)
       Quality:        of outstanding physical beauty, in face and body,
                       sometimes extending to a moral and spiritual quality; an
                       innocent in the fairy tale sense.

Example:      Miranda (*The Tempest* by Shakespeare)
              Helen of Troy (*Doctor Faustus* by C. Marlowe)
              Mélisande (*Pélléas and Mélisande* by M. Maeterlinck)
              Deirdre (*Deirdre of the Sorrows* by J.M. Synge)
              Maggie (*After the Fall* by A. Miller).
Function:     to dazzle and enchant; to serve as a love object or object
              of purity.
Style:        generally presentational.
Alternative Quality:   experienced and calculating, using beauty as a
              means of seduction and/or enchantment.
Example:      Helen of Troy (*Helen* by Euripides)
              Cleopatra (*Antony and Cleopatra* by Shakespeare)
              Carmen (*Carmen* by H. Meilhac and L. Halevy)
              Lula (*The Dutchman* by LeRoi Jones).
Function:     to seduce.
Style:        presentational and representational.

9.   **Role Type: The Beast** (see Physically Disabled, 12 and Demon, 81)

10.  **Role Type: The Average One**


*Classification: Health*

11.  **Role Type: The Mentally Ill/The Madman/Woman**
     Quality:      unpredictable, irrational, manic and/or depressive,
                   threatening to self or others.
     Example:      Ophelia (*Hamlet* by Shakespeare)
                   King Lear (*King Lear* by Shakespeare)
                   Caligula (*Caligula* by A. Camus)
                   Blanche DuBois (*A Streetcar Named Desire* by T. Williams)
                   Captain Queeg (*The Caine Mutiny Court Martial* by H.
                   Wouk)
                   Mary Tyrone (*Long Day's Journey Into Night* by E. O'Neill)
                   Patients (*Marat/Sade* by P. Weiss).
     Function:     to reveal the psychologically dark, pathological sides of
                   human nature; to challenge a conventional notion of
                   sanity and normality.
     Style:        generally presentational, sometimes representational.

12.  **Role Type: Physically Disabled or Deformed** (see Beast, 9)

13.  **Role Type: The Hypochondriac**

14.  **Role Type: The Doctor**

## II. Domain: Cognitive

### 15.   Role Type: The Simpleton

15.1 Sub-types:   The Fop, the Pedant, the Ideologue

| | |
|---|---|
| Quality: | ignorant and unaware of his/her ignorance; guileless, the butt of humiliation and ridicule. |
| Example: | Bottom (*A Midsummer Night's Dream* by Shakespeare) Bartholomew Cokes (*Bartholomew Fair* by B. Jonson) King Peter of Popo (*Leonce and Lena* by G. Büchner) Judke (*The Treasure* by D. Pinski). |
| Function: | to offer him/herself up for ridicule; to remain unaware and simple, no matter what the consequences. |
| Style: | presentational. |

Alternative Quality:   ignorant, yet pretending to be knowledgeable.

| | |
|---|---|
| Example: | Polonius (*Hamlet* by Shakespeare) Malvolio (*Twelfth Night* by Shakespeare) Edward Kno'well (*Every Man in His Humour* by B. Jonson). |
| Function: | to attempt to play the wise one and thus appear that much more foolish. |
| Style: | presentational. |

15.2 Sub-type:   The Cuckold

| | |
|---|---|
| Quality: | naive and ignorant, humiliated; sexually incompetent, if not impotent. |
| Example: | Pinchwife (*The Country Wife* by W. Wycherley) Boubouroche (*Boubouroche* by G. Courteline) Bruno (*The Magnificent Cuckold* by F. Crommelynck) Casanova (*Camino Real* by T. Williams). |
| Function: | to be humiliated upon discovering what others apparently know – that one's spouse has been sexually unfaithful; comic relief, as one is usually made the fool by virtue of one's ignorance. |
| Style: | generally presentational. |

### 16.   Role Type: The Fool

16.1 Sub-types:   Clown, Buffoon, Clever Servant

16.2 Sub-type:   The Trickster (see also Fairy, 80)

16.3 Sub-type:   The Existential Clown

### 17.   Role Type: The Ambivalent One

### 18.   Role Type: The Critic

19.  **Role Type: The Wise Person**

19.1 Sub-type:    The Intellectual

19.2 Sub-type:    The Pseudo-Intellectual/Pedant (see Simpleton, 15)

## III. Domain: Affective

*Classification: Moral*

20.  **Role Type: The Innocent** (see Beauty, 8)

20.1 Sub-types:   Virgin, Saint, Ingenue, Child (see 1)
      Quality:      pure, virginal, chaste.
      Example:     Antigone (*Antigone* by Sophocles)
                Cordelia (*King Lear* by Shakespeare)
                Justina (*The Wonder-Working Magician* by P. Calderon)
                Agnes (*The School for Wives* by Molière)
                St. Joan (*St. Joan* by G.B. Shaw)
                Consuelo (*He Who Gets Slapped* by L. Andreyev)
                Josie (*A Moon for the Misbegotten* by E. O'Neill)
                Billy Budd (adaptation of Melville story by L. Coxe and
                  R. Chapman)
                Teresa (*The Hostage* by B. Behan).
      Function:    to assert the moral virtue of innocence and expose the
                opposite moral quality of cruelty.
      Style:       presentational.

21.  **Role Type: The Deceiver** (see also Beast, 9, Immoralist, 24 and
                    Demon, 81)

21.1 Sub-types:   Hypocrite, Charlatan, Con Artist, Thief, Traitor

22.  **Role type:  The Villain**

23.  **Role Type: The Moralist** (see Innocent, 20)

23.1 Sub-types:   The Puritan, The Pious

23.2 Sub-type:    The Idealist

24.  **Role Type: The Immoralist**

24.1 Sub-types:   Rogue, Lecher, Courtesan/Prostitute, Pimp

24.2 Sub-type:    Libertine/Hedonist

24.3 Sub-type:    Adulterer/Adulteress

25.  **Role Type: The Victim**

25.1 Sub-types: The Scapegoat, Prisoner, Slave, Hostage

25.2 Sub-type: The Martyr

26. **Role Type: The Opportunist**

26.1 Sub-type: Demagogue

27. **Role Type: The Bigot**

27.1 Sub-types: Racist, Sexist, Misogynist, Misanthrope

28. **Role Type: The Avenger**

29. **Role Type: The Helper**

29.1 Sub-types: Loyal friend, Good Samaritan

30. **Role Type: The Philistine**

30.1 Sub-types: Boor, Idler, Gossip

31. **Role Type: The Miser**

32. **Role Type: The Coward**

32.1 Sub-type: Braggart/Braggart Warrior (see Narcissist, 37.1).

33. **Role Type: The Parasite**

34. **Role Type: The Survivor**


*Classification: Feeling States*

35. **Role Type: The Zombie**
   Quality: emotionally frozen, lifeless, amoral.
   Example: Robots (*R.U.R.* by K. Capek)
       Krapp (*Krapp's Last Tape* by S. Beckett)
       Peter (*The Zoo Story* by E. Albee)
       Charlotte Corday (*Marat/Sade* by P. Weiss).
   Function: to shut down all feeling in order to protect oneself from
       memory and intimacy.
   Style: generally presentational.

36. **Role Type: The Malcontent**

36.1 Sub-type: The Cynic

36.2 Sub-type: The Hothead

36.3 Sub-type: The Shrew

36.4 Sub-type: The Rebel

37. **Role Type: The Lover**

37.1 Sub-type:    The Narcissist/Egotist (see Braggart, 32.1)

38. **Role Type: The Ecstatic One** (see God, 79, Dionysus, 79.1)


## IV. Domain: Social

*Classification: Family*

39. **Role Type: Mother**
    Quality:    moral, loving, caring, nurturing, a survivor.
    Example:    Hecuba (*Hecuba* by Euripides)
                Constance (*King John* by Shakespeare)
                Grusha (*Caucasian Chalk Circle* by B. Brecht)
                Mama (*I Remember Mama* by J. Van Druten)
                Linda Loman (*Death of a Salesman* by A. Miller)
                Thelma (*'Night, Mother* by M. Norman).
    Function:   to protect and nurture the children.
    Style:      representational.
    Alternative Quality:   vengeful, amoral, violent, murderous.
    Example:    Agave (*The Bacchae* by Euripides)
                Medea (*Medea* by Euripides)
                Athaliah (*Athaliah* by J. Racine)
                The Mother (*Blood Wedding* by F. Garcia Lorca)
                Natella Abashwili (*Caucasian Chalk Circle* by B. Brecht).
    Function:   to assert the Dionysian power of women; to destroy their
                children.
    Style:      presentational.
    Alternative Quality:   progressive, revolutionary.
    Example:    Pelagez Vlassova (*The Mother* by B. Brecht)
                Sarah (*Chicken Soup with Barley* by A. Wesker).
    Function:   to envision a new moral and political order and to fight
                for its realization.
    Style:      generally presentational.

40. **Role Type: Wife**

41. **Role Type: Mother-in-law**

42. **Role Type: Widow/Widower**

42.1 Sub-types:  Spinster/Bachelor

43. **Role Type: Father**

44. **Role Type: Husband**

45.  **Role Type: Son**

45.1 Sub-type:    Renegade, Black Sheep, Rebel

45.2 Sub-type:    Bastard son/prodigal son

46.  **Role Type: Daughter**

46.1 Sub-type:    Renegade daughter

46.2 Sub-type:    Bastard daughter

46.3 Sub-type:    Daughter-in-distress/daughter as victim

47.  **Role Type: Sister**

47.1 Sub-type:    Renegade sister

48.  **Role Type: Brother**

48.1 Sub-type:    Renegade brother

49.  **Role Type: Grandparent** (see Elder, 4)

49.1 Sub-type:    The senile or mad old person


*Classification: Politics/Government*

50.  **Role Type: Reactionary**

   Quality:     backward-looking to the extreme; desirous and in active
                pursuit of returning to the past; extremely conservative
                and rigid in thought and behavior; often ruthless and
                brutal in pushing through his/her agenda.

   Example:     Angelo (*Measure for Measure* by Shakespeare)
                Richard III (*Richard III* by Shakespeare)
                Judge Hoffman (*The Chicago Conspiracy Trial* by R. Sossi).

   Function:    to return to some idealized notion of a more perfect past;
                to subjugate all spontaneity and critical thought in the
                pursuit of that aim; to force others to accept that point of
                view.

   Style:       representational and presentational.

51.  **Role Type: Conservative**

52.  **Role Type: Pacifist**

53.  **Role Type: Revolutionary**

53.1 Sub-types:  Agitator, Anarchist, Radical

54.  **Role Type: Head of State**

54.1 Sub-types:   King, Queen.

55.   **Role Type: Minister/Advisor**

56.   **Role Type: Soldier**

56.1 Sub-type:   The cowardly soldier (see Braggart Warrior, 31.1)

57.   **Role Type: Police**

58.   **Role Type: Bureaucrat**

58.1 Sub-type:   Clerk

*Classification: Legal*

59.   **Role Type: Lawyer**

Quality:     protective, moral, intelligent.
Example:     The Grand Inquisitor (*St. Joan* by G.B. Shaw)
             Henry Drummond (*Inherit the Wind* by J. Lawrence and
                R. Lee)
             Otis Baker and Louis Schade (*The Andersonville Trial* by
                S. Levitt)
             Quentin (*After the Fall* by A. Miller)
             Kunstler (*The Chicago Conspiracy Trial* by R. Sossi).
Function:    to defend and protect.
Style:       representational.
Alternative Quality:   greedy, amoral, self-serving.
Example:     Pierre Patelin (*Pierre Patelin*, anonymous)
             Voltore (*Volpone* by B. Jonson)
             Cribbs (*The Drunkard* by W. Smith)
             Mr. Sharp (*Money* by E. Bulwer-Lytton).
Function:    to manipulate justice for his/her own ends.

60.   **Role Type: Judge**

61.   **Role Type: Defendant**

62.   **Role Type: Jury** (see Chorus, 70)

63.   **Role Type: Witness**

64.   **Role Type: Prosecutor/Inquisitor**

*Classification: Socio-Economic Status*

### 65. Role Type: Lower Class

65.1 Sub-type:     Beggar, peasant

      Quality:       poor in material possessions, sometimes in spirit; downtrodden and oppressed, neglected and invisible to those with plenty; sometimes depressed, sometimes ironic and witty, rising above the physical squalor.

      Example:       Beggars (*The Beggar's Opera* by John Gay, *The Three Penny Opera* by B. Brecht)
                      Coolie (*The Exception and the Rule* by B. Brecht)
                      Woyzeck (*Woyzeck* by G. Buchner)
                      The Matchseller (*A Slight Ache* by H. Pinter).

      Function:      to express the conditions and consequences of poverty; to draw attention to the connection between material and spiritual poverty; to challenge the human spirit to transcend the conditions of economic oppression.

      Style:         generally presentational.

### 66. Role Type: Working Class: The Worker

66.1 Sub-type:     Proletarian

### 67. Role Type: Middle Class

67.1 Sub-type:     Bourgeois

67.2 Sub-type:     Nouveau Riche

67.3 Sub-type:     Merchant/Salesperson

### 68. Role Type: Upper Class

68.1 Sub-types:    Aristocrat, Nobility

68.2 Sub-type:     Industrialist/Entrepreneur

68.3 Sub-type:     Socialite

68.4 Sub-type:     Servant to the rich

### 69. Role Type: Pariah

69.1 Sub-types:    Homeless, Beggar, Ethnic Minority

69.2 Sub-type:     The Lost One

### 70. Role Type: Chorus, the Voice of the People

70.1 Sub-types:    Everyman, Narrator/Storyteller

*Classification: Authority/Aggression*

### 71.  **Role Type: Warrior** (see Soldier)

71.1 Sub-types: Conqueror, Victor, Captain

Quality: aggressive and assertive, moral, knows what he/she wants and is willing to fight to get it.

Example: Lysistrata (*Lysistrata* by Aristophanes)

Henry V (*Henry V* by Shakespeare)

Goetz von Berlichingen (*Goetz von Berlichingen* by W. von Goethe)

Adolf (*The Captain* by A. Strindberg).

Function: to engage in physical, moral, or intellectual battle to defeat an opponent and achieve a specified goal.

Style: presentational and representational.

71.2 Sub-type: Tyrant, Bully, Sadist/Masochist

Quality: brutally assertive, despotic and power-hungry, immoral and megalomaniacal; physically and/or psychologically harmful to others or to self.

Example: Menedemus (*The Self-Tormentor* by Terence)

Tamburlaine (*Tamburlaine* by C. Marlowe)

Richard III (*Richard III* by Shakespeare)

Caligula (*Caligula* by A. Camus)

Crown (*Porgy* by D. Heyward)

John Claggart (*Billy Budd*, adaptation of Melville novel by L. Coxe and R. Chapman)

Peron (*Evita* by T. Rice and A. Lloyd Webber).

Function: not only to control others, but to brutalize and humiliate them in order to feel powerful; in the case of the Masochist, that tendency is turned back on one self.

Style: generally presentational.

### 72.  **Role Type: Killer**

72.1 Sub-types: Assassin

72.2 Sub-type: Suicide

72.3 Sub-type: Matricide, Patricide, Infanticide

## V. Domain: Spiritual

*Classification: Natural Beings*

### 73.   Role Type: The Hero

73.1 Sub-types:    The Searcher, Pilgrim, Tragic hero
     Quality:        journeying forth on a spiritual search that will prove in
                      some way to be transformational; moral and open to
                      confronting the unknown.
     Example:      Antigone (*Antigone* by Sophocles)
                      Coriolanus (*Coriolanus* by Shakespeare)
                      Mary Stuart (*Mary Stuart* by F. Schiller)
                      Phaedra (*Phaedra* by J. Racine)
                      Joan of Arc (*St. Joan* by G.B. Shaw)
                      Juno (*Juno and the Paycock* by S. O'Casey)
                      Abe Lincoln (*Abe Lincoln in Illinois* by R. Sherwood).
     Function:     to take a risky spiritual/psychological journey toward
                      understanding.
     Style:         presentational or representational.

73.2 Sub-type:    Faust
     Quality:        restless, inquisitive, assertive, creative – the searcher for
                      ultimate knowledge.
     Example:      Faustus (*Doctor Faustus* by C. Marlowe)
                      Faust (*Faust* by W. von Goethe)
                      John Gabriel Borkman (*John Gabriel Borkman* by H. Ibsen)
                      Peer Gynt (*Peer Gynt* by H. Ibsen).
     Function:     generally, to strive toward the realization of one's full
                      creative potential; moral function of pointing to human
                      limitations;
     Style:         presentational.

73.3 Sub-type:    Anti-hero (see The Lost One)
     Quality:        a modern figure that is the antithesis of the tragic hero; an
                      ordinary person trapped in an ordinary, often dull
                      circumstance. The search for meaning is limited, if at all
                      present.
     Example:      Willy Loman (*Death of a Salesman* by A. Miller)
                      Godo and Didi (*Waiting for Godot* by S. Beckett)
                      Berenger (*Rhinoceros* by E. Ionesco).
     Function:     to endure within an indifferent universe.
     Style:         generally presentational.

73.4 Sub-type:   Post-Modern Anti-Hero.

     Quality:   an emblem, a cipher, an absurdity, a factotum, with few recognizable human qualities.

     Example:   Rhoda (*Rhoda in Potatoland* by Richard Foreman)
Rosencrantz and Guildenstern (*Rosencrantz and Guildenstern are Dead* by T. Stoppard)
Lincoln (*The Civil Wars* by Robert Wilson)
Hamlet and Ophelia (*Hamletmachine* by H. Müller).

     Function:   to signify or point to ideas and concepts, rather than feelings; to serve as a formal element within the performance, deconstructing the text as well as a realistic notion of human behavior and motivation.

74.  **Role Type: Visionary** (see Wise Person, 19)

74.1 Sub-type:   Prophet, Seer.

75.  **Role Type: Orthodox**

75.1 Sub-type:   Fundamentalist

75.2 Sub-type:   Ascetic

76.  **Role Type: Agnostic**

76.1 Sub-type:   Skeptic.

77.  **Role Type: Atheist**

77.1 Sub-types:   Heretic, Infidel.

77.2 Sub-type:   Nihilist.

78.  **Role Type: Cleric**

78.1 Sub-types:   Priest, Rabbi, Nun, Monk, Spiritual Leader.

78.2 Sub-type:   Lapsed Spiritual Leader.

*Classification: Supernatural Beings*

79.  **Role Type: God/Goddess**

     Quality:   magical, moral, prone to influencing natural events to satisfy their godly pleasures.

     Example:   Zeus (*Prometheus Bound* by Aeschylus)
Jupiter (*Amphitryon* by Plautus)
God (*The Tragedy of Job* by anonymous)
Zuss (*J.B.* by A. MacLeish).

     Function:   transcendence: to assert power over life and death.

Style:          Presentational.

Alternative Quality:   ironic, witty, and wise.

Example:        Three Gods (*The Good Woman of Setzuan* by B. Brecht)
                Steambath attendant (*Steambath* by B.J. Friedman).

Function:       comic relief; to provide dramatic irony based upon the
                superior foreknowledge of the gods; to satirize the limits
                of human desires.

Style:          presentational.

79.1 Sub-type:  Dionysus

Quality:        impulsive, ecstatic and irrational; androgenous.

Example:        Dionysus (*The Bacchae* by Euripides; *Dionysus in 69* by R.
                  Schechner)
                Baal (*Baal* by B. Brecht).

Function:       to assert the primal, uninhibited impulses of human beings.

Style:          presentational.

79.2 Sub-type:  Apollo

Quality:        rational, dreamlike, prophetic.

Example:        Apollo (*The Eumenides* by Aeschylus)
                Prospero (*The Tempest* by W. Shakespeare)
                Dr. Dysart (*Equus* by P. Shaffer).

Function:       to assert the principles of order, rationality, beauty, and
                  prophesy.

Style:          presentational and representational.

79.3 Sub-type:  Christ/Saint

Quality:        saintly, suffering and serving others, loving
                unconditionally, moral.

Example:        Christ (*The Passion Play*, anonymous)
                Christ (*Jesus Christ, Superstar* by A.L. Webber)
                Violaine (*The Tidings Brought to Mary* by P. Claudel)
                Archbishop Becket of Canterbury (*Murder in the Cathedral*
                  by T.S. Eliot).

Function:       to teach moral virtues; to provide a model of sacrifice,
                martyrdom and love.

Style:          presentational.

80.   **Role Type: Fairy** (see also Fool, 16)

80.1 Sub-types:  Sprite, Guardian Angel, Good Witch

81.   **Role Type: Demon** (see also Beast, 9 and Deceiver, 21)

81.1 Sub-types:  Furies, Maenads, Mephistopheles, Witch, Ghost

81.2 Sub-type:    Satan

81.3 Sub-type:    Death

82.   **Role Type: Magician**

82.1 Sub-types:   Sorcerer/Sorceress

## VI. Domain: Aesthetic

83.   **Role Type: The Artist**

83.1 Sub-types:   The Poet, Actor, Troubadour
    Quality:      creative, sensitive, easily distracted, often a pariah.
    Example:      Cyrano de Bergerac (*Cyrano de Bergerac* by E. Rostand)
        Manrico (*The Troubadour* by A. Garcia Gutierrez)
        Rubek (*When We Dead Awaken* by H. Ibsen)
        *** (*When Someone Is Somebody* by L. Pirandello)
        Robert and Elizabeth Barrett Browning (*The Barretts of Wimpole Street* by R. Besier)
        Dubedat (*The Doctor's Dilemma* by G.B. Shaw)
        Dearth (*Dear Brutus* by J.M. Barrie)
        Orpheus (*Orpheus* by J. Cocteau)
        Edmund Kean (*Kean* by J.P. Sartre).
    Function:     to assert the creative principle, envisioning or creating new forms or transforming old ones.
    Style:        presentational or representation.

84.   **Role Type: The Dreamer**

84.1 Sub-types:   Idealist, Romantic.

## The Role Method in Drama Therapy

The following section is a discussion of how to apply the taxonomy to treatment. The basic approach through the role method involves eight steps:

1. The invocation of the role.

2. The naming of the role.

3. The playing out/working through of the role.

4. Exploring alternative qualities and sub-roles.

5. Reflecting upon the role-play; discovering role qualities, functions, and styles inherent in the role.

6. Relating the fictional role to everyday life.

7.  The integration of the one role with other roles in one's internal role
    repertory/cast of characters.

8.  Social modeling: discovering ways that the clients' behavior in role
    affects others in their social environment and community. Finding
    effective ways to model the role so that others are given appropriate
    positive opportunities to play out their roles in return.

## The Case of Michael Revisited

Several months after Michael presented the story of 'The Wooden Clogs and
the Rubber Boots,' he offered the following:

> There are many fears in the house. Yet the house is so nice and relaxing.
> It overlooks the river and trees. You'd think you were in a paradise. You
> try to make it your web. In the house a young man comes to fuck an
> older man. The young man felt what it was like to be with someone.
>
> In the house of peace, a scary monster came out of the closet. The young
> man pushed them both into the closet and said: 'Stay in there until you
> can leave me alone! I just want to stay in peace in this house.' From under
> the door came black bugs. They circled the young man.
>
> > 'Help me! Can't you see your fear is getting me? Take
> > them back. I don't want them.'
>
> OLDER MAN:   'You have to let me out of the closet first.'
>
> The young man kicks through the circle of bugs and yanks open the
> closet. But only the older man is there. The bugs have vanished.
>
> OLDER MAN:   'You see, you have nothing to be afraid of. This house
> is a safe house.'
>
> YOUNG MAN:   'I don't trust you anymore. You brought on these
> monsters.'
>
> But the young man couldn't leave because there was a storm outside. He
> didn't want to be touched by the older man.
>
> In the morning it was tranquil. Was this all a nightmare? There were
> only clothes in the closet. The bed was made and it seemed that no one
> had lain in it. The young man got dressed, opened the window and saw
> a slight piece of wing from a black bug. He threw the wing out the
> window and watched it turn over and over, catching the sunlight,
> fluttering until it reached the ground. He felt something in his heart.
> Was it fear? As the wing caught the sun, it turned gold. It wasn't fear
> alone. Just as the young man knew what it was, the sun blinded him and
> made him forget.

So the young man waited for the older man to come back, but he didn't come. He waits and waits and wonders if it really happened at all.

Michael told this story, which he entitled 'The Beat of Black Wings,' after actually spending a night with Bill, an older man who had become Michael's lover. They had satisfying sex, an unusual occurrence for Michael. Long after falling asleep, Bill woke up in a panic, screaming. Michael became very frightened. He got up out of bed and went to the bathroom down the hall, fearful that he would encounter a water bug. When he turned on the bathroom light, a large water bug appeared. Michael became terrified, turned off the light and ran back toward the bedroom, without daring to kill the bug. In his panic, he became aware that someone had turned on the bathroom light. He turned around and saw Bill, who somehow had gotten out of bed and into the bathroom. Michael just wanted to sleep it off. He did not ask Bill about his nightmare. They both eventually fell asleep, without talking about the incident.

In his story, Michael identified the following roles: the Young Man, the Older Man, the monster, bugs, wings. He did not mention the house, the sun or the closet. He called the Young Man a confused searcher, a role that is ambivalent, the spiritual role of hero juxtaposed with that of the adolescent. His purpose is to search for a safe home, a loving place. He is open and trusting but is confused: In the role of confused searcher, Michael says: 'I don't know what I feel. I feel scared. Hurt. Angry. I don't know where this is coming from.'

For Michael, the older man is also a searcher, but he is more complex. He is the hero as fearful searcher, as there is a negative father part of him. On the one hand, according to Michael, he is 'searching for the end of the rainbow'; but, on the other hand, he is the keeper of the scary monster. There is an undercurrent to him; something is not completely safe. Without the older man there would be no scary monster.

The scary monster is somewhat undefined by Michael. All that he says is that the monster knows when to come to the young man and that the young man can call him up at any time. In my own mind, I relate the scary monster back to a role previously created by Michael, The Black Rage, which he sees as the terrifying, demonic, Dionysian power of his father. The screams of Bill might have provoked a reaction in Michael similar to that of the Black Rage, and, if this is the case, such terrors need to be shut up in the closet.

For Michael, the little bit of wing is something left behind by the scary monster bug. It has a mythological power and is part of the terror. Yet, it is also transformed by the sun into something beautiful, 'like a gift or angel trying to show something.' There is a spiritual role at work here, interjecting a healing, transformational power.

Michael also addressed the roles not initially mentioned:

The sun is the healer. It can shine light or make love where it's impossible to be. It can establish trust and impart knowledge where there was once confusion.

The closet is the place where the scary monster lives, the passageway, the gateway between human being and scary monster, fear and trust, the dark and the light room. It is the place where fear lurks and the monster can get you.

As such, the closet is a transitional space, a kind of looking glass. On one side one is safe and intact, but, on the other side, through the looking glass is an unknown and fearful world.

I asked Michael which character he felt closest to. He answered: 'The sun... the safety and the distance that I have now. There's always a bit of black wing.' I asked how the sun served him in his life? He responded: 'I am like the sun, the part that will protect me. Maybe there's too much protection. Maybe that's the black wing... pulling back and opening up, fear versus life.' Going further, Michael wondered if he needed more than protection: 'I want to blame the other one for making me sad and angry and mistrustful, but I don't know. I'm angry that I'm not saved by the sun or the older man. It's gonna be work. I wanna be taken care of.'

Michael was lying on the floor and had assumed the fetal position. He continued: 'I feel that the Black Bug is sexual. Sexual terror.'

Here we see the several bug fears: the actual fear of the deadly AIDS bug and the psychological fear that the father will creep in with his dreaded axe, abusing him, raping him, castrating him.

I asked him to take on the role of the Black Bug, the one role he has neglected to reflect on:

> I don't know. I am the Black Bug. I come out of the darkness. I move very slowly. I'm only looking to fulfill my needs. I come out of the darkness. Looking for... looking for... I don't know what I'm looking for. When you're unprotected, I walk across your arm, across your mouth in your sleep. If you admit that you want it, you might not be afraid. I creep. I'm looking to fulfill my needs. If I touch you, you will not die. I can be beautiful if you look at me. Then you try to kill me and I'm very afraid. I must die because of your fear. To die because of fear – that is my legacy.

The Bug is a repeated role that functions to keep Michael in his fear and in his victim role, that separates him from good sex and real intimacy. The legacy of the Black Bug is the legacy of the Black Rage, one of a paralyzing fear that can kill all chance of sexual and filial love. The Black Rage is a demonic role that fuels several other role types, primarily the father/tyrant and the angry young man. With the role of the bug, however, Michael has provided the possibility of transformation, with the image of the sunlight in the wing. 'I can be beautiful if you look at me,' he says. If he can indeed see fully and admit the powerful role of fear into his life, then the legacy of Black Rage can be transformed into that of another kind. When I asked Michael what it might be, he responded: 'A life of love.' That life remains elusive, but suddenly possible. Bill is not his father and he recognizes this. He knows, too, that he has the power to defeat bugs, or, at the very least, to confront them.

The older man, Bill, is, in fact, a lawyer. And the function of the lawyer role is to protect and defend. This is the good father that Michael so desperately is trying to find, not only in the world, but within himself. In his relationship with his lover/lawyer, he has found a way to transform the negative father/son relationship, with all its fears intact. The father part is still too intrusive – the demonic bugs threaten to keep Michael in the victim role. But the lawyer is there to mediate, as Michael now attempts to play the role of the fearless lover, one who can transform bugs and fears into a thing of beauty. The Dionysian role gives way to the Apollonian. The child gives way to the adult. The roles transform as Michael begins his healing. There are more bugs to transform and more father/son battles to wage, but, for this one moment, God is in his heaven and all is right with the world.

The role method attempts to answer the following questions:

- What are the roles played?
- What are their qualities?
- What do they mean? How do they serve the client in his life (function)?
- How are they played out (style)?
- How do they intersect with other intrapsychic and interpersonal roles?

Drama therapy treatment through the role method will be complete for Michael when the key ambivalent roles of child/adult, son/father, male/female, hero/victim, innocent/demon, gay male/straight world have been played out enough so that a transformed role system is functional and intact. This is not to say that the ambivalences will or should be resolved. Rather, that they transform to the extent that father is not so much in control of the son, the demon is not so much in control of the innocent, the victim is not so much in control of the hero, the straight world is not so much in control of the gay man, and so on. The therapeutic goal, then, is to learn how to live in the role ambivalences so that one powerful role becomes less overpowering to the system of roles.

The role model, based in Hamlet's existential dilemma, 'To be or not to be,' recapitulates the ambivalent reality of the actor who is identified enough with his role in order to give a convincing performance, yet who has so many other roles in reserve that no one part can ultimately threaten to take over the whole. Because of this ambivalence, he lives fully, with the knowledge that he can and will take on new roles and stretch old ones as the situations arise. In drama therapy, too, the role is the thing. And as it is taken on and played out in its endless variations, the client comes to see the ambivalences of being that ultimately respond to the identity question: 'Who am I?'

As Michael grows in his ability to move throughout the taxonomy of roles with some facility, building functional somatic, cognitive, affective, social, spiritual, and aesthetic roles, he, too, becomes a model for others engaged in the same struggle. In the business of acting, there have always been some known as 'actors' actors,' those like Spencer Tracy who provide role models of professional excellence. In the business of daily life, those who can present themselves effectively through role, acknowledging the inevitable ambivalences and contradictions, will likewise provide powerful models for others within their social worlds.

The taxonomy is intended as a blueprint for possibilities of being. It is limited by the specificity of its source, that of theatre. But if theatre is indeed a mirror held up to nature, then the specific source implies a more universal one. As a model, the taxonomy might well be applied in practice, as a means for diagnosis, treatment, and evaluation. It might further serve as a research instrument, generating the kinds of questions germane to the types and styles of enactments that guide us through our lives in the world that is so much like a stage.

# CHAPTER 10

# A Research Agenda for
# the Creative Arts Therapies

Research, whether in the biological or social sciences, humanities or arts, is about a systematic exploration of a problem, stated in such a way as to be subject to that exploration. The kinds of problems stated and the methodologies that researchers will apply in exploring the problems will vary within and among disciplines. This appears to be the case even though many hard-liners within a particular discipline will insist upon one set of questions and one method as *the* path toward establishing research parameters.

As creative arts therapists, we are in both a favored position and a potentially confusing one *vis-à-vis* research. The confusion comes in when we feel inadequate in asserting a unique research agenda separate from but equal to that of the reigning scientific and positivistic approaches applied regularly within the biological and social sciences. For many, the question becomes, do I have a right to carry on a different form of research? Will I then be respected among my peers and among those hard-liners in clinical professions who view my work as suspicious, at best.

But then, as creative arts therapists, we are potentially liberated from the kinds of scientism that often frustrate our colleagues in the social sciences who are drawn to new paradigms of research (Junge and Linesch 1993), but feel compelled to work within more conservative frameworks in order to be taken seriously within their academic faculties, clinical and research facilities. The liberation can come from the fact that we are still a relatively new field of inquiry with the potential to set forth a fresh approach to research that is neither science nor art exclusively, that is not tied to a traditional conception of the scientific method, and that reaches into inadequately explored realms of the body and image and role.

At the heart of the creative arts therapies is the notion that healing occurs because one is involved in a creative process. Thus, although the creative arts therapies are interdisciplinary, they are first and foremost, aesthetically-based. This assumption will effect the ways that researchers set forth their research questions, choose relevant theory and methodologies, and draw conclusions from their data. A research agenda for the field of Creative Arts Therapy, based in this assumption can include the following guidelines:

1.  Framing researchable questions that are germane to the aesthetic nature of the creative arts therapies and that lead to an uncovering of the healing properties of the creative arts.

    1.1 Framing researchable questions that are significant, that is, non-trivial and meaningful to both theorists and practitioners in the field; and timely, addressing issues of present concern to theorists and practitioners.

2.  Demonstrating a need within the field for a particular research project.

3.  Providing a context for the research based upon a review of literature within a particular creative arts therapy discipline and within related fields.

4.  Choosing relevant theory that illuminates the meaning of the research. The theory can come from several areas in the biological and social sciences, humanities and arts. However, creative arts therapy theorists should consider the value of basing theory within their creative art discipline. In each case, theory should focus upon the clarification of an aesthetic process as it facilitates healing.

5.  Choosing relevant methodology that is most appropriate to answering one's research questions and that responds to the aesthetic nature of the creative arts therapies. Junge and Linesch (1993) specify 9 research methodologies: phenomenological, heuristic, hermeneutic, ethnographic, empirical, action research, comparative/historical, theoretical, and evaluation research. I would add aesthetic research as a category, wherein the researcher documents and/or analyzes her creative process while engaged in creating an artwork for therapeutic purposes.

6.  Analyzing or systematically describing data according to criteria derived from one's theory. Again, the means of analysis/description should reflect the aesthetic nature of the research.

7.  Drawing conclusions from the research data that reveal the efficacy of the creative arts in psychotherapy. Placing the specificity of the study in a larger context as it correlates with other creative arts therapies or related disciplines.

The time has come to disseminate and apply knowledge more openly among the fields of art, dance, drama, music, and poetry therapies. The time has come to draw upon the research of colleagues in such related fields as aesthetic education, anthropology, critical theory, and psychodrama, to mention a few, and find new ways to collaborate. The time has come to challenge not only the reigning positivistic approaches to research in the social sciences but also our own limited imaginations in regard to an understanding of research. And the time has come to move out of the shadows of insecurity and publish compelling research that affirms the uniqueness and timeliness of Creative Arts Therapy as well as its continuity with ancient healing traditions.

# CHAPTER 11

# The Child, the Dreamer, the Artist and the Fool

## In Search of Understanding the Meaning of Expressive Therapy[1]

He makes abstract sweeps on his paper with brightly colored markers. His brief compositions want to fly off the page. And he lets this happen, drawing on furniture, walls, and floors. But he still requires a more personal canvas so he turns to his body and finds just the right flourish of red and yellow and green on his legs and arms and nose and forehead. Even his glasses are stained with yellow. Without missing a beat, he dives into an expressionistic dance to the Brazilian street drumming of Paul Simon's 'Rhythm of the Saints.' For a moment, offering up limbs and body in supplication, he is entranced.

She is drawing a picture, one in a repeated series of families of mice. Part of her recent composition includes playing with the letters of her name which assume a hieroglyphic quality. They sometimes look like images in a Miro painting. They fall in an order and in a space that is unpredictable each time she sets out to craft the letters. As she draws, she also experiments with sound. She hoots like an owl, hums, whistles, shrieks, clicks her tongue, blows air bubbles through tight lips, and chants simple Phrases over and over: Mamabear, Usabear, Papabear, Usabear...

These multimedia performance artists are neither Laurie Anderson nor Merideth Monk nor Ping Chong. They are my children, ages two and four respectively. As artists, they are irrepressible.

It is now common knowledge that one of the earliest forms of human expression is aesthetic. By early, I mean both the first years of individual human development and the ancient history of human cultures. The humanity of infants

---

1 This chapter was presented as a Titus Lecture at the Lesley College Colloqium on Expressive Therapies, August, 1993.

is based in large part on their ability to move, to sound, and to communicate with the outside world through images that might seem to the casual viewer random and arbitrary, but are actually ripe with meaning. What does it mean to draw mice families and letters and to chant nonsense syllables? To the parent, it might appear quite unremarkable, signifying a passing of time in harmless play. But to the child artist, it might signify a sense of delight, joy, and accomplishment, an experience outside the realm of time, consequence, and morality.

A significant developmental stage in early life occurs when the child is able to think and act dramatically. By that I mean that the child is able to live simultaneously in two levels of reality – that of everyday life and that of the imagination. This can be best understood by the relationship of actor and role where one playing at being another is also oneself at the same time. The actor, Al Pacino, takes on the role of the Godfather even as he remains Al Pacino.

At 20 months old, my son was able to fake crying. He would look at a book whose pages he had ripped up minutes before and begin a mock cry, knowing well that he had done something wrong and that the book was somehow 'hurt.' In joining in with him, I was affirming the fact that he had indeed hurt the book, but that his actions were within the range of normal baby behavior. Instead of punishment and remorse, he received an invitation to play a role – that of the remorseful one. In playing the role, he lives both in the everyday world where real actions have real consequences, that is, one feels sorry that one has damaged property, and in the imaginary world, where actions in role do not have any real consequences, that is, one can actually *make* fun of the situation and *have* fun doing so.

The child of two is an extraordinarily expressive being, moreso, I would think, than a creative person of any other age. If given free rein to paint, to sing, to dance, to play, to experiment with language, and to dramatize, children will do so spontaneously.

They express themselves aesthetically for a wide variety of reasons: to explore the world and their developing identities, to give shape to their feelings, to amuse themselves and to engage in social interactions with others, to create order and to create disorder, and to play with possibilities. Children also express themselves aesthetically when they are hurt and have no other effective means of expression. Even when children are not free to tell grown-ups that they have been violated in some way, they will most likely express their hurtful and angry feelings in their sounds and movements, in their sketching and scribbling, and in their dramatic play. In infancy and childhood, language is so minimal and direct, simple and image-bound as to be closer to the forms that adult artists struggle for years to create. I think of the operas and songs of Philip Glass, the paintings of Grandma Moses and Red Grooms, the poems of William Blake and Gertrude Stein.

Further, through evidence on the walls of caves, in ancient documents, in depictions discovered on prehistoric pottery, and in traditional ritual practices handed down over many centuries, it becomes clear that some thousands of years ago aboriginal peoples in all continents engaged in aesthetic forms of expression for myriad purposes – to mark significant passages and transitions in the life of a community, to celebrate festive and solemn occasions, to express a feeling, to pray and worship, and to heal the sick.

In his book, *Ur-Drama: The Origins of Theatre*, E.T. Kirby (1975) offered a convincing argument that the art form of theatre originated in the practice of shamanism. By extension, we find in the early shamanic rituals, as well as rituals passed down within current traditional cultures, examples of highly stylized chant, music, dance, mask, and impersonation of spirits, all in the service of healing. Many traditional cultures, removed from the vast imagery of modern technology and spiritual nihilism, still maintain an aesthetically-oriented life-style (see Schechner 1985).

One common denominator of all early individual and cultural creative activity is its propensity to allow the creator to feel integrated while in the act of creation. There is a sense of well-being present when a two-year-old discovers that he can create pleasing forms on his body or when a four-year-old discovers that she can whistle. There is even a sense of well-being present when an infant uses the contents of his diaper, the primal ooze, to create his first finger painting on the walls of his room and the skin of his body, that is, until a horrified and disgusted parent appears. Even so, to the infant, the body provides both the media and the message. The image of the body as supplier and receiver of creative activity is a very powerful one. If I can create both from myself and on myself, am I not, then, creating primarily for myself, regardless of the reception from a sometimes hostile audience? And could it be, by implication, that I am at the same time also creating myself – as a creative being who joyfully plays with the most primal of substances to satisfy a need for expression?

The function of aesthetically-based ritual within communities is also thera-peutic in the sense of creating balance and harmony among a people linked by cultural and blood ties. Richard Schechner (1985) gave a number of examples in his book, *Between Theatre and Anthropology*, referring to such rituals as the deer dance of the Yaquis of Arizona and the 3000-year-old Vedic ritual of the Agnicayana in India. There is ample evidence of the shamanic healing through-out the world, especially in cultures such as Korea, that are in transition between agrarian and technological. In Korea, shamanic ritual healings, involving music, dance, and drama to a large degree, are frequent and well documented (see Kim 1993).

It may well be true that there has always been a healing function inherent in the creative process, whether performed by a child, a shaman, or a fine artist. We in the field of creative arts therapy seem to understand this and take this point one step further. If art implies a natural and unconscious form of healing, then art can be harnessed consciously as a means to heal those who are imbalanced, victimized, and removed from the joys of play and the comforts of ritual.

This chapter is an attempt to clarify the meaning of creative arts therapy, a discipline I see as synonymous with the term, expressive therapy. Although I am more used to the former term, the latter intrigues me. 'Expressive' is rich in implication. It might refer to one who talks a lot or uses a lot of body language to make a point. But this understanding is only about quantity, that is, 'a lot' of expression makes one expressive. Expressive behavior is also about quality. I can express myself without overt and frequent gestures and words, through a drawing, for example, that depicts an image, or a sound that carries a feeling, or a look at another person that calls out a response. 'Expressive,' then, refers to a range of overt and covert actions, presented in word and gesture, sound and image. Expressive actions are enacted by a person, sometimes in the presence of another, for particular purposes, generally, to communicate feelings and thoughts. The specific purposes are varied. I might, for example, express my feelings to you because I want you to like me. When I do this, I often express myself indirectly, for fear that you might judge me for my need to be liked. I am like most people in this way, couching my expressions obliquely and requiring interpretation on the part of the other, or of myself, in order to be understood.

Instead of saying, 'I like you and hope that you will like me back,' we say: 'Where did you get that dress?' or 'How much did you pay for your car?' or 'Will you call me later?' or, in the words of my four-year-old: 'You're a poopy-head, Daddy!' Or, wanting to be liked and uncertain of our self-worth, we might not have the words at all. We might recall a song in private we haven't thought of in a while (see Diaz de Chumaciero 1992). Or we might doodle on a page, unconsciously sketching, trying to find a visual way out of an endless spiral of self-pity or doubt or shame.

In expressive therapy, we encourage the client to commit an expressive act from an often unconscious source as a vehicle for expressing a feeling or thought. Most people who are troubled are not aware of the nature of their troubles. And even those who are clearer about their troubles, those who, for example, are mourning the loss of a parent or recovering from an abuse or trauma of some kind, are not often able to express themselves fully enough in order to recover a sense of balance. The reasons for this are many. We are, for the most part, not educated by parents and teachers for expression other than verbal and cognitive. There is little education for the feelings, other than television and related popular media, often depicting complex emotional problems in simplistic ways. As a culture, we do not value rituals that facilitate expression of hurt or frightened feelings. As a body politic, our expressive models are limited; we are presented endless examples of violence, rage and revenge, but few of compromise and compassion. The sociologist, Tom Scheff provides a convincing analysis of how Western culture offers little but violent alternatives to feelings of shame and rage (see Scheff 1991).

If it is true, as I suggest, that our expressive options are limited, then the discipline of expressive therapy looms even larger as a significant alternative to cycles of hurt and violence. In order to understand expressive therapy, I feel it important to look at the primary sources from which the expressive therapies spring. These sources, which Howard Gardner (1983) might describe as 'Frames of Mind,' seem to me to be most clearly based in the creative forms of art, dance, drama, music, and poetry or literature. Expressive therapy derives from one's ability to draw, to move, to play dramatically, to sound and sing, to compose and speak with a voice rich in imagery. We begin with the assumption, shared by all the arts, that these abilities are healthy. Through such expression we, in a sense, create ourselves anew.

But this assumption is, of course, a generality, which few, I think, would deny. The field of expressive therapy and creative arts therapy must move further into the specifics of why and how the arts are healing. Many theoretical attempts have been made to link aesthetic processes with psychological ones. I would agree with a point stated clearly by Shaun McNiff (1993) that the most fruitful approach to this is to base those explorations first and foremost in the arts.

My own research in drama therapy has taken me to the primary question: how is performance healing? In order to answer that question I needed to discover some very basic concepts and processes involved in the dramatic experience. Throughout several years of research, I concluded that one of the most primary concepts in drama is that of role. Role, a term originally derived from theatre as the scroll-like object that held the lines recited by an actor in a play, represents the imaginative life of the actor. In order for drama to occur, a person must take on a persona or mask or character or other life – in other words, role. Without role, there can be no drama. A child at play is in role as much as an actor on stage. In fact, a number of sociologists have attempted to analyze social life in terms of role-taking and role-playing; the former an internal process of conceiving of oneself as the other, the latter an external process of enactment (see, for example, Mead 1934, and Goffman 1959).

In extrapolating from drama, I concluded that one primary means of self-expression was through role. Before proceeding, let me clarify and summarize my points about the term 'expression' which applies to both quantity, that is, how much expressive behavior one produces, and quality, that is, how deeply connected the expression is with one's feelings and thoughts. The content of one's expression, responding to the question, 'what does one express?' tends to be feelings and thoughts. Methods of expression, responding to the question, 'how does one express oneself?' pertain to those of the art forms and include visual, musical, gestural, dramatic, and verbal means.

In answering the question, 'why does one express oneself?' I have implied that, in general, expression is about the communication of feelings and thoughts. Further, in thinking through the question, 'when does one express oneself?' I would add that expression occurs consciously and unconsciously. We express ourselves consciously when we need or desire to communicate to another, whether the other is in a distanced relationship to us or a more intimate one. We also express covert feelings to these others through our non-verbal behaviors. Further, we also express ourselves to others with whom we do not wish to communicate often through nonverbal means. We express ourselves every day of our lives through day dreams and night dreams, through fantasies and wishes that can either be fully unconscious, dimly perceived, or, with effort, recalled, at least in part. And finally, in response to the question, 'where does one express oneself?' I would say anywhere and everywhere, as long as there is life and hope.

Role, then, is a means or method of expression. One expresses oneself in role in order to communicate feelings and thoughts. Role expression occurs everywhere and at all times. I would be hard-pressed to think of a time or place when and where expression in role does not occur. I dream in the role of the dreamer. In my dream, I appear in the many roles present. In delivering a paper I appear in the role of expert, and my job is to communicate my ideas and feelings to those in the role of audience, viewer, student, colleague.

Behind this notion of dramatic role is a deeper and to some a troubling assumption. If it is true that roles are indeed ubiquitous and that one is always in role, then where is the self or central core of the personality located? Surely there must be a sense of persons separate from their personae. After all, there is always, predictably, a face under a mask (except if you are the invisible man...or woman).

In terms of the dramatic world view, there is ultimately no self or core being, only roles. One might argue that beneath all the roles one plays lies the actor who, in effect, generates all the roles. But, I would argue, the state of being actor is another role. It is that of the performer whose purpose is to spin roles and present him or herself in such a way that they are acknowledged by an audience.

I would further argue that there is no longer a need for a Self, with a capital 'S,' at least in the minds of those who are capable of living with the ambivalences of their existence, with contrary thoughts and feelings, with paradox and, in the words of Blake, 'fearful symmetries.' Those who hold on to the center, believing that the personality has a fixed and constant point, might miss the complexities offered by what I call the dramatic world view. Like those who believe in an unassailable religious or political center, a core of righteousness and dogma, choices become limited.

Within the dramatic world view, the forces of morality clash. Dramatic reality, reflective of that of everyday life, presents the play of opposites. Each complex character, whether Antigone, Hamlet, or Blanche DuBois, is a battle-field unto herself. Each character type, including heroes, victims, and deceivers, endlessly clash within the drama with their counterparts – villains, survivors, and helpers, respectively. Although order may be established at the end of a tragedy, as the young Fortinbras, in role of peacemaker, approaches at the conclusion of *Hamlet* to establish a new political order, there are still a number of dead bodies lying around who, in fact, have died a rather gruesome death. In a psychological sense, there is no real closure in *Hamlet*, only death and destruction.

These dramatic complexities reflect psychological ones that can well be observed as a client is in the process of working through drama therapy. In that process clients begin to reveal the cast of characters that govern their existence and the ways that they have been victimized and continue to victimize themselves. One goal in drama therapy is to help clients uncover a survivor part that is powerful enough to counteract the powerful grip of the victim. The therapist aids clients in empowering a whole internal cast of characters that can ultimately find a way to peacefully coexist.

This world view implies that the personality is peopled by a wide variety of characters, as opposed to a central Self. And it implies that the balanced life is not one where the hero slays the villain and lives happily ever after, but one in which the drama of hero versus villain is a constant that needs to be played out again and again throughout one's life. The therapeutic goal is not to vanquish the villain, but to find a way to live comfortably within the ambivalence of hero/villain, within the framework of knowing that battles will always need to be fought and that if one has an intact hero role within one's internal role repertoire, then one has less to fear when the victim part falls prey to an external villain.

One way to express oneself, drawn from the world of drama, is through role. The human personality, conceived through the lens of drama, is a compilation of personae, a system of roles, which, although interrelated, often stand in opposition to one another, creating a certain creative tension within an individual.

Through some years of research I posed the question, again drawn from theatre: What roles are available to take on and play out? To answer that question, I began an exploration of Western dramatic literature, from the pre-Greek times through the present. I extrapolated repeated character types throughout, distilling them again and again as new types surfaced and old ones seemed to blend together. I invited colleagues and students to comment upon these types and compared them with other typologies drawn from archetypal psychology (see Jung 1971), transactional analysis (see Berne 1961), literature (see Propp 1968) and religion (see Riso 1987). In the final analysis, I settled on 84 role types which I organized into six domains: somatic, cognitive, affective, social, spiritual, and aesthetic. My most daunting task was to substantiate this system and to demonstrate how it might serve as a map of the human personality from the dramatic point of view of role.

Today, my task is somewhat more modest. I have extracted four role types from the taxonomy – Child, Dreamer, Artist, and Fool – and will argue that these can be seen as central figures who can speak to the meaning of expressive therapy. That is, if we were to listen to these figures, they might collectively tell us something about the field we are all here to study and to practice, the basis of which has to do with interrelated forms of creative expression.

Earlier in the chapter, I offered a picture of two children, one two years old, the other four. The child was presented as 'an extraordinarily expressive being.' I spoke of my children as if they were performance artists, which they are, in part. In fact, my intention was to fool you into believing that I wasn't describing children at all, but actual performance artists. Let me give voice to the child, that is, the Child with a capital 'C', as type. These voices are my own inventions.

CHILD:     You know me. Some people have made a lot of
           money selling you books about how I am really inside of
           you, you know, your 'inner child?' Well, here I am. You
           can decide for yourself if you're like me. I'm a very
           expressive type, you know. Some say I'm innocent, but I
           don't know what that means. I live to please myself, have
           a good time. They tell me I'm spontaneous. I don't know
           what that means either. I just do what I feel like most of
           the time. Sometimes when I start to run I feel like I could
           go on forever. And if a car came by on the road, I'd just
           jump up in the air and sail right over. Some grown-ups
           get mad at me a lot. They make me cry sometimes. They
           hurt me. When I feel like it I talk back to them, kick
           them and call them doody-head and things like that.
           Then I play quiet. With my dolls. I talk to them and tell
           them how I am feeling. I tell them Cinderella stories, like
           one time she fell and had a cut and had to go to the
           doctor and one time her brother ran out into the street
           and got hit by a car and went to the hospital and died
           and then was an angel. The fairy godmother takes care of
           him just like Cinderella. I'm a good painter, you wanna
           see? Here's one I did of my whole family. My brother's
           the one who looks like a bird, but he's really an angel. He
           can fly in the sky and the Fairy Godmother will take care
           of him. She can fly, too. She takes care of everybody who
           gets hurt. She's a good helper. I like her a lot.

Let me switch roles. As I presented it, the child is endearing, playful, and guileless, maybe too cute at times, at least from an adult point of view. And the child, confronted with external realities, is always trying to make sense of the world, based in her observation and imagination. When confronted with a crisis, such as the injury and death of a sibling, the child turns to the imaginary world as a source of explanation and comfort. Developmentally speaking, children four years old and under, for the most part, are not fully able to make clear distinctions between reality and imagination, that is, their reality is one very much linked to their imaginations. In crisis, children need expression; they turn to their dolls and tell a story; they paint a picture of the now transformed family. In storytelling and painting they have expressed their feelings and thoughts. Many children, when supported in this by sympathetic and loving adults, can work through their various minor and major life crises, from cuts to death. But only if expression is allowed and encouraged, as long as it takes to work through the pain. When the child shuts down, the caring adult figure needs to intervene in some way, to help facilitate an opening of the expressive channels.

Some children, who have been severely abused or who suffer an acute form of autism or developmental disability, need to be taught how to play. This is hard work, but imperative if they are to assume the role of child which, by definition, is one whose life is characterized by the ability to play.

The child tells us the importance of expression as a means of healing, provides a model of healing through the arts, even gives us the seeds of a theory about aesthetic distancing by moving away from the actual event of a brother's death and transforming it into images within a story and a painting. The image of the brother as angel, who will soar above the family, is more acceptable than that of the brother as casualty, who will be buried in the ground. But the child at the same time knows the stark reality, even if conscious awareness is limited. The child exemplifies, then, the actor who lives simultaneously in the two realities of the everyday and the imagination. As such, the child actor provides a powerful model for the expressive therapist who helps clients move in and out of the two realities as a means of both working through a problem and, when developmentally appropriate, reflecting upon it.

On the other side of the Child is the Adult, whom, as I have mentioned, can be a helper and caretaker of the child when she is in need. As antithesis of the child, the adult also can block the spontaneity and playfulness of childhood, providing, at times, an overpowering dose of rationality and morality. When in balance the roles of child and adult provide one's inner life with a sense of order. A balance would imply that a person is able to be both playful and rational, both spontaneous and reflective, both innocent and experienced. Not that all these qualities need to counterbalance each other all of the time, but that, from the point of view of the expressive therapist, an ideal balance would allow people to express their child part when they are too rational and uptight, and the adult part when they are too irresponsibly playful and boundaryless.

The next voice is that of the Dreamer, which again I will translate in my own way:

DREAMER:  It's good to get this body to slow down and stay put
for awhile. It's good to get the eyes moving behind
closed lids, for then I let my visions appear. I have so
many stories to tell, the most wonderful stories in the
world. Some are scary, some are even boring, but all are
about you. Do you remember Romeo? His nightmares
proved prophetic, even though his friend Mercutio called
them 'the children of an idle brain,/begot of nothing but
vain fantasy;/Which is as thin of substance as the
air,/And more inconstant than the wind.' I bring you
messages, despite the words of the doubters. When you
are troubled, I can bring you face-to-face with the
troubles. I can depict them for you in colors and shapes
that you can read, if you so choose. But you must do the
work, because I often appear disguised. My creations are
dreams. As dream, I can take any shape I want; I can be
your mother or your father or your sister or a strange
room you think you have seen before, or I can be God or
a disembodied spirit or Death. I can be a part of your
body or a mountain or a bird or a bed the size of a large
yard. And the strange thing about me is that I might be
real or fake. It depends upon how you see me, *if* you see
me. As dream, I can be your fantasy and take you far
away from your troubles, feeding into all your needs for
escape and avoidance. Or I can be a beacon, illuminating
your existence and showing you a way out or even a way
in. I am a salve for lovers and romantics and escape artists
of all kind; and I am a guide for visionaries and artists
and all searchers for new solutions to old problems. I am
hardly the child of an idle brain; I spring from an active
mind that even when at rest, spins my visions. I have
many stories to tell. Use them as you will.

The dreamer, then, is two things – idealistic and romantic, leading one to
escapist fantasies; and visionary and creative, leading one to search for new
forms and new insights. As a role type, the dreamer is a potential guide. But
the direction that one chooses to take under its sway is of great significance –
whether moving away from one's problems and thus avoiding to look at one's
inner life, or moving toward some sense of understanding and perhaps,
transformation.

As you know, dreams have served as the cornerstone of many forms of
psychotherapy, especially analytic forms. One could well argue that Freud's
major literary contribution was *The Interpretation of Dreams*. Many schools of
therapy claim to have valid approaches to interpreting dreams, conceived of as

embodying archetypes of the unconscious, wish fulfillments, split-off object relations or Gestalts.

The dream as story told by the dreamer as storyteller offers an expressive approach to dreamwork. As clients narrate their dreams they will actually be telling stories about their lives from the point of view of the dream images. I take a broad view of storytelling. Stories can be told verbally, of course, but also through drawing or sculpting or singing or dancing.

An interpretation of dreams must suitable to the expressive therapies, I think, is that of the dream figures as roles of the dreamer. Each figure of the dream can, in fact, be given a voice (or a visual or gestural image) and can be listened to. Let me give you an example of a dream narrated to me by a client some years ago. He called the dream, 'The Double':

> There is a monster, a controlling force that lives in my bedroom. I see it as a chain that hangs in 3 parts over my bed. The bed is my parents' bed. There is a cross in the center of the chains. I play the monster's role and speak for him in a hoarse voice. I call out: 'René! René!' We have little dialogues and I don't know whether I'm him or I'm me. He controls me and I'm not really free. Sometimes when I come home late from a date, I'm in the role of the woman I went out with. He doesn't say anything, but I know he's there. He's always there. I go to the bathroom where it's dirty. I wash everything down. I am washing him out of everything, ridding myself of him, washing him out. I'm afraid to go to therapy, ashamed to let others know that I am possessed.

That was all he remembered. As you know, doubling is a method used in psychodrama. It is also a concept pertaining to a kind of alter-ego that has appeared in drama and literature for hundreds of years. It has been most widely used in modern literature by such exemplars as Doestoyevsky and Conrad. It is well exemplified in the classic stories by Edgar Allen Poe and Robert Louis Stevenson, 'William Wilson' and 'Dr. Jekyll and Mr. Hyde.'

I asked this client, whom I will call Barry, to take on the role of monster and that of himself as narrator, as René, as woman, and as cleaner. He did this by moving from one chair, which represented the monster, to another, which represented the other characters, and engaging in a dialogue. He then sculpted his body into the shapes of each character. I asked him, finally, to find appropriate movements for each character. As the monster, he looked old and tired, slumped over with a poor posture. He didn't at all appear frightening to me.

Following the enactment, he recalled another part of the dream, which he verbalized:

> The monster is my father. I'm asking him questions and he's telling me stories about the war and about famous people he knew. I'm very close

to him, crawling between his legs, wanting the contact so very much, but afraid of the closeness of his body.

In completing the session, it became clear that Barry was wrestling with the power of the father upon his life, the father who exists as a terrifying yet somewhat pitiful force within his psyche. At this early point in his treatment, Barry was one who merged too easily with others. He spoke of the religious connection between his father and himself, represented by the chains and the cross, and of his need to separate himself from his father for fear of being engulfed by this double. He also spoke of his shame around the issue of desiring physical contact with his father but being so frightened by his powerful maleness.

Through the therapy, Barry worked toward reconstructing an internal father role that could help him work through his frightening and shameful feelings and do what a father is supposed to do, that is, pass on a male legacy to his son and offer a model of how to father himself.

In mobilizing the dreamer role, Barry received psychological information in the form of disguised imagery, e.g., father as double and monster, which once deciphered, led him toward a new vision of himself. This is what the role of dreamer can give the expressive therapist – a way of understanding dreams as parts of the dreamer, and a way of working with the dreams creatively, giving them voices and shapes so that the dreamer can envision new possibilities of being. In one sense, all dream images are doubles of the dreamer.

On the other side of the dreamer is the grounded one, the realist. This realist attends to the daily business of life, making sure there is food on the table and that the garbage is taken out. When in balance, the dreamer and the realist allow one to indulge in visionary and romantic activity while at the same time taking care of material needs. Many individuals who seek expressive therapy are artistically inclined. They choose expressive therapy because it provides a comfortable and familiar way of self-exploration. In working toward a balance of dreamer/realist, they are able to discover a way of co-existing within the paradoxical dramatic realities of world and stage, the everyday and the imaginary.

This same kind of balance is desired by people working through the artist role. Like the dreamer, the artist is visionary and creative, searching for new forms and new insights. But rather than escaping, the artist often commits a radical act of exploration. Artists may escape from the world of things for a while, but only to enter another world of images or of emptiness – a blank canvas, an empty space, a blinking prompt on a barren computer screen. In confronting their resistances, they ready themselves to leap into the act of creation. One specific type of Artist is the performing artist or performer. Let us listen to that voice:

PERFORMER:   I can't tell you how many times I've had that same
dream, you probably know it well – 'the actor's
nightmare.' I'm on the stage, I've been given my cue, I
open my mouth to speak, but nothing comes out. I
don't know my words. I don't even know the play I'm
in. I look around. The other actors are staring at me.
The audience is out there waiting, but I am lost,
totally lost. I am ashamed and so sorry. I need
attention, you know. I want you to like me for all the
tricks I can do. My talents are limitless. I have studied
for years with the best voice and mime and dance
coaches in the city. I have been to Japan and Bali and
India to learn the classical Eastern forms. I can execute
leaps and intricate gestures. I can sing falsetto and I
can cry real tears. When you see me like this, you will
cry too, or laugh, and you will applaud – Bravo!
bravo... Don't get me wrong, I don't want to hold
your attention completely, I mean, I don't want you to
only see me up there. There are others who can leap
just as high and cry just as well as I can. Look at
them, too. They are wonderful, marvelous performers!
But don't forget me, please, don't forget me. When
you talk about the play, the dance, the singing, on
your way home from the theatre, when you send your
congratulations in the mail for a job well done, and
write your reviews, please, please, don't forget me.
Even if you need to consult your program, you must
remember my name... Wait a minute... It's here
somewhere... Where is it? Ah, here – the Second
Gravedigger...the Second Player...the Second
Fiddle...that's me!... Hey, there are no small parts,
only small actors... Or is it the other way around?

The performing artist, although appearing to be in control, removed from an
audience, safely ensconced on a stage, is often quite vulnerable and needy of
recognition and praise. Performance anxiety is pretty much a universal fact of
a performer's life. Further, the performer often engages in a balancing act while
on-stage, wanting desperately to be seen and praised, the others be damned,
while at the same time wishing to be generous in sharing the stage or at extreme
times, wishing to disappear.

The image of the performer offers the expressive therapist a glimpse of
certain ambivalences confronted by most all clients, that of the need for
acknowledgement as opposed to the need to remain distant and anonymous,
that of the need to risk tempered by the fear of failure. These ambivalences,

when clearly present, might even be the motivating force that drives people into therapy, especially narcissistic people whose needs to be acknowledged can become all-consuming. Standard statements heard early in therapy, common to the concerns of the performer, are: nobody understands me; I feel invisible; or, my life is too controlled; or, I always seem to risk too much emotionally and get hurt by it.

A recurring dream of one of my clients, an aspiring actor, concerned a sense of himself in foreign lands without a role to play. Without the clarity and definition provided by the role, he was lost, unrecognized and unseen by anyone, including himself. And shortly after retiring from a distinguished baseball career, Mickey Mantle was plagued by a dream of hearing his name called by an announcer: 'And playing center field for the New York Yankees, Number 7, Mickey Mantle.' The fans applaud but he stands outside the stadium, locked-out, with no hope of ever again taking-on his hallowed status.

This existential state of estrangement, so prevalent in technocratic cultures, can lead some individuals to seek careers in the performing arts or professional sports in the hope of being 'discovered,' not necessarily in the sense of making it as a celebrity, but simply being seen, recognized, validated. Clients in expressive therapy often desire the same effect from their creative activity, that is, a recognition of value as a person.

In group therapy, a central issue for members is often how much of the group's time to take up as they 'perform' themselves through verbal and non-verbal means. Most groups will have those who appear to 'show-off' and constantly demand attention and those who appear to blend in with the scenery. Through an effective therapeutic process, the group can learn to find its own balance and provide effective critical feedback as to when one is too large or too small for his performer role.

On the other side of the artist and performer is the one who feels empty, who plays it safe, risks little, and expresses less. This persona can be characterized as the lost one, like my client in his dream of being faraway from home without a role, and like Mickey Mantle locked out of his stadium. Again, this state of being is one that often drives people into therapy. Performers who are lost would be excellent candidates for expressive therapy in that this form of treatment concerns the relationship between performers and their performance, whether through visual, verbal, musical, or physical means. The lost one and the artist/performer well compliment one another in that each authentic act of creation implies a struggle with the void, the unknown, the empty space. Should one give in to the emptiness, one takes on the role of lost one. Should one commit to working through the emptiness, then one makes the journey toward expression hand-in-hand with the dual roles of artist and lost one.

In the act of expressive therapy, therapists are well aware of the seduction of the role of Lost One, both for their clients and for themselves. In the twists and turns of another's expressive journey, therapists can easily lose their capacity to guide. So too can they easily become flooded with their own needs for expression when clients perform issues too close to home. Thus, if the expressive therapists are artists, e.g. director, conductor, choreographer, as artists they must be aware of their own tendencies toward feeling lost, so that they may model for a client a way of living within the paradox of creation and nihilism.

The final role I wish to discuss is perhaps the most complex of all in that it contains bits and pieces of the other roles, yet is far greater than the sum of these parts. It is the Fool who has much wisdom to share with those of us in the field of expressive therapy. Let us listen to this fool:

FOOL:      You know, the funniest thing about me is that I'm not as dumb as I look. Don't confuse me with that other fool, the idiot, the guy with half a brain in his head. He's the one who every hustler in the world can't wait to rip off. They get him on three card monte, the shell game, and every other scam you can think of. One time I saw him get off a bus at Port Authority, he's wearing plaid golf pants with a T-shirt that says: R.J.'s Pasta Factory, Tulsa, Oklahoma, or some place like that. So I bumped into him, you know, accidentally on purpose, and I go: 'You new in town, cowboy?' or something like that. And I tell him I work for the housing authority, like I, myself, am an authority on all the available rent-controlled apartments in the city, that it's up to me to check them out and make sure they're legit. He buys it and is about to pay me my modest fee of $100 cash or traveler's checks when he pulls out this badge from around his neck. He's an undercover cop and the joke's on me. It cost me a total of 525 bucks in fines to get out of that one. So who's the fool?... I'm really not such a bad guy; in fact most people get a real kick out of me because I'm able to lighten things up, you know, like Woody Allen used to do in the old days when he was just a little neurotic schmuck trying to find sex and God, but always tripping up on his own insecurities. Now look at him. All the wit and charm and cash in the world can't get him out of the mess of public humiliation. What a fool! He should've stuck to acting out all his adolescent fantasies in the movies!... I don't know, call me crazy, but I'm just having a good time. I get most kicks beating up on the rich and powerful guys bigger than me, you know, the ones who thinks they're on top of the world. I'll do anything – carry their bags, shine their shoes, chauffeur their cars – but when they begin to pontificate and seduce, I'll be there, and I'll be sure to get them. Bring me the presidents and I'll find means to shame them for the way they cut their hair or screw up political appointments; bring me the super-moralistic southern Senators and I'll have them publicly referring to some Supreme Court nominee on national television as 'Long Dong Silver'; bring me superstar athletes and I'll have them run out of town for throwing firecrackers at babies; bring me Judges of great power, wisdom and sagacity and I will have them cut down by sex scandals. And you should watch yourselves, too, my friends, for the lust and the shame that you think is safely hidden away in your heart of hearts is just on the surface, waiting for the likes of me to prick that thin membrane and let it all out, just when you are feeling most powerful and in control. Tie your shoelaces, fools, and adjust your underwear! I am near-by, waiting to humiliate you. Resist me not, fools, for I am mightier than you are, and much, much smarter! Look around you. The person seated to your left might actually be me in disguise… But relax. Take a nice, deep breath. I'm only fooling. Nothing that I said was true. I'm the fool, not you.

Let me de-role from this very powerful character. I mentioned before that the fool role contains qualities of the others already discussed. The Fool is certainly childlike in the sense of having a highly playful attitude toward life that is often endearing, at least from the point of view of one who is not the butt of the Fool's jokes. Like the dreamer and artist, the Fool is a highly original and creative type, even though fools may use their creativity in the service of ridiculing others. The Fool is also a paradoxical creature, paradoxical in the sense that one ordinarily thinks of fools as simpletons and dupes. Actually, the Fool character in mythology, often seen as the trickster, and in drama, seen as the clever servant or the harlequin or the philosophical, postmodern clown, displays a certain cunning and wisdom as to the ways of the world.

In relationship to expressive therapy, a central component of the role type is the fool's propensity to humiliate and be humiliated. There is a large part of this character that is based in shame, stemming from the fact that when being fooled or when playing the fool, one often feels diminished in the eyes of others. Our culture demands the formula that success equals control. A political or religious figure, for example, must appear to be the antithesis of the Fool, which is, as I have suggested, the one who is in control. Popes and Presidents can ill afford to play the fool without fully covering their tracks.

But part of the stuff that defines most mere mortals is our capacity to be fooled, tricked, humiliated and compelled to face our human frailties. In becoming foolish, we have the opportunity to allow a healthier sense of ourselves to emerge. That is, unless we can express the foolish parts of ourselves, we risk engulfment in the authoritarian, controlling parts of our psyches.

As expressive therapists, we encourage clients to play imaginatively, believing that through such creative activity, a sense of emotional restoration can occur. Imaginative play of all kinds must allow the Fool in as a player. The Fool inspires clients to laugh at themselves and not take themselves too seriously. The Fool serves all kinds of liminal and transitional functions in that it moves between dualities of physical form, that is, the trickster as fool can be male or female and can assume many disguises; it moves between dualities of cognition, that is, this type can appear as wise fool and foolish wise person; and it moves between dualities of affect, in that the Fool can provide both pleasure through wit and pain through shame.

It seems to me that expressive therapists are well suited to help clients work through these and related paradoxes in that they work through art forms that bring clients in and out of the dual realities of the everyday and the imagination. In helping overly-controlled people to fool around, the expressive therapist moves toward a significant therapeutic goal. In helping those too possessed by their foolish tendencies to take more control of their often childish wishes, the therapist also helps one move toward a balance of roles so essential for effective treatment through the arts. The Fool informs the expressive therapist that life is heavy and light at the same time, a knowledge well documented in the novel and film, *The Unbearable Lightness of Being* (see Kundera 1984). How valuable a goal for all to achieve a way of living through desperate times lighter and through frivolous times wittier. The wisdom of the Fool can be had by entering into the fool's paradox.

The expressive therapist can also be seen as a kind of fool, one who seems to assume an inferior role to that of the client and takes on the shapes and disguises within the transference as is necessary to explore particular issues. The foolish wisdom of the therapist, when expressed in an indirect, tricky or playful way, can lead clients toward an understanding of their own tendencies to feel foolish and ashamed. In some ways the whole idea of expressive therapy is foolish, in the sense that therapist and client play together, assume disguises on purpose, try to trick one another into believing their own point of view is valid, attempt to lighten or at least distance the painful burden one brings into therapy, and ultimately explore images of shame and humiliation in order to discover a way to live in the paradoxes represented by the Fool.

Taken together, the child, the dreamer, the artist, and the fool tell us much about how and why and when our profession works. The Child provides a method of creative treatment, the play way (see Cook 1917), a means of making sense through pretense, of removing oneself from reality and playing with it for the purpose of discovering meaning therein. This is a primary understanding and treatment strategy inherent in expressive therapy where the blank sheet of paper, the empty space or the unplayed instrument invites the client to enter into the imaginative realm and play.

The Dreamer also invites one to play in an imaginative realm. As a role type it provides the expressive therapist with a goal – to encourage clients to envision new forms and new insights and to struggle with their tendencies to escape. The dreamer further provides the expressive therapist with an understanding of dreams and, by implication, of images. They are parts of the dreamer, the one with the active imagination, and working through the creative arts therapies, we are able to help the dreamer give voice to them and then integrate these highly expressive images.

The Artist is a state of being that often characterizes both client and therapist in expressive therapy in their attempts to wrestle with the void and create meaning through their music, drawing, dance, writing, and drama. The paradox of the performer offers an understanding for expressive therapists of a daunting task, that is, to help others (and themselves) work through the need to be seen and acknowledged on the one hand, and to remain anonymous and sheltered on the other. Further, the role of the performer reminds expressive therapists what they must do – guide clients in and out of their sense of alienation by means of performing images of themselves on paper and in space and through rhythm and time.

And finally, the Fool tells us all not to take ourselves too seriously; it's all a dream anyway, this dance of healing – a lie, a fabrication, an artifice. Like Puck at the end of *A Midsummer Night's Dream*, the fool tells us:

> If we shadows have offended
> Think but this, and all is mended –
> That you have but slumb'red here
> While these visions did appear. (v, i, 418–21)

All tricks, dreams, fantasies, wishes, visions are fake, Puck seems to be saying, and if they are presented in a way that is too disturbing, then let them go, for they are unreal. So I tell my clients when they rip the head off a doll or plunge a knife into the genitals of a puppet: 'You can perform these outrageous actions because this is all trickery, stuff of the theatre.' But Puck knows better, as does Shakespeare, as do we all. Dreams and fantasies are real, but in a different way than everyday life. They represent our inner lives of feeling and thought not easily accessible. We often fear these kinds of expressions, especially those that carry a burden of violence and shame.

So we, who are trained to use dreams and visions for healing purposes, unapologetically encourage clients to enter into their own midsummer or winter or autumnal dreams safely. In the enchanted forest of the imagination, all is permitted, but only in the safety of the concurrent knowledge that one takes the journey inward to the imagination in order to discover a way back home, back into the world. The expressive therapist is the guide, the Puck figure who will trick clients into acting foolishly, then help them back into the familiar world, transformed in some significant way by the experience.

Puck embodies many qualities of the Child, the Dreamer, the Artist, and the Fool. In this sense, he (or she) is the consummate expressive therapist who knows how to live within the two realities of the imagination and the everyday, who understands how to instill and interpret dreams, who knows the effects of disguise, foolish wisdom, and shame. Above all, this Puck figure comprehends the endless complexities of paradox as it applies to art, everyday life, and healing.

The meaning of expressive therapy is contained in expressive acts that are performed for healing purposes. I suggest a dramatic approach as one way of understanding these performances. Performers make performances. They do so in role. The roles of Child, Dreamer, Artist and Fool might be compelling enough to offer a sense of how and why and when performances are healing.

The final role I would like to take on is that of Puck. I might have offended some of you with my words. Some people don't like to hear me say that there is no self. Others might not like other things I have said or my method of presentation. To you, I apologize. Anyway, I didn't really say those offensive things at all. They were just the wanderings of a weak and idle mind, no more than a dream.

> So, good night unto you all.
> Give me a hand, if we be friends,
> And Robert shall restore amends.

# CHAPTER 12

# Three Scenarios for
# the Future of Drama Therapy

The following remarks were given in a speech to members of the National Association for Drama Therapy (NADT) at the 14th annual conference in Chicago entitled, 'The Winds of Change.' In preparing the speech, I initially wondered what the conference planners had in mind by 'The Winds of Change.' Were they referring to the present as a time of change or the future as a time when change might occur? And what changes did they have in mind? Changes in practice and theory from within the field? Changes in governance of the field? Changes in the field's relationship to other disciplines and systems of law, education, and mental health?

In my puzzlement, I focused on the images of winds and of change. I immediately thought that for the present, the field of drama therapy seemed becalmed and sedentary rather than stormy. I also thought that this state of affairs was temporary and there was much hope that the winds could be coaxed into blowing again.

In that the conference was to begin by taking a look backward to the founding of NADT, I, too, thought about the past and the beginnings of this most promising field. But what came to mind was not the initial coterie gathered in New Haven to assist in a birth, but rather an image of Shakespeare's King Lear on the heath. This king who was once so powerful and in control, was later to appear ranting on that barren heath half-naked, pitiful, humiliated, drenched to the bone, attempting to assert his control over a thunderstorm. Lear's rantings began:

> Blow winds, and crack your cheeks.
>> Rage, blow,
> You cataracts, and hurricanoes, spout
>
> Till you have drenched our steeples,
>> drowned the cocks,
> You sulphurous and thought-executing
>> fires,

Vaunt-couriers of oak-cleaving thunderbolts,
Singe my white head. And thou
  all-shaking thunder,
Strike flat the thick rotundity o' th' world,
Crack nature's moulds, all germens spill
  at once,
That makes ingrateful man...
I tax not you, you elements, with unkindness.
I never gave you kingdom, called you
  children;
You owe me no subscription. Then let fall
Your horrible pleasure. Here I stand your
  slave,
A poor infirm, weak and despised old man...
  O! O 'tis foul. (III, ii, 1–9, 16–21, 25)

Lear had changed from powerful king to impotent madman, from providing father to groveling babe. His inner turmoil took the shape of a terrible storm that racked his soul.

Many years ago I worked as an actor with the Utah Shakespeare Festival. At the beginning of the season we all had to present an audition scene. All were required to audition by the producer, even those who would play walk-on roles. Most of the untrained actors chose simple scenes with minimal physical and emotional demands. The auditions occured in alphabetical order and the last to be called was Worrell F. Zefman, a teenager from Provo, Utah. He chose Lear's mad scene on the heath. He turned his back to the audience, stood as far away from us as he could get and began in a flat monotone: 'Blow winds...' The audience fought hard to control its near hysteria that needed to be released after three grueling days of competition for choice Shakespearian roles. Zefman ingrained himself in my memory forever. He was a very sweet, kind person with no understanding of how inappropriate his choice was. He didn't aspire to Lear but to being a messenger in 'The Comedy of Errors'. But he needed to do a dramatic audition scene and so he chose one of the best. In some ways, he was becalmed in the great storm and in that great venerable role which requires not only aspiration, but considerable talent, understanding, and depth – or at least a sense of irony. Worrell was not a satirist, nor did he intend a humorous reading. He was a naive person who meant well, but came off foolishly as he was light years away from a role the size of Lear.

The field of drama therapy began a lot like Worrell F. Zefman, trying to take on a large role before developing the substance necessary to fill it. Among the drama therapy pioneers, there were a number of highly gifted individuals of known substance who had already established themselves in clinical and educational circles, and, to a lesser extent, in theatrical fields. But in the mid-to late-1970s in the United States, drama therapy was to clinical psychology as Worrell F. Zefman was to King Lear. It certainly was possible that Worrell might grow up to be a brilliant Lear. Likewise, a handful of pioneers hoped that the field of drama therapy would grow up to be a significant part of clinical psychotherapy.

It is my opinion that, with some notable exceptions, the hope of drama therapy has not been realized. At the 14th annual conference of the NADT in Chicago, there appeared to be too much similarity with the previous 13 meetings. There are still just two approved training programs in the United States. The profession still features the same kind of workshops and presentations done primarily by the same people (including myself). One notable exception is the inclusion of more colleagues from psychodrama. Presenters tend to preach to the converted, a practice which provides a small venue and few opportunities for criticism and dialogue. The professional organization struggles to keep up with its self-imposed bureaucratic tasks, but hardly seems to be leading or even guiding a movement beyond its growing conservatism and incipient apathy. Membership in NADT is not growing. Few links have been maintained with those interested in lobbying and affecting legislative action.

Of those who graduate from approved Masters degree programs, some choose to leave the field; others remain in clinical positions but tend to get lost in clinical settings with psychodynamic or behavioral orientations, without the support of colleagues in the creative arts therapies.

There has been a movement afoot to mentor recent graduates. But it seems questionable whether there are sufficient mentors available in the field, or, for that matter, whether mentors should be confined to the field of drama therapy or, even yet, the value of a mentor system within a culture that values individualism and narcissism above cooperation and dialogue.

In many ways, as I look at the field of drama therapy at the time of its 14th annual conference, I see few winds of change. I feel, rather, becalmed even though I, like Worrell F. Zefman, would like to feel differently. I would like to think that the students I and others have trained have effected change – that they have begun new programs, lobbied in state capitals for recognition, carried on effective practices and research and publication. I would like to feel that colleagues throughout this country have done the same. There are certainly breezes blowing from the Pacific and both sides of the Atlantic with new books by Sue Jennings and Alida Gersie, Renee Emunah and Penny Lewis, to mention a few. But in my position as Editor-in-Chief of *The Arts in Psychotherapy*, I receive few articles on drama therapy practice, fewer on any aspect of drama therapy research, which leads me to believe that little research is being done. The field is developing techniques and concepts and even differing theoretical orientations. But the winds are not raging.

Even though a small number of relatively young pioneers still develop their ideas, there is such little movement generally in the field. It is easy to blame this state of affairs on outside realities, such as the low status of creative arts therapy within large bureaucratic systems of medicine and psychology. It is harder but more significant to look for reasons inside the field. Let me take a shot – it could be a narcissism on the part of many in the field, a sense that 'I can do King Lear and I can do it now, by myself – I can treat people better than the doctors and the analysts and the counselors and the social workers and even better than the other creative arts therapists!' On the other side of this point of view is the fear that I have nothing to say.

Not only do I feel that this is a false, defensive position, but I also feel it must be challenged if the field is to change. After more than 20 years in the field, I am convinced that drama therapy alone is not going to forge a revolution. Its leaders, as competent as they may be, need to branch out. Bridges rather than trenches need to be constructed. The NADT needs new leadership with fresh ideas and an openness to press beyond narcissistic and bureaucratic structures. The Masters degree training programs need to look at their missions within and beyond the field, within and beyond the university and the society.

With this in mind, let me now offer three alternative scenarios for the field that might at least provoke dialogue, and at best might give us all a sense of possibility along with a breath of fresh air. My aim is to challenge our profession to avoid the fate of King Lear, ranting, naked on the heath, alternately blaming others and pitying himself for his profound loss of power and promise.

## Scenario 1: Theatre

When the first two drama therapy programs in the United States began, the one at Antioch was part of a Psychology Department and the one at New York University was part of Educational Theatre. Both psychology and theatre still, to my way of thinking, represent two larger containers within which drama therapy can exist and expand.

I begin with theatre because, of the two, theatre is the art form that provides drama therapy with its uniqueness among other forms of healing. A logical question at this point might be, 'Hey, I thought you were talking about the future of drama therapy – why turn to the past?' My answer – I am trying to identify the essence of the field, that is, its rootedness within an existing framework. I am also attempting to uncover a larger vision and connection with preexisting disciplines that appear to be open to revision and inclusion.

Theatre and its generic, drama, began as healing performance. At its best, it continues to address ways that people destroy and create themselves. Through-out the history of dramatic literature, dramatic play, and related forms of social and personal performance, drama has revealed a range of role types that, when closely analyzed, seem to conform to the kinds of roles we play out in our everyday lives (see Landy 1993b). And when working in drama therapy, it is also possible to move toward healing by accessing, working through, and transforming those roles that are painful and discordant.

The problem with the scenario of envisioning drama therapy as part of theatre is that established disciplines tend to be entrenched and conservative. Paradoxically, they hold onto the past without fully remembering it. Drama began in healing, not in Rogers and Hammerstein or, for that matter, Robert Wilson. The new kid in town has to prove himself before he will be acceptable to the reigning cliques. From the point of view of most theatre departments, theatre companies, and educational theatre organizations, there is no room for drama therapy. For some, drama therapy is threatening; for others, it is not threatening enough and thus dismissable.

But there is a larger dramatic vision possible – a sense of inclusion, a sense of the power of the dramatic act in ritual, play, performance, popular culture, education, and healing. Some, like Richard Schechner and his colleagues in performance studies, have picked up on this point of view, but their conception is also limited. Heavily influenced by the work of Grotowski, Victor Turner and other prominent anthropologists, it tends to embrace a limited post-modernist aesthetic and adhere to an academic prejudice against that which smacks of education and therapy.

But prejudices can be changed when one has met the assumed enemy and learns that there are common interests and concerns and ways of making sense of the world. For this scenario to be implemented, drama therapists and theatre people must engage in productive dialogue through face-to-face meetings and exchanges of articles and artworks. The common interests and concerns are noted in such questions as: Why do people perform? How do people perform? Where and when do people perform? How can the performance of text and story illuminate the human condition even as it entertains?

Drama therapists like others in the dramatic field, make sense of the world through observing and facilitating acts of performance. They share a common purpose – to make meaningful and joyful performances; and a common method – to perform through taking on roles and telling stories in role. Their differences are also significant as some aim toward healing, others toward entertaining, still others toward educating. Yet within a culture of theatre or drama workers, all devoted to making sense of the performed act and applying it to these and related aims, a powerful sense of shared meaning could arise.

Drama therapy is an offspring of drama/theatre. But will it or should it return home? And if so, will its parents recognize it as one of their own? The fate of this scenario lies in answers to these questions.

## Scenario 2: Psychology

As theatre artists raise the question of the legitimacy of drama therapy: 'Yeah, but is it art?' psychologists and psychotherapists raise the question, 'Yeah, but is it science?' This second scenario thus comes with all the problems of acceptability as in the first scenario. It seems logical that drama therapy would join its sister healing disciplines loosely arranged under the heading, psychology. Yet logic has a way of escaping otherwise logical thinkers when the issue at hand is the protection of turf and the defense of one's own professional self-worth.

Some psychologists I have known have told me, 'Yeah, this is great stuff, very creative, I use it all the time.'

'How?' I ask, incredulously.

'I have them role-play.'

'Right,' I say, 'but for what purpose?'

'You know,' they respond.

'No, I don't,' I say.

'To loosen things up, to break through the resistance…so we can talk better.'

'Ahh!' I say, 'You use drama so you can talk better with your clients.'

'Right,' they say, 'I know all about what you do.'

At that point, I find myself getting a little hot around the collar. If I feel particularly brave, I say, 'No you don't. You haven't even asked me what I do.' And if I feel secure enough to venture further I say, 'Would you like to find out? Maybe we can talk about how our work is similar and how it's different. Maybe I can show you mine and you can show me yours.'

Again, dialogue is the healer. This scenario, like the first can only work within the confines of an open exchange of information. But even assuming that such an exchange were possible and that psychologists and even psychiatrists would refer clients to drama therapists and support the research, treatment, and theoretical musings of drama therapists – would this be desirable for drama therapists? What's in it for us?

For one, credibility. Drama therapy has shown the tendency, from time to time, to become soft around the edges, too easily associated with imprecise thought, too quick to shun or reject research as a way of knowing. Certainly, one could make the same claims for other forms of psychotherapy practiced solely as workshops to help men become wild or women become assertive and all to discover their inner child or inner something. But with these forms of pop psychotherapy, there is still the wider framework of psychology, the mix of art and science, the endless departments and faculties that spin out research articles, M.A.s and Ph.D.s, and professionals who are licensable and who will be welcomed without question in clinics and laboratories throughout the country.

Drama therapists might also wish to join the psychology club because they conceive of themselves primarily as clinical practitioners, as psychotherapists whose skills are similar to those of other trained clinicians, even if their techniques are somewhat different. A strong argument could be made for training all therapists within a clinical psychology program at the M.A., Ph.D. or Psy.D. level that addresses the basic issues of normal psychological development, psychopathology, personality theory, theory and practice of individual and group psychotherapy and the like. Certainly such a core curriculum would apply to counselors, clinical psychologists, clinical social workers as well as creative arts therapists.

Given this scenario, drama therapists could join in the political struggle to gain respectability for many alternative forms of legitimate and credible psychotherapies. The recent success of Bill Moyer's PBS series on 'Healing and the Mind' will be followed up with another on 'The Arts and Healing.' If the arts could be seen as an important piece of the psychotherapeutic pie, as a significant applied arm of psychology, then the credibility problem might be solved. If drama therapists could see themselves as psychotherapists with a core training fully equivalent to that of their peers in social work, counseling psychology and clinical psychology, then their identity problem might be closer to being resolved.

The problem of art versus science is rampant within psychology, with the dominant branch becoming even more experimentally inclined, even more aligned with the mainstream of biological and medical research. The other branch that tends toward developing alternatives to the reigning culture of scientism and quantification has much to offer drama therapy which, as a field, has a long way to go *vis-à-vis* research and publication. Within the structure of a form of psychology based upon phenomenological principles that embrace art as a way of knowing and as a way of healing, drama therapy might well find itself a home.

Both theatre and psychology have a rich aesthetic and intellectual history. Both respond to the dual nature of drama therapy. Although many in both fields are entrenched in traditional perspectives of performance and healing, others share a vision of alternative forms that provide further sustenance to the whole. These first two scenarios could be realized only when those others embrace the potential of drama therapy as a powerful means of healing performance.

## Scenario 3: Expressive Therapies/Creative Arts Therapies

In this third case, drama therapy would not lose its individuality to psychology or theatre, but would fully embrace its most intimate relatives in art, dance, music, poetry, and literature. At the center of this model would be the creative process of art-making.

David Johnson (1991) has written eloquently about the need for collaboration among the creative arts therapies. The National Coalition of Arts Therapy Associations (NCATA) has been hopeful at times in fostering this position, but primarily at convention time. There have been many lean years of in-fighting over turf and frustration at the inability to share resources and a larger, grander vision of expressive therapy.

But it is not necessarily at the bureaucratic level where this kind of collaboration can and must happen. It is already in process in varying degrees at Hahnemann in Philadelphia and Lesley College in Cambridge. Even in the entrenched system at New York University, we are making some headway with a new course in collaboration among the creative arts therapies and with a series of colloquia and meetings designed to move the creative arts therapies into closer proximity and collaboration.

It would seem to me that this option, Scenario Three, holds the greatest promise for a number of reasons. First, it is arts-based and shares the position of the artist as healer among all the sister disciplines. Second, a shared vision of creative arts therapy invites a joining of many disciplines weakened by a lack of political clout in universities, hospitals, clinics and state and national legislatures. Indeed there is power in numbers. Third, each art therapy would retain its connection to its art form and a more general connection to psychology. Yet at the same time, in collaborating with the other arts therapies, a unique and powerful vision of the arts as healing would emerge. This whole vision would be greater than the sum of its parts.

The forthcoming American health care plan is a great unknown. Many doctors and lawyers are worried that the Clinton administration will jeopardize their earning potential. The situation is much more critical for creative arts therapists. The new plan might overlook our profession entirely, simply because we have yet to make a strong-enough, united stand. Our acts of research, publication, clinical treatment, political organizing, agitating, and lobbying have simply not, with some notable exceptions, been sufficient to warrant attention.

It is time to crash through the self-love of drama therapy or any other singular creative arts therapy. After 14 years of conferences it is time to face the fact that alone we cannot fill the shoes of King Lear. Worrell F. Zefman can no longer stand in as our prototype. It is time to realize that our adolescence and innocence are long gone. If we don't grow further, we will continue to stagnate.

Perhaps we don't need more drama therapy programs and drama therapy theories and methods of treatment. Perhaps we need more creative arts therapy training programs that look to ways of building collaborative strategies in treatment and theory and research and legislation. That may be the hardest road of all to follow because it requires that we give up something that many of us have struggled for many years to build. I, for one, would be willing to shed my beloved attachment to the one and only creative art therapy of drama if, in return, I were to participate in a larger community of like-minded individuals who would work to get the wind machines moving again. I want to play Lear, but I am afraid that I am not ready. For much of my life I've played the role of Worrell F. Zefman and it has cushioned me.

Now it is time to move on – beyond the naivety, beyond the dependent and freewheeling spirit of adolescence, beyond the doubts and insecurities of being different from everybody else, beyond the complacency of self-satisfaction and the need to indulge in given bureaucracies and mediocrities – it is time to stand up and confront those forces that appear so intractable, those winds that bow to no master. It is time to fight against the calm, the resignation within us all. And it is also time to play the version of Lear that remains after the raging, after the narcissistic indulgence in his own sense of victimization. It is time to enact the survivor and seer, the one who dares to take on the elements and then equally dares to acknowledge his hubris, his sense of humanity.

I began this chapter with an indictment of our field and what I perceive as its limitations. I do this in the spirit of hope for a real change in the way we perceive ourselves as a profession and in the way we proceed to present our vision of healing through the arts. I intend this as a wake-up call. We need to grow and change and yes, we need to rage on the heath a little or suffer the consequences of the calm.

I don't know where Worrell F. Zefman is today. But I can't help wondering if he has found a part of Lear within himself. I hope he has learned along the way that daring to play the fool was an act of courage that has deeply affected at least one drama therapist. Only an old fool would take on Nature. Only a young fool would take on Lear. Only a fool would take on the established systems of education, medicine, psychotherapy, insurance, and government.

In 1968, in the streets and parks of Chicago outside the Democratic National Convention, a group of fools gathered – Yippies, Hippies, and other concerned but unaffiliated individuals. In Chicago in 1968, they committed an act of revolution posing as theatre. Among other things, they staged a mock nomination of a pig for President of the United States. This was the pinnacle of the Youth Movement, an attempt to topple a joyless establishment of old, tired, bureaucratic white men.

The serious antics were crushed on the streets of Chicago by the brutal force of the police, spurred on by Mayor Richard Daley. Some would argue that this attack and the subsequent trial of the Chicago Seven, an incredible travesty of justice, were key events leading to the decimation of the several liberation movements that seemed so hopeful in the 1960s.

But do not despair. The spirit of the fool, who dares to attempt the insurmountable by ridiculing and challenging those of much power but little means, lives on. In the spirit of King Lear raging on the heath, Worrell F. Zefman wandering on the stage, Abbie Hoffman laughing through the flames — I challenge you to demand better of yourselves and of those who seem to be in more powerful places. I challenge you to find ways of bringing this field, not only of drama therapy, but of creative arts therapy to a greater degree of visibility, credibility, and excellence.

# CHAPTER 13

# The Dramatic World View

## Reflections on the Roles Taken and Played by Young Children

## Introduction

During a thunderstorm late at night, Georgie, age four, woke up and cried. She was frightened by the noise and the flashes of thunder. Her brother, Mackey, age two, slept through it all. In the morning, the two spoke:

GEORGIE:   Mack, are you afraid of storms?

MACKEY:   Yes.

GEORGIE:   But you didn't wake up last night.

MACKEY:   I wasn't outside.

In overhearing the conversation, I thought of Alice's adventures in wonderland and through the looking glass (see Green 1965) where logic is turned on its head. Or, perhaps more apt, a different logic is at work. Alice's fictional adventures are reflective of the world view of many young children whose sense of reality is quite different from that of grown-ups. Although I eschew Lewis Carroll's romantic conception of childhood, I agree with him that the early years in one's life are highly dramatic and imaginative. I also believe that one way of understanding early childhood development is to accept the unique logic of children on its own terms. As one who conceptualizes personality as a system of interrelated roles and social life as in interplay of character types, I offer a dramatic conception of childhood.

The dramatic world view implies that:

1.  In everyday life, as in drama/theatre, persons or actors take on and play out personae or roles in order to express a sense of who they are and what they want. Role taking is an imaginative process of identifying with a role model and internalizing several of its qualities. For example, if I see my father as a victim, I might take on his propensity to feel victimized and begin to view myself as a victim.

Role playing is an external process of enactment where, for example, I enact the role of victim in relation to some real or imagined victimizer in my life.

2. Each role taken or played represents one part of the person, rather than a total personality.

3. There is a paradoxical relationship between an actor and a role, a person and a persona (Landy 1993b). When an actor, such as Vivien Leigh, takes on a role, such as Scarlet O'Hara, she is both herself (Leigh) and not herself (Scarlet) at the same time. In a like manner, a child playing doctor is both the child (not doctor) and the doctor (not child) at the same time.

4. When in balance, the relationship and tension between actor and role promotes creativity, spontaneity, and healthy development. When the actor is too merged with a role or too distant from a role, a sense of confusion as to one's identity subsists.

5. Roles exist in relationship to one another. Each one taken or played often implies the possibility of the role not taken. Thus, each time one chooses (or is chosen) to be a victim, the possibility also exists of becoming a victor (survivor) or victimizer.

6. People make sense of themselves (and others) by taking on and playing out roles and communicating that sense to others through stories. Each story contains views of individual people or generalized groups of people as told from the perspective of a particular storyteller.

This chapter, applying the dramatic world view, attempts to examine primarily the early development of roles. The cast of characters to be explored is small, including the two introduced at the beginning, Georgie and Mackey, my children.

To allow myself the appropriate aesthetic distance, I needed to confront certain methodological problems. Certainly my objectivity would be impaired. Unlike Piaget, who formulated some of his developmental theory through observation of his children, I was studying my children in a non-scientific way. I engage with my children in an often random, imaginative fashion, telling stories and playing roles with them as a way of building my sense of father and of participant observer. My years of notes do not add up to a scientific understanding of role development. They read more like a diary written by a novelist or poet or painter, noting striking observations about phenomena. (For an application of such an approach, see Hillman 1983.)

Furthermore, as I was taking notes, I was in the process of developing observational criteria regarding role taking and role playing, a process that is still developing. I still raise the same questions that I asked four years ago: is it possible to know when one has taken on a role? What is the relationship between role taking and role playing? Although one can see a role as it is played, how does one know what to call it? What do we call, for example, the four-year-old who is afraid of storms – the fearful one? The coward? Is there some system of roles or role types to refer to? When observing role play, what aspects does one need to look at? And on a larger, philosophical plane, where do roles come from? Are they inherited? Taken on from the social world? Generated through an individual creative act?

These and many related questions guided my research process for the past several years. My methodology is, in many ways, a work in progress. As such, I cannot claim that my findings are either reliable or generalizable in a scientific sense. Their value will lie in their uncovering of individual moments that, if well described and substantiated, touch on a more universal experience. This is the method of art.

My research findings also added to a theoretical understanding of role development. In an earlier publication (1993b), I devised a system of understanding role in terms of role type or universal form, similar to Jung's notion of archetype; role quality or descriptive aspects of role; role function or the reason that one plays a role; and style of role playing, or degree of affect and cognition, verisimilitude and abstraction. Also, I devised a taxonomy of roles identifying and categorizing role types that subsist throughout theatre history and in everyday life. The taxonomy includes 84 role types organized into six domains: somatic, cognitive, affective, social, spiritual, and aesthetic.

In looking at the early development of roles, reference will be made to these recent conceptual findings. My primary approach, however, will be anecdotal and interpretive. As such, I offer a number of stories about Georgie and Mackey and examples of their expressive activities, both visual and verbal. This information should provide a view of how and when roles are taken on and played out. I offer a way of knowing about roles that is quite different from the cognitive schemes presented by Piaget and his colleagues. This is a dramatic method, a story method, a way of knowing through telling. It differs from a more scientific method not in its rigor and intention, but in its vision of who we are as human beings and how we make sense of our existence.

## Georgie

As early as one-year-old, Georgie was eager for stories. She would ask that each story told by her mother or father be repeated endlessly. By two, she would do the same although she preferred that they read picture books to her. Georgie was a wonderful audience to their stories but would rarely venture out into the storyteller role herself. At least, that's how it appeared to her parents.

The other side of her social reticence was the fact that she seemed to have a rich imaginative life. By one, she would gather her stuffed animals and other soft objects and arrange them in various pleasing tableaux. They would appear to be audience to her storyteller role. In that role she would talk to them at length in an apparently non-sensical, sing-song fashion. Even though she was unwilling to 'perform' for parents and friends, she had nonetheless taken on the role of storyteller at one year old and practiced it within her arranged world.

Georgie told her stories in many ways – by 'speaking' to her dolls; by setting up tableaux, which in themselves embodied a story; and, as she became older, pushing three, by drawing pictures. Her pictures revealed a complex narrative that often helped her make sense of real or imaginary experiences.

For example, at three, Georgie drew a picture which she characterized as a faraway place where people are different. She noted the following characters in the picture: two gypsies, a bride and groom, a baby, and a faraway house.

This picture was quite clear to both her parents as it depicted not only several basic role types that Georgie took on at an early age, but also a significant experience in her young life. When Georgie was eight months old, she and her parents moved to Portugal for half a year, where her father was a Fulbright lecturer at the University of Lisbon. The experience of being in a foreign culture where babies are treated reverently and playfully by most everyone, including passers-by on the street, left a strong impression upon Georgie. To be a baby meant to be unconditionally lovable and desirable. Even though her actual memory of Portugal was limited, she continued to look at photographs and request 'Olà stories,' tales of her adventures in a faraway land where babies rule the roost, the sun always shines, and playground and beach are a five minute jaunt from the apartment.

Each day out, whether to the city, the beach, or the market, the family would see gypsies and Georgie's attention was often drawn to them. The gypsies were pariah figures who looked and behaved differently from the others. Some dressed flamboyantly and exuded an air of fierce independence and sensuality. Sometimes the gypsy women were beggars and would be dressed in rags and would carry babies who appeared equally ragged and desperate. Other times, they would coach their young children, like the Peachums in *The Threepenny Opera*, to look pathetic and beg for small change. There were many rumors, told everywhere, of how the gypsies would intentionally maim their children so they would appear even more pitiful on the streets. Georgie's parents were used to aggressive homeless people on the streets of New York, but this was more exotic, more primal. Who were these people and where did they come from? What dark rituals did they practice? Were they actors wearing elaborate disguises or were they simply as they appeared – poor, oppressed outcasts who no-one really wanted. Did they choose to be pariahs or did others cast them in this role?

At eight months Georgie was, of course, oblivious to these questions. But she was well attuned to her parents' reactions to this faraway culture. She came to know gypsies through her parents' eyes. In many ways her parents were gauging their own sense of rootlessness, alienation, and strangeness through their attention to the gypsies. So, too, were they weighing their own sense as parents who needed to guard against any impulse to use or abuse their children. They were wrestling with two images of parents and children – the first, observed in this faraway culture, unconditionally loving parents exceedingly attentive to their radiant children; the second, the distant or absent father and pariah-like mother, imposing an attitude of mendacity upon their oppressed children.

It was curious that Georgie drew two gypsies. When asked why, she had no explanation. Maybe they were mother and child, as they so often appeared on the streets. Maybe they were simply another variation on mother and father, a prominent theme in Georgie's drawings at three years old.

Where did Georgie's sense of gypsies come from? There were no photographs of gypsies at home nor did her parents speak of them in the house. At three, it was hard to imagine that Georgie remembered seeing them or hearing talk about them when she was barely one. Could it be that Georgie had internalized a gypsy role? If this were so, it might not be based on her memory of actual gypsies but on the part of her parents that identified with the rootlessness and romance of the gypsies.

The fact that gypsies appear in Georgie's picture of a faraway place is significant. It could be that each expressive act of a child embodies one or more roles. We can assume that the gypsy role is taken on by Georgie from an early cultural experience as filtered through the experience of her parents. If this is so, then Georgie will have available certain gypsy qualities, as mentioned above. She may enact this role for a number of purposes, e.g. to express her sense of romance and passion (in fact, since the age of two she has taken great pleasure in dressing up or dressing up her dolls, and in dancing with abandon) and to express her own sense of disconnection or defiance of the conventional order (which she has done frequently since the age of two and has been noted by both parents as an ongoing issue). The latter qualities are characterized in the taxonomy or roles as aspects of the pariah who is assigned to the fringes of society and functions as a challenge to the established order, a reminder that all is not well (see Landy 1993b).

From her parents, Georgie may have internalized two images of herself: as a gypsy street child, conditionally lovable, based upon her ability to please her mother, and as Olà baby, a child of the sunny side of Portugal where all babies are unconditionally lovable.

The bride and groom have been important figures for Georgie since she was one, when she would create marriage scenes with her dolls and respond intently to any image of marriage encountered in everyday life. Generally, the roles of bride and groom were interchangeable with those of Mommy and Daddy. These, very clearly, were two of the earliest roles she had taken on.

I give the example elsewhere (Landy 1993b) of behavior at 17 months when Georgie moved back and forth between her parents, touching each one and chanting: 'Mommy, Mommy, Mommy,' and 'Daddy, Daddy, Daddy.' Then she retreated to her dolls and spoke to them, as if to tell a story of who she was in relationship to her parents. Through her play, Georgie was not only taking on the roles of mother and father, but also staking out her own territory as child in relation to them.

In a faraway land, the parents as bride and groom are a foil for the gypsies. The parents must be stable, married, and connected, unconditionally nurturing, unlike their counterparts who are strangers in a strange land and who might mistreat their children in order to feed themselves.

Even at eight months old, Georgie made distinctions between the bride/mother and the groom/father. The father had clearer boundaries. He worked in the house and was not to be disturbed when working. The mother, however, was less clear. She wanted to be unconditionally available but could not, due both to circumstances, e.g. illness and work, and temperament, in that she felt ill-equipped to amuse an infant twelve hours a day. That ambivalence often caused her anxiety and guilt. Georgie could not and would not leave her mother alone. She constantly tested her, demanding extra feedings of breast milk, refusing to eat much solid food, denying her privacy or time alone.

Role theory tells a story of family legacies. Role types and qualities seem to be passed on from one generation to another. The Jungians take the idea much further in suggesting that archetypes which are unconscious, collective forms of being embedded in the psyche, are ubiquitous not only in families over generations, but also across cultures throughout history. Although there appears to be much validity in this point of view, it doesn't address the specific ways that children take on and play out the roles of mother and father. Georgie's conception of mother appears to be that of one who wishes to be unconditionally loving but cannot always be so. The mother role that Georgie takes on well reflects her mother Katherine's reality as she attempts to be a 'good enough' mother for her daughter. In truth, Katherine has taken on her conception of mother from her own narcissistic mother. Through therapy and years of reflection, she has become aware that she was mothered by a person who always put her own needs before her childrens' and demanded to be mothered by others, e.g. husband and children, to protect her from maternal responsibilities.

The narcissistic mother breeds children who are unclear as to how they are to play out their child roles (should they mother their mothers?) and how they are to take on the mother role. When they are young, their children will play out these confusions in relationship to their dolls, friends, and others in their social world. When they are grown and become mothers themselves, they are often faced with the kind of ambivalence experienced by Georgie's mother.

Of the two parents, the mother is the most significant for Georgie. She is the first one she goes to when hurt or sad or lonely or needy. She is the primary feeder, teacher, moral figure, and punisher. In Georgie's imagination she takes on many incarnations as bride, fairy godmother, queen. As bride, she is endlessly hopeful, a fairy tale figure who may well live happily ever after.

This image of the bride is reflected in many of the stories Georgie reads and films she watches at three years old. The figures of Cinderella, Ariel (from the Disney film, *The Little Mermaid*), and Belle (from the Disney film, *Beauty and the Beast*) all become brides and as brides will be endlessly happy. This is the mother Georgie so very much wants to have and to become. Less than this, which is reality, is often unacceptable and cause for disappointment, resistance, and anger. In taking on the romantic role of bride, Georgie plays with her fantasies. She tells her dolls and stuffed animals that she will marry the prince, that this is what grown-ups do. Georgie also sees that these female figures have to endure hardship before their transformation into bride. Cinderella, for example, is endlessly humiliated by her step-sisters and step-mother, that is, until she meets her savior in the figure of the fairy godmother, a perfect helper who will allow her to transcend her squalor and find the perfect life of brides.

In playing out the bride, dressed in a yellow gown at four or an Afghan at three or a ragged towel at two, Georgie enacts the ritual of trial, transformation, and perfection. While in role there is a clear end in sight and that vision steers her through the hardships of biting brothers and scolding, demanding parents. The function of the bride role, then, is to provide a sense not only of romance, but also of a happy ending to the difficulties of living among demanding and self-involved people.

As I am writing about the bride role, I notice that with each attempt to write the word 'bride,' I instead write down (in long hand) 'bridge.' In fact, it happened so often that I could not dismiss it as a typographical error. How then, I ask myself, is the 'bride' a 'bridge?' It seems to me that for Georgie, the bride is a bridge between the drudgery of everyday life, as in Cinderella's burden of virtual slavery, and the fantasy of a perfect relationship or marriage with a savior figure, whether mother, as in fairy godmother, or father/husband, as in prince. The wish for a perfect mother, father, and husband, all of whom can magically fulfill her needs, is a very comforting one for a child who has not too long ago lost her mother's breast and her mother's body as an endless supply of sustenance and identity.

In standing alone at two years old, Georgie, like other children, needs bridges or, in D.W. Winnicott's (1971) terms, transitional objects, to help her cross the dangerous waters of separation and individuation (See Mahler 1975). In this deeper sense, the bridge serves as a transition between a merged identity with the mother and a separate identity as a girl who will grow up and 'marry' other roles, that is, take on those roles that are needed to further her developmental journey.

In normal development, the roles taken will further the process of individuation and allow for effective marriages with others in their complementary roles. In abnormal development, the individual unable to separate from the mother will seek others with whom to merge or to mother. Thus, one's own identity will become submerged in another and one will use the other as a kind of skin to enter in order to feel whole. For this kind of woman, the husband would be seen as a romantic figure, a prince whose function is to save her both from the drudgery of everyday life and the need to become an independent human being in her own right. While it is normal for a three-year-old girl to wish for a prince on a white horse to whisk her away, it is not so for a 30-year-old woman whose bride role has remained marooned on one psychologically primitive shore with no bridge available to help her across.

For Georgie, the groom is a less prominent figure than the bride. In all her expressive activity, especially her drawings, the groom is generally smaller than the bride. It would appear that this figure represents the father role. As a role model, Georgie's father has been paradoxically present and distant. As an academic, he has always spent a lot of time at home and has participated fully in the tasks of raising Georgie. While in Portugal, this was particularly true. Yet, especially in Portugal, he was troubled and professionally stuck, feeling both alienated from the new culture and angry that there was not enough recognition forthcoming from students and colleagues. This was his sabbatical and he was unable to rest. Thus, although he was available to his eight-month-old daughter, he was also self-involved and often emotionally unavailable.

This image of the father, so unlike the prince with the glass slipper, must have caused some ambivalence for Georgie. In taking on the father role, she might well have internalized this ambivalence. It was later, at the age of two, when she became aware of other kinds of 'grooms,' that is, fathers-to-be, who were unambivalent rescuers. Like the image of the bride, the groom might also have served Georgie as a bridge between the imperfect father who was present and absent at the same time, and the perfect lover/husband who would save her from a life of ambivalence.

Through Georgie's first four years, the father has remained smaller in stature than the mother. Many times at four, Georgie exclaimed: 'Mommy is smart; Daddy is silly.' For Georgie, the smart one is more desirable. Taking on the mother role will give her more wisdom and power. As mother, she will be ultimately able to nurture herself and know what it means to be female.

The silly father, although more distant than the mother, takes on another significance. This kind of father likes to play the fool and Georgie likes to engage with the foolish figure who tells stories and acts childlike and makes up silly songs. The father/fool role is also worthy of taking on as it, too, offers a wisdom, although one more indirect than that of the wise mother.

In the taxonomy of roles, I refer to the function of the father as protecting the family and providing a positive masculine role model; and that of the husband as providing for the wife and maintaining an aura of strength and stability. The role of father and husband that Georgie internalizes during the first four years of her life is much more complex than this. He does provide a sense of safety and stability. But he is also an ambivalent figure. He is masculine, but he also expresses his feminine side; as the mother is one who easily expresses her masculine side.

At four years old, it is unclear how Georgie will sort this all out. In her play, it becomes clear that she wishes for a happy, perfect marriage of bride and groom, father and mother, who will be unconditionally loving and accepting of one another. She, too, looks to these figures for an understanding of how to play out her complimentary role of child. The gender ambivalence that Georgie internalizes might prove to be confusing in the sense of not knowing what men and women are supposed to do. On the other hand, it might well help her in constructing a non-sexist attitude toward masculine and feminine roles.

Back to the drawing, we find another important figure in the baby. This is the most prominent role of the eight-month-old Georgie, one given at birth. This role has also been socially determined by all the adults who endowed her with the rights, privileges, and sometimes, scorn attached to their conceptions of how a baby should behave. Thus, the baby is one of the earliest visible roles taken on by a human being. In the first days of life, it is played out automatically, given the infant's biological need for care and nurturance and her psychological need for merging with the mother. As the weeks and months pass, the baby role is highly influenced by parents and other intimate adult figures, and Georgie learned further how to be a baby as she took on those adult points of view. Also, by taking on the generalized role of parents (on the generalized other, see Mead 1934), she learned what a baby is supposed to do in relation to parents.

As Georgie has developed throughout her first four years, the baby role has remained prominent. Generally speaking, the baby is dependent, needy, ego-centric, curious, spontaneous, sensual, and playful. As the infant becomes a toddler and child, these qualities tend to diminish as she experiences a sense of decentering (see Piaget 1977), that is, a movement from egocentricity toward sociability. In Georgie's case, many of the baby qualities lingered into her third and fourth years. She was reluctant to give up her dependence upon her mother. She was reluctant to leave her self-contained egocentric world.

There are many explanations for why one needs to hold onto a particular role beyond its apparent developmentally appropriate time span. For one, people hold on to roles because they provide a way to meet their needs. One plays the baby because of needs to avoid the responsibilities and demands of a later stage of development. Further, picking up on Hamlet's reminder that 'readiness is all,' individuals can let go of one role and embrace another only when they are psychologically and physiologically prepared to do so. Some may never feel ready to decenter and take on the responsibilities of growing up. In this extreme, individuals would certainly have difficulties within a conventional society and might seek out relationships or a sub-culture that would support their needs to remain dependent and delay the responsible life.

In Georgie's case, her reluctance to give up the baby role might be based in a fear of losing her mother's unconditional love and attention. The psychologically greatest blow in her young life came with the birth of her brother when she was two years old. Suddenly there was another baby to take her place. Her reaction was extreme. She refused any contact with her mother in the hospital and, for several weeks after the birth of her brother, she remained distant and angry. Her only connection to her mother was through a transitional object, a large stuffed dog which her mother gave her in the hospital as a present. She became focused on her mother's breast and would demand a feeding herself when her mother was nursing her brother. She would find other ways to regress throughout the two to four years to assure herself that her mother still loved her, even though she had forever lost the role of the baby of the family. All these regressions were duly noted by her parents who used stories, drawings, and other projective means to help her bridge the gap between baby and child, with the knowledge that both roles are lovable.

The function of the baby role for Georgie was to remain tied to her mother and to delay her fall into a more grown-up, responsible state of being. When an 'Olà baby' in a culture that adored babies, and when an only child with no competitors, she was well reinforced in her role playing. But upon her return to a more 'baby neutral' culture and the realization that she was growing up and had been relegated to the role of big sister, the baby role lost its effectiveness. Because of the realities and demands of family and society, Georgie needed to find a way to let go of her baby role or force it into a mold that no longer fit. Well aware that the latter decision would cause her anxiety, Georgie's parents did all they could to help her through this difficult transition.

By four years old, Georgie's drawings of babies had diminished significantly. Much of her prolific output of artwork concerned depictions of the family, most especially of sister and brother. She had, in many ways, diminished the power of the baby role, which is not to say that she had transcended or extinguished it. Roles once taken are not then banished from one's personality, which I have conceived of as a system of roles (see Landy 1993b). Rather, they are inflated or deflated as necessary, to serve particular individual needs. Georgie will always have a baby role available within her internal role system. It will surface at times when she feels most vulnerable, isolated, and unlovable. But as she develops other age-appropriate roles, as well as roles concerning secure feeling states, it will have less control over her. Further, as she grows up, she will discover positive ways to use her baby role, perhaps to counteract the peer pressure to act grown-up before she feels ready, perhaps as a safety valve to help release hurt feelings that have built up within a relationship or environment that disallows such 'infantile' expression. And should she continue to express herself aesthetically, the baby part might well counteract a burgeoning grown-up tendency to be overly rational and critical.

The final figure in Georgie's drawing is that of the faraway house. As noted above, this represents the new apartment in Portugal, far removed from Georgie's home across the ocean. Although not literally a role, the notion of being removed, separated from home, is a powerful one with many psychological implications. In some ways it connects with the role type, the lost one, defined in the taxonomy as: 'estranged and alienated, lacking a sense of purpose or understanding of one's place in the universe' (Landy 1993b, p.201).

Most people take on this role either from a powerful role model who exemplifies these qualities, or from an experience of being removed or separated from home, whether by divorce or war or fire or poverty or, in some cases, a psychologically difficult move from the familiar to the faraway. In some ways the reality is less important than the way that the individual internalizes such disruptions. Some will move on from disaster with minimal psychological turmoil, having developed an intact survivor role. Others, with little ability to play the survivor, will experience considerable distress when temporarily moving to a 'faraway' house or when permanently moving from one house to another.

The ability to be a survivor as opposed to a lost one will again depend upon many factors. For many children, change of routine causes much anxiety. But some adjust to change well. One explanation of this, applying to an understanding of why any role seems to be prominent within a person's psyche, is that roles, like temperament, are to a large part genetically determined. The fact that some will survive disasters and others will fall apart when moving to a new town, speaks to the way people are individuated genetically. Another explanation is that if one's parents take change and movement in stride, they provide strong role models for their children who, if genetically and temperamentally suited, will take on the survivor role and act accordingly.

Georgie, exposed to her parents' difficulties living and working in a foreign culture, might take on her father's ambivalence which might surface later on when she is confronted with a similar situation. She, like her father, might have a propensity for playing the lost one. That is not to say that the survivor role will be squelched. Her parents are also survivors. But like her father, caught between the roles of survivor and lost one, Georgie might also be likely to take on that particular ambivalence.

I have gone on at length extrapolating from a single drawing made by Georgie at three years old, referring back to an episode in the month preceding her first birthday. The several roles of gypsy/pariah, bride/mother, groom/father, baby, and lost one/survivor have been explored. Let me now turn to the source of Georgie's fall from grace, her brother, Mackey, and his early acquisition of roles. In my discussion of Mackey, I will also focus upon the relationship of brother and sister as it impacts upon role acquisition and development.

## Mackey

When Mackey was born Georgie was two years old. As noted above, she had a difficult time accepting her diminished status from only child to big sister. Like most older siblings, she feared that she would lose attention and affection from her parents. In some ways, with the birth of her brother, she began to assume the role of orphan, at least temporarily.

There was some real cause for Georgie's concern. Although Mackey experienced a normal and healthy birth, after several weeks it became apparent to his mother that his ability to respond was impaired in some way. He was not smiling like other newborns. His eyes seemed vacant or moved in odd patterns. Further, he quickly developed colic and screamed inconsolably each evening from six to midnight. His mother became anxious and his father became distant. Both were exhausted from the evening ordeal of attempting to mollify the frightening screams and hysteria. Nothing seemed to work – neither breast nor pacifier, neither swaddling nor any of several ways of holding suggested by the books. To his parents, Mackey appeared to be in great pain each evening.

Who, then, was Mackey in his first weeks of life? He was a beautiful child with a beast-like disposition. Even during his placid moments, something seemed off – he wasn't connecting. Like Georgie, Mackey was breast-fed from the beginning, but he had a harder time staying on the breast. He often seemed to lose it and became easily frustrated. Yet when he first arrived home from the hospital, only days before the colic would hit, Mackey appeared to his father to be fully content in his own body and contained space of bassinet and basket. His father predicted, in fact, that Mackey would be a mellow child, a 'sunny boy'.

Many of the early roles that one takes on spring from a common source – one's parents or caretakers. As parents view a baby, a baby, in some essential ways, will come to view itself. According to this formula which, like most formulas, is imperfect, Mackey will take on a paradoxical sense of himself as beauty and beast, lovable and terrible, mellow and hysterical, attached and detached, healthy and sick.

From a future point of view, Mackey at two and a half-years-old, having long since left the colic behind, appears to play out the more positive role qualities, confirming his father's prophesy of the 'sunny boy.' But the journey from colic to contentment, from the darkness of the moon to the light of the sun, was a very long one indeed.

At four months old, after consultations with a number of specialists in the field of ophthalmology, it was determined that Mackey was not seeing anything. Light was passing through his eyes, but for some unknown reason, he had no visual response. His prognosis was uncertain. His parents were suddenly confronted with the reality of having a blind child and the possibility that this condition was uncorrectable.

Mackey, who had just about recovered from his colic and was shedding his hysteria, was again thrust into a disabled role. The doctors were stumped until one retinal specialist made his pronouncement: Mackey had albinism; the prognosis, although guarded, was hopeful. Mackey would see the world, but how much he would take in was still to be determined.

The images of blind men with white canes, blind blues singers with dark glasses, and old men with seeing-eye dogs selling pencils in the street vanished from the mind's eye of Mackey's parents. Mackey's mother now imagined her son as Johnny and Edgar Winter, albino rock musicians with pure white hair and pink eyes. But Mackey's appearance was not that harsh: he could 'pass' as a light-skinned boy with sunglasses.

The 'sick' role that had been imposed upon Mackey by the doctors and parents began to shift by five months. He had been working twice a week with Joanne, a gifted teacher from the Lighthouse, a state funded organization that, among other things, sends teachers into the homes of visually impaired children. Within a short time, Mackey was responding to the various visual stimuli presented by Joanne. His parents, instructed by Joanne, implemented the exercises each day and as Mackey responded more and more, another level of bonding was taking place. Over several months, Mackey became quite responsive. His parents began to see him as less disabled and Mackey picked this up.

During these months of visual education, Mackey became attached to a stuffed animal, a tiger, which he later named 'Tigo.' Tigo became his transitional object which he held and slept with daily through his first two and a half years. A major function of Tigo was clear – to help Mackey move from the physically ill, disabled person who could not take in the world through his eyes, to the healthy, self-contained 'sunny boy,' who could take in the multi-faceted imagery and roles and direct his external play accordingly.

With his improving eyesight, Mackey developed motor, cognitive, and verbal skills normally. His capacity to learn and use language actually developed early, as he began to speak shortly after his first birthday. So, too, did he begin to develop a sense of himself as a male differentiated from his mother and sister. Even though he was born with a genetic disability that affected his vision, Mackey was able to move beyond the role of the disabled, having internalized from his parents and teacher the sense that he was worthy and lovable and that he would get better.

Aside from his parents, Mackey's primary role model was Georgie. He imitated her laughter, gestures, dress, and routines. He even attempted to take on her fears, even though he had not fully internalized them. As an example, Georgie developed a fear of fire sirens which sometimes went off several times a day in the small town where she lived. One day, Mackey, shortly before his second birthday, was playing on his fire truck. The siren went off. Georgie was nowhere to be found. Mackey stopped his play and looked up as if to say:

'Should I be scared?' He came toward his father who asked: 'Are you scared?' Mackey replied: 'I scared.' Again his father asked: 'Is Mackey scared?' 'Georgie scared,' he replied.

Indeed, Mackey was thinking about his sister's reaction and attempting to take on her role as frightened one. But because Mackey was indeed undaunted by the noise, he could not fully take on her role this time. Despite this, he was still ever ready to take on the many roles of Georgie in so many other ways, to swallow her whole if necessary, even if some of the pieces did not go down too well.

Mackey's wholesale imitative behavior allowed Georgie to role-reverse, taking on the baby role, herself, and hoping for the inherent gratification stemming from being dependent and helpless. Role-reversal, which appears frequently during the early years, is part of normal development. Young siblings, like Georgie and Mackey at four and two, reverse roles in order to either practice new roles or seek gratification from older ones. When the taking on of appropriate roles becomes blocked in later years, role-reversal can be employed as a technique to help individuals recognize another point of view.

At two, Georgie would revert to baby talk. At three, she would either pretend to cry or find occasions to justify crying for the purpose of keeping herself tied to the baby role. In her play at four and a half she would cast Mackey in the role of Mommy and demand that he change her diaper, even though she was long since toilet trained and Mackey, at two and a half was not. This was joyful play as the two would laugh gleefully each time they played out their family roles.

The following anecdote of Georgie at four and Mackey at two offers another role-reversal, this time as the father takes on the role of baby and the children act out different versions of parents:

> It is late in the afternoon and Georgie is in an ornery mood as she is often at this time of day since she gave up her afternoon nap. Her father is exercising and accidentally kicks her with his foot. She is not really hurt but pauses a bit to weigh the moment. She cries, in a strained fashion. She goes to her mother and whines: 'Daddy kicked me!' Her mother assures her that it was an accident. Then she turns to her father: 'You're a baby, Daddy! Daddy's a baby!'
>
> Her father takes on the role of baby and responds, childishly: 'I'm not a baby.'
>
> Georgie counters: 'You are! You are a baby!'
>
> Her father whines and says: 'I want a bottle!'
>
> Georgie hits her father several times. Mackey, who has become interested in this interaction, joins in. The father cries some more in an exaggerated fashion and both children are amused. Georgie continues to hit, playing

out a punitive version of a parent. When she hits too hard, her father pretends to be hurt. He cries more realistically, asking for comfort – a hug, a kiss, a nice word. Mackey becomes concerned that his father is really hurt. At two, he has less ability than his sister to separate out play from reality. He comes over and gives his father a kiss and a hug. He demonstrates his ability to role-reverse with his father and to play out the nurturing parent when needed.

Georgie stops hitting her father and moves away, feigning disinterest. For her, the role play is over. She has been upstaged by her brother who played a more kindly parental role than she did. Unlike Mackey, she knew all the time that this was a game.

Where did each child's version of the parent come from? Could it be that both have internalized the generalized role of parent differently? I think not. The answer may be that Georgie, at an older age, more mindful of the differences between playing and reality, uses the play as a way to express her ornery mood. She projects her mood upon her role of parent and aggressively acts out toward her father. Mackey, caught up in the reality of his father as sad and hurt, plays out the role he would want for himself if he were hurt, that is, the nurturing parent. Each child's version, then, is based upon his/her own needs at a particular developmental stage.

## Georgie and Mackey

If it is true that genetics has a profound effect on the kind of roles we will take on and play out, we should be able to view this state of affairs at an early age. Georgie and Mackey both seemed to be predisposed to certain roles and certain ways of playing them out. Georgie often would take on either hurt or aggressive roles at three and four years old. Mackey, on the other hand, at two would take on more conciliatory roles.

When asked to compare their two children, both parents would agree that Georgie was very sensitive to slight physical discomforts, such as a splinter in her finger, and tended to panic at loud noises. She was generally more difficult and resistant. Mackey, on the other hand, once free of colic and severe visual impairment, seemed less resistant, more light and quick to bounce back from physical pain and disappointment.

It appeared to both parents that these genetically-based traits affected the childrens' choice of role taking and role playing. And yet the genetic explanation of when and how roles develop is limited. As we have seen, roles are also strongly based on social factors. Georgie, for example, took on gentle and nurturing roles as Mackey took on aggressive and resistant ones from their role models. This is more in keeping with conventional social and cultural expectations regarding gender. The following are examples of these more conventional behaviors in role:

> Georgie at three is sitting in her mother's lap in the morning. She opens the front of her mother's nightgown and exposes her breast. She examines it attentively and touches it in a very serious way, paying particular attention to the nipple. Her mother says: 'Do you remember when you were a baby and you had your milk from Mommy breasts?' Georgie replies: 'When I am a Mommy and you are a baby then I will feed you on my breasts.'

In experimenting with the role of nurturing mother, Georgie imagines a time when she will nurse her own babies. In doing so, she casts her mother in the role of baby, a role that she has only recently left behind.

> Mackey at two is with his father at the lake. He climbs on a large rock and straddles it. His father is nearby, watching. A four-year-old boy approaches Mackey and makes threatening gestures, growling like a tiger. Mackey stands his ground and says, forcefully: 'No!' The boy growls again, even louder. Mackey counters with a more aggressive 'No!!' He then climbs down and sneaks up on his father who is lying on a towel. He growls, trying to frighten his father. He circles around and growls even louder. The father feigns surprise and fear and both father and son laugh heartily. But Mackey goes a bit too far, hitting his father in the face. The father tells Mackey not to hit, but Mackey continues. The father becomes more forceful. Soon Mackey grows tired of his play and moves off.

Mackey in this case is testing out his power at both defending himself against an aggressor and playing the aggressor, seeing how far he can go. In his aggressive play with his father, Mackey enacts the same scene he had just experienced on the rock. The difference is that in the first instance he was cast by the older boy in a victim role. But he refused to take on that role and stood up to the aggressor. Feeling victorious, he did a role-reversal playing out the aggressor role in a safe context, that is, toward his father. In playing out a frightened role (in a comic, stylized way), the father signals to the son that he is impressed by the son's display of power. This provokes Mackey to act out more aggressively, perhaps catharting his own sense of fear when confronted by the older boy. By standing up to Mackey's aggression, the father causes the aggressive play to stop. Even this mirrors the previous scene where Mackey caused the aggressive tiger behavior to stop by standing up to the older boy. Mackey has internalized the understanding that aggression can sometimes be stopped by a forceful and aggressive response.

The genesis of aggression is a powerful topic that has been the source of research by philosophers, scientists, and artists for many centuries. In this case, we may speculate that aggressive roles come from two basic sources: genetic, despite the fact that Mackey tends to appear 'sunny' and conciliatory; and social, based upon known and sometimes unknown role models. According to the work of Jung (1964) and his many colleagues, aggressive roles, as well as those of sexuality and other identity factors, are archetypal, that is, embedded in the racial experience of all human beings. This point of view is reflected in my own work developing a taxonomy of roles (Landy 1993b).

It is hardly startling that Georgie would play out nurturing roles and Mackey would play out aggressive ones. In fact, children from birth to four are developing a universe of often contradictory roles from archetypal, genetic, and social sources. In terms of gender identification, Mackey at one and two had little trouble expressing his anima or feminine side (see Jung 1964) as Georgie at two had scant difficulty expressing her animus or masculine side.

At four, however, Georgie is more connected to the trappings of a feminine identity exemplified in her choice of clothes and toys and identification with such characters as Cinderella and Beauty, and most important, in her attachment to her mother. The latter point, however, offers a further complexity as to role development. Georgie's mother is temperamentally quite aggressive and outspoken. Through her identification with these traits of her mother, Georgie, too, plays out her own sense of aggression and power. Some of this is positive, as she learns to assert herself in groups of peers; and some is negative, as she aims her newly learned hurtful language at often unsuspecting targets, such as her brother, parents, and friends.

Certainly Georgie's aggressive role comes from many sources other than her mother. Even though her father's aggression is less visible than her mother's, it tends to explode at times and she internalizes that method of expressing anger as well. As she approached four years old, Georgie began to pick up aggressive words and actions from her peers. At that time, she became more aware of aggressive images in the media, such as guns, and aggressive characters, such as tyrants and killers.

Long before her fourth birthday, Georgie had demonstrated a clear attraction to evil characters in stories – witches, hunters, and bullies. In an astonishing statement directed to her father three days before turning four, she integrated several of these images:

> I don't love you, Dad, I'm gonna get a gun and kill you. I want to poop on your head.

This role of rebellious, murderous daughter serves several functions. It helps Georgie release her negative, angry feelings in a safe way, as she offers up her pronouncement in a matter-of-fact fashion. It helps her continue to test the limits of her own worth as a lovable daughter to her father. In a reversal of the 'Electra complex,' it implies an alternative story of a daughter's parricide so that she might have the mother all to herself. And finally, by playing out the killer in a scatological fashion, Georgie tries out her newly learned words and roles safely, knowing that her father will not strike back in a punitive way. She assures this by choosing a style of presentation that is emotionally neutral and non-threatening.

Mackey's style of aggression at one and two is much different as was noted in the previous example. He has yet to take in the world of guns and killers. He picks up his sister's reference to 'poop' and will imitate her speech, but his style is without much commitment to the shock value of such imagery. Mackey's aggression at home is confined to fights with his sister, occasional tantrums of screaming and flailing when his needs are not immediately gratified, and imaginary dialogues with rocks and cups which he occasionally sets up to receive his wrath. His words: 'I'm very angry at you!' or 'You're a bad boy!' are taken from his parents who occasionally express their displeasure toward him in similar phrases. When overwhelmed by anger coming from either his parents or himself, Mackey reaches for Tigo, holds it tightly up in front of his face, and sucks his thumb. He then knows he is safe.

At four and a half, Georgie became aware of death and the possible consequences of unchecked aggression. She is not introduced to death stemming from aggression, but from illness. In her four years she had been exposed to two hospitalizations of her father and much anxiety on the part of her mother. And one day, she discovered a photograph of a dog on her mother's dresser. When asked about it, her mother replied: 'This was Cheecha, my dog.'

'What happened to Cheecha?' asked Georgie.

'She died.'

'I'm very sad, Mommy.'

'Why?'

'Because Cheecha died.'

'Cheecha was a wonderful dog,' said her mother. 'We had great times together. But she got very old and died.'

'I'm very sad,' said Georgie.

For some weeks, Georgie transferred her sadness and fear of this terribly complicated death role upon Cheecha. All the while she held onto her own stuffed dog, the present from her mother in the hospital when Mackey was born. The following conversation helped calm her ultimate four and a half-year-old fear, that of losing her mother to death. It was provoked when Georgie overheard her mother say that she was feeling very old:

GEORGIE:  Mommy, are you deading soon?

MOTHER:  You mean, are you going to die soon?

GEORGIE:  Yes, like Cheecha.

MOTHER:  No, not until I'm very old. Cheecha was very old and lived a long, long life. I need to see you get bigger and go to school and get married and have your own babies. Only then will I feel ready to rest and die.

GEORGIE:  But you said you're old.

MOTHER:  Sometimes I say I feel old, but that's just an expression. It's like people saying they're so hungry they could eat a horse... I'm not really old.

GEORGIE:  For real?

MOTHER:  For real.

The role of death is formidable. In the taxonomy of roles it is listed as a sub-type of demon, a dark inhabitant of the spirit world who is magical and evil, threatening and powerful. Death is also seen as one of the earliest roles personified in ancient dramatic rituals.

It could be that when the role of death appears early in one's life, one lives close to the world of magic and spirits on the far side of the looking glass. Thus at four, death is more acceptable as a persona than at 24 or 44 or 64, as one comes to reject a magical world view and begin to accept the inevitability of death.

For Georgie, taking on the role of death, personified in a dog, is sad. But there is room for it in her world. Each day, she sets up her stuffed animals, including the transitional dog, and tells them stories. Through these stories, she comes to know her inner world whose magic will diminish as she grows older and accepts more adult, logical explanations for unfathomable events. When her mother explains that she won't die until Georgie becomes an adult and she grows old, Georgie responds: 'For real?' In the asking, she begins to acquire the sense of reality that exists in a realm different from magic. This looking glass is not a window through which one can enter a new world, but a mirror, reflecting back an image of oneself.

Mackey at two still lives in the realm of windows. Many of the roles he has taken on still retain a magical quality. He sees the world as animistic. When he is angry, he scolds the rocks. When he is naughty, he calls his father a bad boy. When he is lonely, he throws Tigo out of the crib and cries for his mother to return it at once.

When his father returned home from the hospital, recovering from back surgery, Mackey, at two, came into the bedroom to greet him. He could see that his father was in pain and was told that it was time for his father to take a nap. Before saying goodbye, Mackey lifted the covers and placed Tigo gently next to his father's wound. For that moment, all distinctions between reality and magic were dissolved, all pain was gone. Mackey had taken on the role of healer. And all was right with the world.

## Conclusion

It could be that roles are pre-existent forms, archetypes in a Jungian sense, dramatic artifacts in an aesthetic sense, that subsist throughout history, culture, and theatrical literature. As such, they are inherited, given as a birthright. By implication, newborns would have the potential universe of roles within their psyches.

It might also be true that roles pre-exist in a culture and society and are, in part, culturally and socially determined. From this perspective, newborns acquire roles as they interact with those in their cultural and social spheres.

So, too, might roles be inherited genetically both as a means of survival – as, for example, a newborn assumes the somatic role of eater – and as a series of predispositions that will determine the kinds of roles to be taken on and the ways those roles will be played out.

Despite the archetypal, dramatic, social, and genetic determining factors, human beings are still creators of their own identities, at least in part. Georgie and Mackey in the many examples above were pictured as active players of their various roles, rather than passive takers of some predetermined substance. Implicit in dramatic playing is the sense of the player as creative (see Winnicott 1971). Even if roles are, to a large degree, predetermined, each individual must still choose those roles that are most appropriate to a given circumstance and most meaningful to that individual. Each role chosen and played must be done so for a purpose, whether to survive, express a feeling, or meet a need. And each act of role taking and role playing is creative in the sense that one is building a piece of one's identity. Like theatrical actors, actors in everyday life receive a predetermined script that includes the substance of particular roles. Their artistry comes in humanizing those roles, filling in the personae with the breathe of life that is unique to each particular person.

Throughout this chapter we have looked at ways that early roles develop. I have chosen to focus most especially upon the genesis of family roles, as well as those concerning physical ability and disability, fear, aggression, and gender identity. The examples of Georgie and Mackey are typical in the sense that most all children from birth to four will take on and play out similar roles of parents and siblings, aggressors and victims, males and females. Yet each one will do so in a unique way and not necessarily within the same time span as Georgie and Mackey.

Some children who are severely emotionally disturbed will not be able to play and thus will not be able to take on or play out a variety of roles. Others, with less severe forms of disturbance or disability, will be able to take on and generate roles, but in a somewhat limited way. Still others, who appear normal by most measures of mental and physical health, will experience trauma through any number of physical, environmental, or psychological circumstances. In such cases, they, too, might experience a diminished capacity to take on and play out roles.

With such children, a treatment through drama therapy based in an attempt to build new roles or restore old ones might well be indicated. Elsewhere, I have outlined a method of diagnosis, treatment and evaluation of such individuals using a role method (Landy 1993b).

Any attempt to understand the ways and means of presenting oneself in role requires a view of young children as they begin to assert their identities through play. This view through the looking glass is one all of us have experienced once upon a time. And this view is one most of us have forgotten. If we try hard, we may begin to recall images. As there are in Wordsworth's terms, 'intimations of immortality' (see Wordsworth 1807/1965), there are also intimations of infancy that can be accessed in visions of white rabbits, gypsies, and stuffed animals named Tigo.

If our own memory fails, we can observe the children around us and even those within us who seem to embody the primal dramas of individual identity and family, of power and loss, of sex and death. In their struggles with role lie the seeds of our struggles as adults who live on the other side of the looking glass but sometimes imagine what it would be like to venture forth again through that magical window.

# CHAPTER 14

# A Short-Term Model of Drama Therapy Through the Role Method

The role method was developed by Landy (1993b) as a means to treat clients in drama therapy. It is based in a theory of role which views the act of performance as one of role taking and role playing wherein the performer experiences a paradoxical state of living within two simultaneous realities, the fictional and the non-fictional, and two simultaneous identities, me and not-me. In drama therapy, the therapist aims to help the client live within these paradoxes and discover a balanced system of interdependent roles.

To date, the role method has been used with several populations, as follows:

1. With graduate students in drama therapy as a means of education and training;

2. With groups of normal neurotic adults, as a means of group therapy;

3. With normal neurotic individuals experiencing issues of anxiety, alienation, identity and relationship;

4. With individuals experiencing specific emotional problems (e.g. bipolar disorder, anorexia nervosa, and various mood disorders).

Most of the treatment with these individuals has been medium-term (i.e. approximately six months) or long-term (from six months to several years). The purpose of this chapter is to examine the application of the role method to short-term drama therapy with a variety of populations. I will begin by reviewing the role method of treatment and offering a rationale of why it would be appropriate as a short-term treatment modality. Then I will delineate the kinds of disorders or problems that seem most amenable to this kind of treatment, offering brief clinical examples. Within this section, I will also discuss treatment goals. Finally, I will discuss issues germane to assessment through the role method.

## What Is the Role Method?

The role method is a means of treatment wherein clients are asked to engage in the primary task of actors in the theatre – that is, to imagine themselves as fictional characters and to act as if they were another. The purpose of the role method, unlike that of theatre, is to illuminate the everyday life of clients as it is reflected in the their dramatic fiction.

The role method proceeds in eight steps, as follows:

1.  Invoking the role.

2.  Naming the role.

3.  Playing out/working through of the role.

4.  Exploring alternative qualities and sub-roles.

5.  Reflecting upon the role-play: discovering role qualities, functions, and styles inherent in the role.

6.  Relating the fictional role to everyday life.

7.  Integrating roles to create a functional role system.

8.  Social modeling: discovering ways that the clients' behavior in role affects others in their social environments.

**Steps one and two** comprise the warm-up to a session, whereby the client is asked to engage a particular role and provide specificity through naming it. Roles can be invoked in a variety of ways from sources both outside and inside the client. For example, after telling a story, either fictional or non-fictional, the client can be asked to choose one character or object from the story and give it a name. Or clients can be asked to close their eyes and to imagine a particular neutral scene, identifying people and objects therein. By choosing one and naming it, the client has both invoked and named a role from an internal source.

Roles from external sources can be invoked by asking clients to reach out and specify who they are reaching for, to push away or to pull in, again specifying the object of their action.

**Steps three and four** involve the action part of a session and concern an improvisational process of enactment through the given role. This can be done as an individual plays in role or as group members play out their roles in relation to others also in role. In step four, the therapist might freeze the action and ask the clients either to reverse roles with someone else or to play out an alternative quality of a given role. For example, in one group, an improvisation was set up concerning a long-distance telephone conversation filtered through an operator who was overwhelmed and disinclined to connect the callers. All were talking at once at a frantic pace so that no one person could be heard. The therapist froze the scene and asked all to slow down and find a way both to express their own feelings and communicate them to another. By altering the frantic, angry qualities of their roles, all were able to express and communicate their feelings.

**Steps five and six** occur during closure. They involve two levels of reflection, the first, step five, upon attempting to make sense of the role as a fiction, as existing outside the client. Thus, the long-distance operator would reflect upon the qualities of her role, as opposed to those of herself in everyday life. By *qualities*, I refer to six domains (see Landy 1993b):

1.  somatic, pertaining to the body;

2.  cognitive, pertaining to the capacity for understanding and awareness;

3.  affective, pertaining to moral and feeling states;

4.  social, pertaining to status and stature within family and society;

5.  spiritual, pertaining to one's relation to transpersonal forces;

6.  aesthetic, pertaining to one's creative capacities.

In **step five**, the client also looks at the *function* of a role, that is, the way the role serves the role-player, satisfying a need or wish. For example, the long-distance operator might have felt disconnected from others in the improvisation. The purpose of assuming the kind of operator she portrayed, then, was to impose that feeling upon the others, insuring that they, too, would be unable to connect, express, and communicate. Certain roles tend to be associated with certain prescribed functions (e.g. the mother nurtures, the lover yearns, the victim gives up control). These functions have become codified through universal exemplification within cultural practices, mythologies, and personal experience (Jung 1964).

The *style* of role enactment refers to the degree of cognition and affect presented in role. Theoretically, the more stylized one's role enactment, the more cognitive one tends to be. The tendency toward reality-based performance implies more feeling on the part of the actor. As the long-distance operator, the actor exaggerated her actions, thus presenting a somewhat distanced portrayal of her character. Yet, in reflecting on her improvisation, she was able to present a more feelingful sense of her role. In some ways, the style helped her from becoming too emotional. In portraying a stylized version of the operator, she operated at aesthetic distance (see Landy 1983), allowing a balance of feeling and thought.

In **step six**, the second level of reflection, the client moves from the fiction of the role to its counterpart in everyday life. This step usually leads to a deepening of the drama experience by linking it to the person's daily existence. Some, like the woman as operator, who have used the role in a balanced way, welcome the connection as it reveals certain qualities of their lives. Others, more resistant and needing to be supported in their defenses, are either unable or unready to see the dreaded connections.

**Step seven** attempts to link the one role with its various counterparts within an individual personality. I have written elsewhere (Landy 1993b) that the personality can be conceived as a system of interrelated roles and that when one becomes too under-powered or over-powering, the role method can help to restore a balance among roles. This step implies an internal process, a reconfiguring of images that one holds of one's identity. Role integration can be compared to that of a balanced *dramatis personae* within a play where villains serve as foils for heroes, survivors balance out victims, and ignorance struggles with wisdom.

**Step eight**, the final step, that of social modeling, generally occurs outside of the actual drama therapy sessions. The point is that individual change is necessary but not sufficient for a transformed society. After one has found a greater degree of balance, the next step is for that individual to model his newly transformed role system for others. Presumably, once victims are no longer obsessed with playing out that specific role, they can help others to understand that each victim has the potential to take on and play out the role of victor or survivor (see, for example, the cases of Michael and Ann in Landy 1993b).

## Why is the Role Method Appropriate for Short-Term Treatment?

Increasingly, the mental health system is moving toward short-term models of treatment. This move is based upon a philosophy of de-institutionalization of mentally ill individuals and a concomitant cutback of funds within various health care systems. Although the re-integration of hospitalized and incarcerated individuals into their communities is a noble aim, it is more often than not fueled by economic expediency and not necessarily based upon the best interests of either clients or communities. Given this reality, those offering psychotherapy through a number of modalities need to develop appropriate models to treat a number of populations in need.

Drama therapy is derivative, in part, from several psychotherapeutic sources (Landy 1994), among them analytic and psychodynamic approaches, Gestalt and psychodramatic approaches, and behavioral and cognitive approaches. Many drama therapists have modeled their work after their psychodynamically-oriented colleagues. Some, including Eleanor Irwin (1985) and Elaine Portner (Irwin and Malloy 1975), have identified themselves more as psychoanalysts than as drama therapists. As such, they tend to practice at least a medium-term form of therapy, if not long-term. As a general principle, the more one approaches the inner life of clients, the more time it takes for the process to develop.

The training of drama therapists also tends to support depth approaches as students are introduced to projective ways of examining the inner life of clients through their play, role enactments, and projections onto such objects as masks and puppets.

Training and practice in drama therapy has tended to shy away from those approaches that are generally short-term by virtue of their more external orientation. Behavioral approaches, for example, are shunned by drama therapists as they seem to deny the image and the metaphor as central ways of making meaning in one's life. On the other hand, some short-term approaches, such as psychodrama, are depth-oriented, quickly touching on inner experience. This complicates the issue because short-term treatment should not open up too much of one's inner life. Once un-covered, the client is too vulnerable, requiring time to re-cover.

The drama therapist can make use of short-term rationales from behaviorists (see, for example, Wolpe 1990) who focus upon the external lives of clients, and psychodramatists (see Moreno 1946, 1959), who focus upon the inner lives of clients. Like the behaviorist, drama therapists can take care not to open up too much inner process, and like the psychodramatist, they can take care effectively to close a psychic rent. One way they can do this is through the role method which is both externally and internally oriented. Before discussing why this approach seems most efficacious, let us examine several principles guiding short-term treatment of emotional and existential problems.

By definition, short-term treatment implies a brief encounter between client and therapist. Brief might be defined as a single meeting or a series of meetings up to a contracted number, decided upon by either the therapist or the therapist in consultation with the client. Short-term treatment is generally based in the solution to a given problem often brought about by a crisis in a client's life.

Short-term treatment is usually centered in the here-and-now rather than in historical life experience and offers support of a client's defenses, rather than challenging the defensive structure or ego integrity. The treatment therefore avoids the tendency to delve deeply into unconscious experience, as this focus is associated with psychodynamic, longer-term models.

In short-term treatment, the therapist takes a fairly active role in helping the client to define problems and move toward solutions. This tends to circumvent intense transference and countertransferential attachments and reactions.

Therapists working through short-term models attempt to contain intense emotional experience and help clients regain a sense of emotional equilibrium within a short period of time. These therapists focus upon discrete aspects of a person (e.g. a single problem or a pattern of behavior), rather than upon the totality of the personality.

The client enters short-term treatment in the hopes of finding a quick solution to an often embedded problem. For some, affected only by a particular and sudden crisis, that solution can be found quickly. For others whose crisis might be simply the latest manifestation of a deeper characterological problem, a quick solution may be illusive.

## Specific Characteristics of the Role Method in Short-Term Drama Therapy

The role method is based in solving a problem, the problem being an imbalance within one's role system which has been brought about by a sudden crisis, such as divorce, death, illness, war, abuse, accident, or loss. When the problem of role imbalance is more embedded, the role method can and should be used over a longer period of time in a more psychodynamic fashion. Further, as mentioned above, the role method helps people access a part of their personalities in the here-and-now, even though in working through that part, people can come face to face with their past. Yet the invocation of a role occurs fully in the present and concerns a person's sense of that role at the time it is invoked.

The role method is non-confrontational and does not shake up a person's defenses. If clients are resistant, then they are asked to stay with the role of the resistant one. If they are defensive, then that quality becomes translated into a role. Thus, the method begins at whatever level the client might be functioning. All images are valued as a statement of the present reality of the client, or, more to the point, of the present reality of a persona that is not the client. This point is most germane to the dramatic nature of role as fiction. The role method insures the safety of clients who in taking on a role are allowed to leave their everyday skin behind and pretend that they are someone else.

It is moot whether or not clients consciously choose roles when engaged in the role method. When telling a story or playing with objects in a sandtray or recounting the figures in a dream, clients work with images, touching upon experience that may very well be beyond their immediate consciousness. Unconscious experience is, thus, generated through the role method. However, when working through role, the therapist should be wary of uncovering too much embedded imagery and focus, instead, upon that which appears to be more available to consciousness. In working short-term with an individual recently recovering from abuse, for example, one would not attempt to uncover certain dark, demonic figures from the unconscious life. Rather, the therapist might focus upon more direct, reality-based roles that could help clients both tell a story expressively and discover further ways to protect themselves from reexperiencing the recent trauma and other traumas from the past.

The position of therapists working through the role method is of facilitator and guide. Sometimes they will engage in the role-play with a client, but more often than not, they will lead the client toward an identification, sharpening, working through, and integrating of the role. In short-term work, therapists may even take on the role of teacher, providing information about alternative roles or helping clients learn about the roles they have been cast in by virtue of being in the wrong place at the wrong time, for example. Rather than dwelling on the transferences between client and therapist, the focus of short-term drama therapy is more on the solution to a life problem as crystallized within a particular role.

By offering the containment of the role, the drama therapist working through the role method is also able to contain overwhelming expressions of emotion. Working with an understanding that cathartic experience is about the confluence of thought and feeling, the drama therapist uses the role to remind clients that they are indeed not the parts that they seem to be playing. Thus, the role of abused person is seen to also be that – a part, a role. Even though one does not generally choose to take on that role, one can choose to move away from it, at least after the fact. Survivors of physical abuse often hold onto their roles of victim long after their physical liberation from an abusive situation. Even though it may cause a sense of alienation and anxiety, the victim role at least provides purpose to the lives of those who feel that any sense of purpose was brutally taken away from them.

Yet even small parts of such a person's role repertoire can be resuscitated and filled up with feeling. This can only happen if the person has given life to alternative roles through calling them up and naming them.

In the case of a survivor of incest or torture, the experience of playing with roles of victim, victimizer, and survivor can be very powerful. Many seek short-term treatment because they feel incapable of survival, of getting on with their lives. The role method helps them see that this sense of dis-ease and stagnation is a part of them that perhaps has temporarily blighted other parts of the personality. As noted above, with short-term treatment, the goal is not to restructure the whole personality, but simply to help clients understand that within themselves lies the means of healing. Within the person who feels utterly humiliated is the potential for a feeling of self-worth, embodied in the roles of warrior, hero and survivor. Within the overly critical person lurks the lover. Within the immoralist lurks the puritan. The role method proceeds through an attention to parts of the person. As such it is suitable to short-term treatment. Yet paradoxically, as it focuses upon single parts, it points to the possibilities of others, alternative personae that can move the person out of a desperate and hopeless condition.

## Who Can Best Benefit from Short-term Treatment through the Role Method?

The ideal candidates for short-term treatment through the role method are those who have been thrust into crisis by some significant deviation from the expected flow of everyday life. The sudden death of an intimate, an abusive incident in a relationship, or a random act of violence can all trigger disturbing emotions and lead toward therapy. In treating such individuals, the drama therapist helps the client to invoke and name one or several related roles germane to the particular incident, then work with the roles through a fictional enactment. If re-experiencing the incident proves too overwhelming, the drama therapist might help the client approach it in a more distanced way (i.e. from the point of view of watching someone else experience an act of violence, rather than experiencing it herself).

Finally, depending upon the amount of time contracted by client and therapist, the client would begin to explore the qualities, functions, and styles of the dreaded role(s). From the therapist's point of view, clients will be searching for ways to integrate the experience and live in the paradox of knowing that although they might have been innocent victims of a rape or a beating, roles exist within their psyches that recapitulate the qualities of both the abused and the abuser. At the heart of the role method is the assumption that all human experience, both violent and gentle, is universal. The violence in Rwanda and Bosnia is not an aberration particular to Africa or the Balkans, but a quality inherited, learned, and generated by all human beings, at least subliminally.

### Example

Herb, a 40-year-old account executive, had moved down south, faraway from his family. He moved to join a group of people who were devoted to a particular guru whom I will call Jen. Herb procured a well-paying job and lived alone in a rented apartment, spending most of his free time in the presence of Jen and his followers. For the first time in his life, Herb felt a sublime sense of peace. He became devoted to Jen. Like the others, he willingly gave Jen a large portion of his salary. Ten years passed and Jen became ill and suddenly died. Herb was devastated and began to travel aimlessly, contemplating suicide in every new town. Finally, he sought help on the recommendation of an old friend.

Herb's treatment lasted four weeks, for a total of eight sessions. His most poignant work was with two related roles, that of the lamb and that of the tiger. Herb conceived of the lamb as a gentle creature, close to the gods. He was innocent and in need of an object of worship. Without that object, he felt lost and despondent. Alone, he wanted to die. Herb's version of the tiger was strong and ferocious. He needed neither human nor god but stood alone and intact. He frightened others and enjoyed his power immensely.

Through playing out these roles in story, drawing, sand and role play, Herb began to see that he had qualities of both the lamb and the tiger. He realized for the first time that the dreaded tiger had qualities that he desired – independence and power. Like the tiger, he stood alone. Like the tiger, he was special, sometimes even feared by others because of his singular choice to be unique among creatures. He began to discover a new purpose in his life – to stand up and allow himself to be seen, even at the risk of frightening others away.

Herb was not willing to let go of the qualities that he shared with the lamb. He recognized his extreme vulnerability and innocence and his need to remain within the compass of a loving mentor or group. He would use the strength of the tiger to search for that community.

As Herb was about to leave for a new home and new job, I brought in the Blake poems, 'The Lamb' and 'The Tyger.' He knew of them both, but did not remember the line from 'The Tyger': 'What immortal hand or eye/Could frame thy fearful symmetry?' When Jen died, all sense of balance seemed forever lost. Through creating his roles and reflecting upon those created by Blake some 200 years earlier, Herb embraced his own contradictory pulls toward submission and dominance, toward living the life of the lamb and the tiger. He choose, finally, the role of survivor. But from Herb's point of view, the survivor was a delicate creature who exists in a fearful symmetry, attempting to control and hold on to that which is ultimately beyond control, yearning for eternal love and eternal life even in the shadow of abandonment and death.

In working with Herb, my goal was to help him recognize that he had become locked into a single role for 10 years, that of the devoted worshiper. When that role was taken away, Herb could only conceive of one other role choice – that of the suicide. By creating and acknowledging alternative roles (e.g. lamb and tiger), he was able to recognize alternative ways of being and chose the survivor over the suicide.

Others will seek short-term treatment based upon a particular fear or a particular problem that needs to be resolved. The anticipation of needing to confront a fear might drive some people into therapy. For example, a woman who has lived her life in the city is terrified of spiders and large insects. She is about to take a trip to a rain forest where she is certain to encounter some exotic forms of insect life. Before her trip, she consults a therapist for the purpose of alleviating some of her anxiety. Or, a man terrified of commitment has been dating a woman whom he loves dearly. She informs him that if he does not commit to marriage, she will leave him. He, too, consults a therapist. Or, a woman who has never left her mother has fallen in love. Her mother recently suffered a debilitating stroke and needed her daughter to care for her. The man she loves wants to marry her but only if she moves away from her mother and lives with him. She seeks out a form of short-term therapy to help resolve her dilemma.

*Example*

The following example is of an actor who was living in a foreign country temporarily and was about to return home. As the day of her return trip approached, she became desperately anxious. She attributed her anxiety to a fear of flying. Being a creative person, she sought out a creative form of treatment. When she called for an appointment, she made it clear that she could only see me for one session.

When working with the actor, whom I shall call June, I intended to help her find a role that could guide her through her journey, rather than one that would bring her to the cause of her anxiety. Our communication was difficult as we spoke different languages and depended upon the few expressions we knew in common. Working non-verbally, I led her to a sandtray and introduced an array of miniature objects. She placed her hands in the sandtray and began moving them in circles, creating a mound of sand imbedded with concentric rings. As she was doing this, she suddenly became flooded with emotion. I asked her to stay with her creation and add whatever objects she wished. A miniature airplane appeared and then a small boy. She named him Le Petit Prince, the character in St. Exupéry's popular book about a lost boy searching for meaning on a planet far away from home.

By working through the role of The Little Prince, June indeed found a compatriot. The fictional lost searcher became her guide. Without much language, June made it clear that she, too, was lost but ambivalent about returning home. She feared that she could no longer connect to her family and colleagues. She saw herself as different and estranged both at home and abroad. At the conclusion of the session, she recognized her connection to The Little Prince and was grateful that she had found this figure only vaguely recalled from her childhood. Although she feared that he would crash and disappear in the cosmos, never to find his home, she felt more prepared to return to hers with St. Exupéry's hero as co-pilot, brother, companion, and guide, reminding her that she was not alone.

Short-term treatment through the role method is not for everyone in need. Some, experiencing the immediacy of a crisis, will be unwilling to work in fiction, needing rather to talk through the moment of reality. Others, suffering long-standing illnesses, will need a great deal of time and support to work through their issues. Still others, with iron-clad defenses that have separated them from intimacy and joy throughout their lives, would need a more intensive form of treatment. But for those who are able and motivated to work through the fictional boundaries created by roles for the purpose of moving through a particular crisis point, the role method might well be indicated.

## Assessment Through the Role Method

I have discussed elsewhere (Landy 1993b) how the role method can be used in assessment. Let me add here some further thoughts about assessment as it applies to short-term treatment. While treating a client briefly for a particular problem, the drama therapist might also offer some thoughts on assessing the client's abilities to take on and play out roles. Given the structure of the role method, the therapist would assess the following:

1. The client's ability to invoke one or several roles.

2. The client's ability to name one or several roles.

3. The client's ability to take on and play out the role(s) in a fictional context.

4. The client's ability to discover alternative qualities of the roles taken on.

5. The client's ability to attribute qualities, functions, and styles to the role play.

6. The client's ability to connect the fictional role play to everyday life.

7. The client's ability to recognize the connection between one role and others that he has played or could play.

Clients who are able to invoke and name roles, to play them out and reflect upon them as fictions and as parts of themselves, would be well within the normal range of functioning. Any significant deviation from this range would indicate a truncated role system. The therapist and client can determine whether the role system can be brought back into balance through short-term treatment or whether a longer course of treatment is required. Further, they can determine if the role method or, indeed, drama therapy is the best way to proceed.

As referred to earlier, short-term therapy might serve as a form of education. Some people come to brief therapy to learn something about themselves that has eluded them. In terms of the role method, some may not be aware of the kinds of roles available to take on and play out. Through an assessment, the therapist might inform them that they seem to be familiar with a very limited number of roles or, perhaps, just one role. For some, characterized as one-dimensional, that one role might be the victim. For others, that role might be the lost one or the nurturing mother or the beauty or the beast. The educational component might be for the therapist to inform them of other role choices: the victim can experiment with the role of survivor; the nurturing mother with the narcissist, etc. The therapist can be guided by the taxonomy of roles (see Landy 1993b) which, though derived from theatre, classifies and enumerates the kinds of roles available to be taken on in everyday life.

Although an assessment instrument based in the role method has not been fully developed, such an approach offers the potential to assess a person in need and offer a plan of treatment intended to develop the quantity and quality of role taking and role playing. Whether used for assessment or treatment, the role method offers a directed and structured way to treat a person in need of short-term therapy by focusing upon a potentially large crisis or problem in terms of more contained and discrete units, those of its associated roles. By naming and characterizing the roles, by playing them out, and reflecting upon them, the client can discover a specificity and focus which can remain in the here-and-now, which can support his defenses and contain intense emotional experience.

In the long run, the therapy is successful when clients are able to see the roles named, played, and reflected upon as parts of themselves and when they are able to recognize that they, indeed, have other parts in reserve which they can call upon when needed. But to get there, in the short-term, clients need to first view problematic roles as outside themselves, existing in the world as potential victimizers and malevolent forces who can randomly suck the life and goodness from innocent victims. Once roles are situated outside, transforming shadow to substance, image to character, they can be captured and concretized.

At the center of the role method is this paradox – the fiction and the fact are one. That which is not-me is also me. By fashioning and recognizing that which is not-me, I return to myself with a deeper and more secure sense of recognition.

# CHAPTER 15

# Isolation and Collaboration in the Creative Arts Therapies
## The Implications of Crossing Borders[1]

Once upon a time, very long ago, people protected themselves by constructing stone walls around their villages and towns. The good townspeople did this for good reasons: to keep out invaders and foreigners and, in many cases, to stop the exodus of their own citizens and slaves who might feel the need to search for a better life on the outside.

But these very protectors all eventually learned the same lesson: no border is impenetrable; no wall is high enough or thick enough to keep the enemy out or the malcontent in. And yet, even though generations of protectors have accepted this common knowledge, they still continue to repeat the same defensive patterns to this very day.

Some, however, in their abundant sagacity, held an alternative point of view. If you can neither keep the enemy out or the malcontent in, then let them all go where they will. Perhaps then these invaders, undesirables and pariahs will either go away or find a peaceful place among more accepting neighbors. Over time, these peacemakers noted some contradictory evidence. Sometimes, when the walls went down, an intermingling of peoples and ideas helped nurture the land and people lived in peace. But other times, foreigners exploited, raped, and maimed the land and its people. Sometimes, when the walls went down, people left to find more desirable lands or when faced with the choice of leaving, decided to stay and make a better life for themselves. But other times, people left in droves, depleting the resources of their native land or, when confronted with a choice, stayed out of fear of the unknown and grew old and bitter with regret.

---

1 This chapter was presented as a keynote lecture at the third European Arts Therapies Conference in Ferrara, Italy

In my profession as a drama therapist, I often ask people to make up stories and, if possible, to reflect upon them, drawing parallels between the fictions that arise spontaneously and their everyday lives. I try to help them discover the nature of their problems as embedded in characters and themes created in their fictions. Theoretically, I am not a follower of Freud, Jung, Laing, Winnicott, Laçan, Skinner, Perls, Moreno, Minushin, Stanislavki, Artaud, Brecht and countless others, even though I have drawn sustenance from all. My thinking is closest to the early 19th century poet and illustrator, William Blake, whose striking images can best be described as paradoxical, as existing in 'fearful symmetry,' one to another. This point of view is well illustrated in the qualities of divine beauty and savage ferocity co-existing within the form of the tiger, found in Blake's 'Songs of Experience.' And the tiger, itself, becomes the antithesis of the lamb, a Christ-like figure in Blake's 'Songs of Innocence.'

In the opening story, I refer to the protectors, those who defend the need to construct borders, and the peace-makers, those who wish to remove boundaries in the hopes of reconciliation and freedom of movement. As a parable, this story is about the implications of crossing borders. And this story sets the stage for the following remarks on the creative art therapies. My thinking has certainly been influenced by the many sectarian political and military struggles in the former Yugoslavia and Soviet Union, in Israel and the Middle East, in Northern Ireland and South Africa, in Rwanda and Zaire, and closer to home, in Cuba, who recently opened its tightly shut doors and tens of thousands spilled out in search of a better life.

As a creative arts therapist I will aim my remarks at a profession that I see as at a crossroad. Some of the road signs point in a hopeful direction: there is a European consortium for creative arts therapists that fosters dialogue among the arts therapy disciplines and among various cultures; there is an American association that has been on a similar mission, the National Coalition of Arts Therapy Associations (NCATA); there are significant international attempts at research and publication (e.g. the journal, *The Arts in Psychotherapy*, and the developing list of offerings by the British publisher, Jessica Kingsley). There are also examples of links between the creative arts therapies and medicine (see Aldridge and Brandt 1991), collaborations between therapists from different art modalities and different cultures (see Jennings and Minde 1993), and attempts to create an integrated theoretical sense of how and why the aesthetic process is healing (see *The Arts in Psychotherapy*, special edition on Aesthetics 1992; Landy 1993a; Knill 1994).

But the signs that point to another road are less sanguine. This path leads to the domain of the protectors and isolates. This is the path of bureaucratic, entrenched mental health systems. When on this road, the traveler is fearful of real and imagined dangers: cutbacks in funds for medium and long-term treatment of clients; cutbacks in funds for research; difficulties in achieving professional credibility through licensure and hierarchical systems; suspiciousness in the mental health establishment and the public at large of alternative models of healing; fear that the profession one has chosen is discredited, scientifically unverifiable, frivolous, and even shameful (see Johnson 1994). When on this path some develop grandiose fantasies, splitting off from their colleagues in related arts modalities, believing that music or dance or art or drama or poetry is the best way of healing. Others go further, splitting their disciplines into smaller pieces, touting Guided Imagery through Music (GIM) or authentic movement or the developmental method of drama therapy as the preferred trail. As these borders grow thicker and higher, within, between, and among individuals, possibilities for reconciliation diminish. Differences are indeed important and provide uniqueness to practitioners. But when differences become dogma, the borders become impenetrable.

As a creative arts therapist, I have stood at this crossroad many times and still, when there, always need to consider which path to take. In preparing and even now, in delivering this chapter, I stand at that crossroad. There is part of me that wants to reach out openly and let in the mix of voices and experiences surrounding me. And there is part of me that wants to shut the gates and assume my position in the field as superior and thus in need of defending.

The defender part experiences a sense of isolation and insecurity. I am an American among Europeans. I am a drama therapist (two words) amongst only a handful of dramatherapists (one word). I am neither a medical doctor nor a research scientist. I have no hard data to report. In my many years of work reporting the effects of drama therapy on a variety of client populations, I can boast neither reliability nor validity. In my country, because of my credentials, or lack thereof, my clients cannot claim insurance reimbursement.

The more open part of me wants reconciliation and connection. I am a fellow creative arts therapist. I work with images, metaphors, roles, and fictions, just like most of you. The national borders and differences among our modalities of treatment are ultimately insignificant for, as professionals, we are more alike than different. Like many of you I am and was a creative artist first and therapist second who believes that the aesthetic act is an inherently healing one and who verifies my work through qualitative means.

I do not think that my position is particularly unique. It seems to me that one very human struggle on a personal and professional level pits the forces of isolation against those of collaboration. It seems to me that as a profession with interior borders dividing our arts disciplines and exterior borders separating our profession from other healing arts and sciences (e.g. medicine, psychology and psychiatry, social work and occupational therapy), we need to find a way to live in the paradox of collaboration and isolation. In many ways, my personal attempt to reconcile these two positions is what has led me to Blake and to a paradoxical frame of reference in which to better understand my professional responsibilities. This frame can be seen as a dialogical one.

At New York University, we offer an advanced graduate course called Collaboration in the Creative Arts Therapies. The course is teamtaught by an art, music and drama therapist and includes an equal number of students from all three disciplines. Dance and poetry are excluded because neither field is offered at our university. As teachers of the course, we aim to help students discover how they can collaborate with others in related disciplines. Our hope is that they will bring these collaborative skills into their clinical environments when they become professional. Throughout the course, we also urge students to listen to and express the inner voice of isolation, that part of themselves that resists an art form, a process of treatment, and a theoretical point of view that is not their own.

In our initial attempt to insist that artists sing and that musicians act, and that actors draw, we learned to listen to the many voices of resistance. For one, many were uncomfortable with the others' media. Some had negative childhood experiences with rigid teachers who insisted that there was only one right way to draw a tree or recite a Shakespearian monologue or who forced young people to perform to an audience long before they were ready. Some, although well trained in one art form were afraid to try another – performing in front of others through voice or movement was terrifying, clay and oil were too messy and regressive.

Further, art therapists were trained to work primarily with individuals. Drama therapists were trained primarily to work with groups. The art people were generally steeped in analytical models; the other two in a range of theoretical positions including humanistic, sociological, and aesthetic frameworks.

Yet despite the differences in approach and theory, the group struggled on. Individuals spoke to each other through their common language of images, the most powerful one created repeatedly through musical improvisation. We collectively discovered that when the group seemed most isolated and defensive, we would turn to an array of musical instruments and improvise. We ended many meetings with drumming and found that in doing so, the needs to create individually and collectively, to expose and to conceal, to magnify and to reduce were all served.

The collective voice of the drums, however, could not and, for that matter, should not drown out the critical need to remain alone in the silence of meditation, resistance, isolation. In this group, as in all effective groups striving for dialogue, these voices all require a means of expression. We were left with a number of unanswered questions: is there a unifying aesthetic applicable to all the creative arts therapies? How much do I need to know of the other's modality in order to be an effective collaborator? Is creative expression enough to heal or is interpretation also needed? How far do I go in crossing the border of my collaborator's aesthetic or therapeutic approach?

The collaborative part of me would foolishly argue that borders are artificial, that as creative arts therapists we do indeed have a common language of images and a common goal of leading others to express themselves through their images, transforming their pain as they do so. These transformative images are present universally, I would add. There is not a British version of drama therapy that is so different from a Dutch or French version, or an Italian or American or a German version.

And yet, another part of me would challenge that point of view. There are cultural and theoretical differences and they comprise necessary borders. Many parts of the world are disinterested in creative arts therapy. Some cultures or sub-cultures dismiss the idea of therapy categorically. And there are significant differences among the arts therapies – this, too, is a border. Why should artists sing or singers draw? Why should actors mold clay and sculptors play Juliet? Why should I embrace your outdated or untested or post-post modernist ideas and why should you embrace mine? I want to be left alone with my work and my students and my clients. Why must I come so far away from home to convince you that I know better?

I try to listen to all my voices, even the ones that have the power to humiliate me. There is indeed part of me that wants to build walls and protect myself from ideas that are too old or too new, too embedded in traditions different from mine, too difficult for me to grasp. And there is part of me that yearns for new colleagues across new borders, willing to look at our common concerns as therapists who are artists and artists who are therapists. In maneuvering between the two parts, I recognize that it is not enough to set up an either/or proposition, a polite dialogue between two intrapsychic adversaries. Rather, both voices have validity and often stand in fearful symmetry, one to the other. Whenever I stand authentically before my colleagues in drama therapy or in other creative arts therapies I try to be aware of my jealousies, grandiosities, and fears of shaming myself for lack of power or wisdom. This awareness creates an edge.

And it is that edge that propels me toward communication and ultimately collaboration. I cross borders to be closer to the realities of new ideas on the outside and to confront my inner need to isolate and create firmer borders. This intrapsychic struggle can have implications for all of us who must try harder to cross all the borders separating our arts modalities, theoretical perspectives, methods of treatment, and tendencies to split and isolate and defend.

Like the immigrant and refugee, we have left the safer shores of more conventional fields to practice a new discipline. As a consequence, many of us feel isolated. We need community with those of our colleagues who have taken a similar journey. Yet in our quest for a unified field of creative arts therapy, let us not abandon our borders and our walls. Just let them be neither too high nor too thick. Let the mortar be made of paradox and let us search for ways to break through even as we retain.

# CHAPTER 16

# In Search of the Muse

Let me know, Muse, of the many wanderings
    of the godlike Odysseus...

Homer, *The Odyssey*

O for a Muse of fire, that would
    ascend
The brightest heaven of invention:

Shakespeare, *Henry V* (Prologue, 1–2)

Sing Heav'nly Muse...What in me is dark
Illumine, what is low raise and support...

Hail holy Light...
Shine inward...that I may see and tell
Of things invisible to mortal sight.

J. Milton, *Paradise Lost* (pp.211–212, 257–259)

I celebrate myself and sing myself,
And what I assume you shall assume...

W. Whitman, *Song of Myself*

Moloch! Moloch! Nightmare of Moloch! Moloch the
    loveless!
Mental Moloch! Moloch the heavy judger of men!

A. Ginsberg, *Howl*

In the classic literary traditions of many cultures, the poet begins his work with an invocation of the muse. The muse is a spirit, a god, capable of granting the poet the power to create. The implication is that a mortal is limited in expression, not up to the task of creating sublime and transcendent images. He can only approach his art with the help of a guide whose function is not only to pilot but also to inspire and to sustain.

For the most part, the muse of antiquity was a divine figure of beauty, grace, and harmony – often female. In modern times, the figure changes. In many instances, the muse descends, appearing, at times, as the subject of the art work. Walt Whitman, in *Song of Myself*, seems to locate the muse within – the poet becomes his own object of worship and inspiration. And Allen Ginsberg, in *Howl*, creates another sense of the muse as a dark, destructive figure, a purveyor of chaos. Moloch, to whom Ginsberg sings, is the god of the ancient Phoenicians to whom children were sacrificed by burning at the stake.

As a drama therapist, I try to help people discover the source of their inspiration, whether it is located within the mind or in the world of nature or spirits, whether it is luminous and balanced or dark and chaotic. It is my hope that this figure will guide them to the parts of their psyches that need exhumation and examination. Further, I believe, the muse will activate the role of the artist, one who can express that which is located underground. In many years of working through the role method of drama therapy, I have developed an approach which begins with the invocation of a role (Landy 1993b). The role invoked serves as a guide and inspiration that, muse-like, can lead clients toward a creative uncovering of disturbing aspects of their existence.

Before I became a drama therapist, I was a theatre artist. I wrote plays that were inspired by a range of characters. I invoked the patriarchs of my father's family, Old Testament-like denizens of sweat shops in New York City's Lower Broadway. I wrote of Odysseus and James Boswell, of children forced into slave labor at the turn of the century, and the heroic political tricksters who challenged the social order of the late 1960's. When I became a drama therapist, I realized that these inspirational figures were very much parts of myself and that by telling their stories, I was exploring undigested fragments of my own experience. The faraway muses of antiquity were coming closer and closer. The inspiration I so sorely needed was often literally within my grasp, emanating from my fingertips onto the keyboard.

This chapter is about my struggle as a creative arts therapist to stay connected to my art even while I drift away and enter into the arts and minds of others. In recognizing my tendency to drift, I acknowledge the need of an anchor in the creative process that led me to the field of creative arts therapy in the first place. That grounding is especially important when in the act of inspiring others. Time and again, as therapist and theorist, I have lost my muse and stood in fear that she might never return.

In my latest return, very much in need of inspiration, I invoked Hetty Green, referred to by journalists, none too affectionately, as 'the Witch of Wall Street.' She died in 1916 worth more than $100 million. Most people have not heard of her because she contributed nothing to any philanthropic or socially useful cause, lived the life of an unrepentant miser, and wrecked the emotional health of her two children who remained childless, devoting themselves to burying the name of their mother. Hetty Green was forged in the mold of Moloch, as she symbolically sacrificed her children to the gods of greed. In telling her story aesthetically, I hoped to uncover a therapeutic question – why did I choose such a dark figure as a guide?

I stumbled upon Hetty Green while reading a history of my home town, Hoboken, New Jersey, which I returned to at the age of 35. It seems that she lived in Hoboken, a working-class immigrant town, to avoid the New York City tax collectors and to reap the benefits of low-cost housing. Around the turn of the century, with more than $60 million in cash, Hetty lived in a cold water flat for $19 a month.

The last of my old Hoboken relatives were in their dotage, and my two great aunts remembered running errands around the turn of the century for Hetty Green who gave them each a penny for their daily labors. I surely had a sentimental attachment to this daunting figure who played a minor role in my family's history. And as I have always been attracted to the dramatic, the bizarre, and the unexplained, Hetty Green well fit the bill.

With a modest awareness of my motivation to dramatize the life of Hetty Green, I rushed through a draft of the play. It was voluminous, unfocused, and sprawling. Recalling an early meeting with a professional writer who told me that she wrote about everything she knew in each new piece, I threw in everything I had on my mind – moral and ironic songs, lyrical choruses, critiques of academics, doctors, lawyers, and a meditation on greed. At the centerpiece was a battle for the estate of Hetty's aunt and the ensuing legal case. From my reading of the historical records, it seemed pretty clear that Hetty manipulated her aged aunt to write a will favorable to herself. But when her aunt challenged her power, Hetty resorted to illegal means – forging her aunt's name on a fabricated will that left her everything.

After sending this version around to various producers and directors and receiving as many rejections, I joined a new theatre company and foisted my play upon my colleagues. We were scheduled for production when my co-directors staged a coup, sending both Hetty and I out the door. It was a temporary setback. I was wounded but undaunted.

Several years later, I teamed up with a director from New Orleans, a place most tolerant of the dramatic, unexplained and bizarre, and produced a completely re-written version of the play. The New Orleans experience was a collaboration and the director, a gifted and strong-willed person, had definite ideas about Hetty and her exploits. This version became lean, cold and cruel – I let go of all extraneous characters and scenes. The new version became a tirade from a pathological person who destroyed all those in her way, even as she destroyed herself. I added two children – a young, innocent Hetty Green, and a young, wounded Ned Green, her son whose leg was amputated because of an infection that set in after his mother refused to pay a doctor's fee following a sledding accident. The children, though cute, were impossible to direct, and I secretly wished they would disappear from the script. At the end of the experience, the director said: 'OK, let's really find this play now. Let's get the re-writes done and take it to New York.' I said, 'Sure,' shuffled some pages for some months, then remaindered Hetty to a drawer in a black filing cabinet in my basement for ten years. The play was lost to me. More significantly, Hetty Green, the one who inspired my creative efforts, was gone, unknowable.

During the ensuing ten years, I all but abandoned my creative work in the theatre. Hetty Green, I thought, was the final blow. When I lost a sense of her character and the play that bore her name, I felt stuck with nowhere to go. Fortunately, I had a retreat – a fortress that could protect me from the wounds of Hetty Green and the creative life. I called my fortress drama therapy and nurtured it very carefully, renovating its rooms and expanding its walls. I didn't abandon writing, but its qualities shifted. This was my time for expository writing, academic and critical writing. I was creating theory and discussing matters of research, training, applications, and clinical outcomes. Near the end of those ten years, I found myself drawn back to the creative impulse, having completed a complex theatrically-based structure, a taxonomy of roles, categorizing 84 role types drawn from the history of Western dramatic literature (see Landy 1993b).

My academic writing began to shift. I found myself wanting to tell stories again. The music that I had stopped writing also began to surface. I realized I hadn't listened to music, except as a background to some other activity, in many years. I started playing the piano again. I found myself searching for the original songs I had written for the play and discovered 'Money Is An End In Itself,' which begins:

> What is it about money,
> That makes us all desire it,
> That makes us all want more and more,
> And not tire of acquiring it?

> Money is not very pretty,
> Like stamps and plants and art,
> It's green or brown or silver hue,
> Cannot, itself, please me or you,
> It must be something more to do,
> With things of the mind and the heart.

Approaching my fiftieth birthday, some 15 years after completing my first draft, and ready to return to New Orleans for a drama therapy conference, Hetty Green returned with a vengeance. She called herself up in me and, as usual, her power was too compelling to ignore. The unasked and unanswered questions kept surfacing: who is this greedy, controlling, horrifying witch? Why have I resuscitated her? What part of me is Hetty Green? Guided by these questions and with my muse clearly visible within my mind's eye, I began to write a third draft.

In the New Orleans version, Hetty's daughter, Sylvia, was mute, a defeated shadow of her mother. In the new version, she speaks. In the New Orleans version, Hetty's son, Ned, was impotent and foolish. He could only confront his mother as she lay dead, and only then in a brief, fleeting way. In the new version he demonstrates flashes of insight and strength. There are no more children in the play; only childish qualities of all the players. These are adults coping with a force more powerful than themselves, struggling to find a way, however small, to feel victorious. In the earlier version they began and ended as victims, helpless against such a formidable demon.

In the new version, I even found some way to humanize Hetty. Toward the end of the play, she is alone in a bank vault, surrounded by mountains of her cash. She is old and has a painful hernia that requires medical attention. She summons a doctor to the vault and is alone with him:

DOCTOR: I don't usually pay house calls.

HETTY: I have no house.

DOCTOR: Bank calls, then. Vaults.

HETTY: I'm not dead yet, Doctor.

*(Hetty hides her ledgers from him.)*

DOCTOR: One fact we can both agree upon. Why did you call me here?

HETTY: Why did ye come?

DOCTOR: I like challenges.

HETTY: What kind of challenges ye have in mind?

DOCTOR: The healing of the truly sick and needy.

HETTY: There aren't enough in yer free clinics?

DOCTOR: Too many. An endless supply of diseases out there. New strains everyday, all of the same origin – poverty. Yours is different.

HETTY: No, Doctor. Not different at all. Not now. I am a poor victim, don't ye see. Of scarcity. My poor flesh and bones have rebelled. I need to be made straight before my mission is complete. Do ye understand?

DOCTOR: I'm afraid I'm at a complete loss.

HETTY: Don't be afraid. Come closer. My body is poor and ye are a healer of the poor. Come closer.

*(She takes his hand and puts it on her groin.)*

HETTY: Can ye fix me?

*(A stick falls to the ground from under Hetty's dress. The Doctor is astonished.)*

HETTY:      Ye never see a stick before? I use it to hold up my hernia. Ye can put yer eyes back in yer head, Doctor. How much will ye charge to operate?

DOCTOR:     I must examine you first, Mrs. Green.

HETTY:      What for? I have a mean hernia. Plain and simple. She's out of control. Strains to push her head through my groin. I think she wants to be born.

DOCTOR:     How long have you experienced pain?

HETTY:      20 years. Maybe more. She's finally caught up with me.

DOCTOR:     I would advise an operation as soon as possible.

HETTY:      What'll it cost?

DOCTOR:     $150. That's my fee. The hospital will charge you extra for the room, medicine, nurses...

HETTY:      Art thou mad?

DOCTOR:     You think about it.

HETTY:      $150 to make a few cuts!?

            *(Hetty grabs his hand, striking out with it in the air, making pretend cuts. She then doubles over in pain.)*

DOCTOR:     Or the pain, Mrs. Green. It's your choice.

HETTY:      What kind of choice is that, Doctor?

DOCTOR:     What possible use could all this money be to you? If you were to live to 100 and spend a million dollars a month, you would still have millions left over.

HETTY:      *(pushing him back)* Get out.

DOCTOR:     *(holding her by the arms)* What is your mission?

HETTY:      Get out now!

DOCTOR:     To hoard, to squeeze the poor, to keep it all for your own greedy

            *(She pulls away from him.)*

HETTY:      To keep it from the dirty hands of doctors who are supposed to heal and lawyers who are supposed to defend and blood relatives who are supposed to love. Ye are the greedy ones, don't ye know. Ye steal our health, our God-given sense of justice, our childhood. Don't ye see – it all comes out in every silver dollar, ever shred of legal tender. The lie is plain to see. In God we trust. If we did, we wouldn't need yer kind of whoring – ye pays yer money, ye gets yer wish. The truth, it's staring at ye every time ye lock eyes with that bald eagle, shining like the sun. Every abuse from every rotten father, every silence from every self-hating, sickly mother, every golden, stinking drop of our worthlessness – it's there. It's our only real mirror, that shekel.

DOCTOR: When one looks in the mirror, Mrs. Green, one sees the reverse of what is real.

HETTY: In that silver dollar I see myself as straight and pure and powerful. It is my correction, that silvered glass, my justice. After I have collected all the booty on the face of the earth, then can I rest assured that I am the fairest of them all. No more vanity. What is my mission, ye ask? To do business and to do it right. Do ye get it now?

This scene is as close as Hetty gets to making sense of herself as victim, one who feels powerless and therefore needs to victimize others in order to feel powerful. I couldn't have written it before, because I didn't fully understand this dynamic. In fact, my particular obsession with Hetty Green was just beginning to make sense. If this fictional character was a mirror, then she reflected back those parts of my psyche that are miserly and controlling, that are simultaneously powerless and powerful.

A friend, having read the current version of the play, mentioned that I was able to complete it because I finally resolved the wound of growing up with a confusing, narcissistic mother, one who claimed the right of victim even as she exerted the cold control of victimizer. There were times growing up when I felt as weak as Ned Green struggling desperately to shake off the insatiable mother.

But this sense of Hetty Green as mother, I thought, was only part of the picture. Hetty Green was also me. She is my tendency to hoard feelings, to hurt others who represent those who have hurt me, to hate in the name of love, to rage against the injustices of the healers and judges and lovers instead of facing my own limitations in all three roles, and to believe that it is possible to rise above vanity by thrift and modesty. Hetty Green is my shadow, my dark double, the other side of the social personae of respectable father, teacher, therapist.

As I finished the play, a synchronistic episode occurred. My apparently tight, loving, extended family split apart based upon a battle over a will left by the last of the Hoboken relatives, one who, as a child, used to run errands for Hetty Green. After a fierce court battle, which involved accusations that one miserly relative illegally manipulated the estate, the shade of Hetty Green seemed very much alive. Could she have been present in this idyllic family all along? Maybe

I had subliminally learned her lessons about greed and covetousness, even while I was taught by the elders to accept the myth of the loving, harmonious family. In that there was no room for Hetty Green within this myth, she managed to sneak in through a basement window and hide in the family shadows, working her dark magic secretly.

Life, I thought, does indeed mirror art. Or is it the other way around? It could be that both sides of the mirror are true indicators of at least a psychological reality. I could complete my art, because I was no longer in denial of my life. I was psychologically ready to face the demonic figure within my psyche who was born and reared within my family of origin. Yet it was hard to face an internal figure with such extreme qualities. Hetty was too angry, too obsessed, too strident, too outrageous and disturbed. But then I realized that it has often been hard for me to see the mean, the balanced and calm, without first exposing myself to the extreme and severe. Sometimes, I thought, it takes an earthquake or maiming, a holocaust or plague to awaken a culture or a psyche from its complacency. Hetty Green was my wake up call. My fear was that if I were to fully embrace her, who is my rage and passion, then I would need to abandon my secure and successful life as a drama therapist and as an academic.

An old writer friend, well into his 70s, who has feared his impending death every day for 65 years, chooses to write about a young, once virile gay man, emaciated and dying of AIDS, who risks all to experience one final moment of erotic pleasure. A client, climbing back up from a series of devastating losses of his family and his mental and physical health, writes about an actor dying of AIDS in a hospital, who is finally able to break through all the lies hidden within the moral fiber of his family and church and say: 'this is who I am and it is OK.' AIDS as a muse, an extreme mask of death and destruction, also unmasks a character's ability to find an inner dwelling where there is no longer a need for self-deception.

It is the creative act – the passionate search for form and order within the chaotic nether regions of mind and heart – that has forged my professional and personal identity. When caught in the creative act, I am wrestling with my demons. Hetty Green is one. But she is more than a demon. In many ways she is indeed my muse, one who inspires me to take on the role of artist. In the taxonomy of roles (Landy 1993b), I write that the function of the artist is: 'to assert the creative principle, envisioning new forms and transforming old ones. Because of the spiritual demands and responsibilities of the aesthetic process, the artist often pays an emotional price.' (p.241)

As her son is fearing the impending loss of his leg, Hetty Green, the visionary artist, urges him to look ahead. These are her chilling words:

> What is a leg, anyway? A nuisance, ye ask me. We'd be better off with better designed parts to get us from place to place – wheels, ha! Why not wheels instead of legs? What do ye say, Ned?..It's our responsibility to live on, son, into the 20th century. A new age is dawning and Hetty

Howland Robinson Green will be there to exploit it! Wheels, wheels instead of whales, that's the modern age!..There are no limits in my 20th century – steam engines, locomotives, transcontinental freight cars, horseless buggies with internal combustion engines, Stanley Steamers and automobiles of all conceivable value, massive steel machines spinning uncontrolled off the assembly lines.

The emotional price paid by Hetty Green is great. In neglecting her son's human needs, she loses his love. This is the pain she must bear. As my muse, Hetty Green is a very horrifying figure. On the surface, she represents all the qualities I have abhorred my entire life – denial, confusion, greed, self-love, coldness, grandiosity, and exploitation. Yet, like Allen Ginsberg evoking Moloch, I ask her to rescue me from a crisis. I seem to be saying, 'help me find my lost creative life.' And she responds by appearing in her dirty, shapeless black dress, veiled, as always, with all her powers of harassment and humiliation intact, ready to pounce. She is a hurricane who destroys all those who get in her way and then wipes the landscape clean. She is relentless and extreme, uncompromising and clear-headed.

If Hetty Green is my muse, no wonder it is so difficult to stay connected to her hateful persona. It becomes so much easier to teach others about her and to help others make peace with their demonic tendencies. Over the years, when I have felt most vulnerable to criticism and most defeated by the world of critics and judges, I have banished my muse and quietly suffered a terrible sense of abandonment and loneliness. In her place I have fashioned personae marked by critical and judgmental qualities. In bringing her back home, I have re-discovered not only my ability to be a passionate artist, but also a more compassionate teacher and therapist. By embracing my furious need to create, I also acknowledge my need to play midwife to those ready to procreate.

And so I welcome this cold wind, this raging fire, this toxin that restores my health. She drives me on my journey, stokes my feelings of rage and outrageousness, points me in the direction of my dark wounds, illuminating them. Hetty Green gives me back my voice and prods me to sing the song of myself with no holds bared. She is my nightmare and judge who challenges me to confront my lovelessness and my alienation. Without her, I can help others and fulfill my professional responsibilities in a good enough way. But in order to help myself reclaim my creativity, I need her.

At 50, I recognize my tendencies to live in dark places. By invoking my dark muse, I am closer to understanding my need for such figures – they turn me back to the light.

# CHAPTER 17

# The Double Life

## A Case Of Bipolar Disorder

## Introduction

Sam, a man in his late 30s, worked through the process of drama therapy for three years, meeting with me on the average of once a week. Much of our work involved playing in role to help Sam reconstruct a balanced role system and learn to live with his many ambivalences. I will present his case generally in terms of role theory (see Landy 1993b), a systematic framework for understanding personality as a system of interdependent roles reflective of types of characters found repeatedly throughout the history of dramatic literature. In discussing this case, I will make reference to the taxonomy of roles (Landy 1993b), a major piece of the overall framework, devised to identify and specify role types in terms of their qualities, functions, and styles. In keeping within the bounds of role theory, Sam's psychiatric condition, bipolar disorder, will be seen as an imbalance of roles and his treatment will be seen as a move toward restoring a balance and discovering a way to live within the ambivalence of opposing tendencies.

Like many, Sam led a double life, caught between many contradictory impulses. He seemed to me to be bipolar more on a metaphorical level than on a clinical one as he attempted to negotiate the north and south of his moods. Even certain facts of his family history supported the polar splits. His maternal grandparents were solid, working class people; his paternal grandparents were wealthy professionals. He was born into two faiths, from a Jewish father and Catholic mother. As we shall see, he attempted to live a moral life of faith, even as he believed himself to be immoral and faithless. A wounded man, Sam suffered not only from a psychological disorder, but also from a chronic congenital arthritic condition that flared up with some regularity. Yet, often in denial of his disability, Sam pushed his body and soul to the limits – alternately overindulging and starving himself. Sam sought therapy because he didn't know how to live with his double tendencies. In the past he sought extreme remedies – 'blowing his mind' through psychedelic drugs or speaking in tongues in a cultist fundamentalist church in the hopes of being born again. He could play Jekyll or Hyde, but could not accept that both roles exist interdependently. When playing Jekyll, he longed for the primitive pleasures of Hyde. When playing Hyde, he experienced anxiety and shame, longing for the security of the good doctor. My therapeutic goal was to help Sam discover an effective way to live the double life, accepting the inevitable tensions born of paradox.

It was the winter of Sam's discontent. His marriage of seven years was going badly. He supported his wife and seven-year-old son as a plumbing contractor. His job was to hire plumbers to work on commercial buildings, and although he did well when he worked, he had difficulty keeping up with the demands to search out new jobs and to collect his fees after a job was completed. Money was tight.

Sam was a highly creative and playful person who spoke with great wit and spontaneity. He was a musician and composer whose dream was to establish himself as a success in the world of jazz. He had played with a number of accomplished musicians who recognized him as a gifted improvisor, but one who seemed unable to sustain the routine of commitment, practice and rehearsal essential to make it professionally. Despite early accolades, he was not able to live out his dream.

Sam's discontents were based in a number of losses. Several years before starting therapy, Sam had committed himself to a fundamentalist church which disbanded when the leader departed. Sam's faith and moral identity hung in the balance. He had committed himself to a marriage with Bonnie, who herself bore wounds from early childhood sexual abuse, but they argued endlessly and couldn't seem to find a way to make peace, even in front of their son, Gabe. He had committed himself to his music, but at the height of his ability, he lost the will to perform. His withdrawal from music occurred as his father lay dying at the age of 55 in a mental hospital. He had committed himself to be a surrogate husband to his mother when his father abandoned the family – Sam was 8 at the time. But as he grew tired of his mother's perfectionism and verbal abuse in the name of kindness, he desired separation.

In the three years we worked together, Sam made a number of painful but profound discoveries that led him to a more balanced state. One of the most painful was to learn that he suffered the same disability as his father. In his search for a legacy from his brilliant and gifted father, a promising criminal lawyer, he discovered that he had inherited the double life that led to his father's demise. This discovery was made in a psychiatric ward, where he was admitted after an unusually severe manic episode.

Bipolar disorder, although occurring with much individual variation in terms of cause and symptoms (see American Psychiatric Association 1995), is generally a disturbance of mood manifested by depressive and/or manic episodes. These episodes can occur infrequently or with some regularity, especially when a person is under considerable stress. When diagnosed, the disorder can be controlled with medication and/or psychotherapy. While in the throes of a depressive or manic episode, an individual is controlled by the disabling qualities of either state.

## The Silent Scream

Early in our work together, Sam reported feelings of depression. When I asked him to embody that feeling, he created a drawing which he called: Mondo Wiley – The Silent Scream of the Hippo. Speaking about the picture, he said: 'The hippo mouth is surrounded by razor wire. It is screaming. He has a bloody eye that was hit. No body. He can go in either direction. Depression as a free-floating eye, detached from myself. There are demons in the stomach. I am watching myself be destructive to myself'. Then he added: 'Thank God my mother didn't understand me. She expects me to achieve, but on her terms.'

This disembodied figure of depression led Sam into talking about his mother, a once gifted and promising artist and teacher, who had given up her career to raise a family and support her husband's ambitions. When abandoned by her husband, she felt betrayed and incapable of resuming her former career. Even as she embraced a Christian orthodoxy, she became moody and controlling. While growing up, Sam saw his role as a fixer of his mother's moods. Fearful that she would spin out of control, he became a martyr who would sacrifice his needs for hers. At many times he felt powerless in her presence, screaming silently for fear of being heard and punished for daring to assert his needs. He often felt detached from his feelings. Like the hippo, an oversized, anachronistic beast with a gigantic mouth that should be able to roar and command respect, he felt silenced and trapped in a threatening, prison-like vortex. He felt alienated from his mother, a potential source of nurturance and comfort, and from parts of himself – his oversized body, his unacceptable feelings, and his voice. Feeling like an imprisoned beast with a bloodied eye that cannot see and an enormous mouth that cannot scream, Sam shut down in the face of his mother.

## The Shrine of Broken Intellect

The following week, Sam's depression expanded, spilling over to thoughts of his father. I asked him if there was a way to express these thoughts. He suggested that he build a box. His box, a rectangular wooded structure, about 30 by 40 inches, resembled an Alexander Calder construction in form. The content, however, was uniquely Sam's.

A small rubber baby boy sat naked on a long screw protruding from between his legs. Sam said: 'He is almost crucified on the screw. He can really live here and have a life. But it requires faith and creativity.' A rubber band was attached

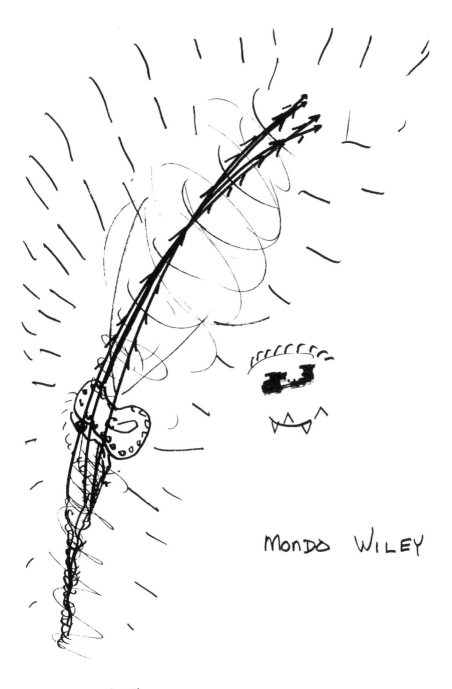

*Figure 17.1 Mondo Wiley*

from the screw to the far end of the box. Sam said: 'This is dangerous. The rubber band could snap and decapitate the baby, just as he is sitting there.'

Sam placed a bible in the box which he called: 'Personal Bible, offering verses of comfort, assurance and salvation.' Alongside the bible was a novelty board with various points labeled: No, Yes, Maybe, Pass the Buck, See Your Analyst, Reorganize. Sam referred to it as a Ouija board, a means of divining the future, of prophesying. He named the board an 'obolynx, a thing that will solve my problems.'

For Sam, pressing the four corners of the box revealed four spiritual laws, defined by Sam as:

1. You're an idiot – you don't understand God and never will.

2. You're a stupid jerk – you've already committed sin.

3. Drop dead – it's better because then you will go to heaven.

4. You're a dope – you should be dopey and doped up.

Two pieces of paper reading: 'Not negotiable,' lay beside the bible, along with pages from Sam's father's memo pad. Sam said that these notes, taken from meetings with his clients, showed his indifference to them. As well as scribblings about a particular law case, the father listed groceries to be bought and errands to be run. Sam referred to these notes as lost pages that have been given to the baby on the screw.

Other items in the box included: broken glass, dried seed pods, a magnifying glass, a sentimental poem about the coming of spring that Sam has copied out of a book in fourth grade, a photographic negative of a cast column labeled 'Joy,' early pornographic slides belonging to his father, and a Christian Science pamphlet entitled: 'Life in a Peaceful New Land.'

Sam referred to the box as 'the shrine of broken intellect.' Why would Sam want to worship broken intellect, I wondered at this early time in our work together? He provided a clue in saying: 'In trying to figure out my father, I can get closer to myself. I want a relationship with him. I want him to help me separate myself from him and him from me.' Sam's father had been dead for more than ten years yet he held Sam close. This man of great intellect and great potential, this contender for the love and respect of his son, had, indeed, failed, ending his days in mental institutions, losing his mind and his dignity, his professional credibility and livelihood, forfeiting his roles of loving husband, father, and friend. Sam was headed in similar directions, with a shaky family life, a precarious mental state, and an inability to realize his potential as an artist or artisan.

Like his father before him, Sam seemed incapable of diverting from the inevitable path of broken intellect. His depression was very much about that incapacity. Despite the messages of hope contained in the box – the child's hopeful poem of the coming of Spring, the fundamentalist vision of a new world, the verses of comfort and salvation – the baby, the most vulnerable and needy part of Sam, was in grave danger. He was naked, without protection, in danger of being crucified, decapitated, castrated. He was surrounded by a message that this state of being is 'Not negotiable.' The spiritual laws reinforced his state of intellectual disintegration – he was an idiot, jerk, and dope. He was surrounded by the errata of his father's failures and further images of emptiness – broken glass and dried seed pods.

Following this session, I had a strong sense that Sam needed an object of worship. His state of alienation might have been about a loss of faith. He was playing out the role of lost one as a result of no longer being able to play the orthodox. The orthodox persona, as specified in the taxonomy of roles (Landy 1993b), is motivated by the need to believe 'fully in the principles of a single faith, practicing its rituals and receiving sustenance from its teachings' (p.233). Having lost his church, about to lose his family, and having long since lost his parents as moral and sustaining role models, Sam required a new object of faith. But in the absence of a reliable orthodoxy, Sam chose to worship its antithesis, the shadow side of a moral belief system, represented by broken intellect and disembodied states of being.

Yet even though Sam was lost, I sensed a glimmer of hope. As became clear in his box construction, Sam's world was rich in paradox. He later entitled his construction, 'Desert Lodge,' which though dry and removed was still a home. The danger and fear in Sam's construction was offset by images of joy and hope. The magnifying glass, Sam reflected, like the photographic negative, turns things around. But the thing itself is still present. 'Joy', the negative photographic image, has a positive counterpart in the world. The magnifying glass, though it distorts, also helps one to see better. The dried seed pods offer the hope for new life. The obolynx which might prophesy 'No,' might also prophesy 'Maybe' or 'Yes.'

Given Sam's openness to contradiction and paradox, I sensed my direction – to help him discover ways to live in the ambivalence of the roles of orthodox believer and nihilist, of lost one and heroic searcher, of artist and artisan, of father and son. My aim was not only to help him separate from painful, destructive relationships, but also to connect with those who might help him nurture and care for himself effectively. Learning to care for himself, I thought, might lead to opening his heart to another.

Sam was angry at many people and directed that anger inwardly, an act which led to further depression. Anger was a quality that was noticeably missing in the various roles he enacted in drama therapy sessions over many months. In moments demanding anger, Sam would often smile, broadly and expansively. In our work together, he would transform anger to forgiveness, a quality he defended by citing verses from scripture. His anger toward Bonnie was building steadily as the relationship dissolved. She was dating other men and openly reminding him of his sexual and psychological failures.

## The Flower Bomb

Sam came into a session talking about feeling angry. But with a smile on his face and a jokey demeanor, he appeared incapable of expressing anger. I asked Sam to draw a picture of anger. He drew a flower. It had a long stem that was attached to a box with a handle. He referred to the handle as a detonator. 'Stupid people like me,' he said, 'would be fooled that this is a flower. It is really an instrument of destruction.'

In juxtaposing an object of beauty with an object of destruction, Sam entered deeper into his internal world of paradox. The meaning of the paradox was clear to him as he said:

> 'I want to fool myself into thinking that anger is a beautiful thing. Life is like that – God creates flowers, but they are really objects to electrocute and detonate. My desire is to be rescued from self-destruction. The bomb is illegal. It's not legitimate to express anger, so it has to be disguised in a pretty form.'

> 'What would happen if you expressed anger? I asked.'

> 'If it came out, it would destroy me, Bonnie, and Gabe, my son. If it came out, it would be too big.'

The metaphor of anger as a flower bomb was very rich. I wondered how and when the bomb would explode. I thought that Sam's disguise of flower child could only last so long. It seemed to be the role that kept him in his depression. Where was the bomb? Was that the manic episode that I was yet to see fully expressed? How could the bomb be justified, legitimized, shrunk in size so as to be more acceptable? It occurred to me that many acts of terrorist bombing are acts of disguise and surprise – a bomb as a piece of mail, a suitcase, a book, a radio or clock. Sam's bomb as a flower was unique. He was fully invested in making things pretty so that he could forestall anger and forget that he was sitting on a detonator that could go off at any moment and blow his cover. And what was he covering up? It seemed to me there were many levels and many roles to uncover. It also seemed to me that the process would take time and trust and that it was not the right time to remove the flower. Sam would proceed petal by petal.

## Cats and Dogs

Two months later, Sam recalled a story about a white cat he found at the SPCA. Although the cat was very frail and crippled, he named her Tiger. It was a time when Sam's father was institutionalized and Sam was living in his apartment near the psychiatric hospital. He was in a wild, almost manic phase and he needed a companion. Tiger fit the bill. According to Sam, she was small, lovable, naive, childlike, with no hostility or bitterness about her. And she was completely attuned to Sam. Sam was supporting himself as a dishwasher but got fired for bursting out in song from the kitchen to entertain the customers. He left town and he and Tiger slept out under the stars. He watched the sky as big black birds circled around the small crippled white cat. Soon, he and Tiger moved back to the city where Tiger grew weaker and frailer. Out of concern, Sam gave her away to friends who lived on a farm upstate. Tiger regained her strength and grew her white fur back. Then one day, two large black dogs happened by. One destroyed the cat.

I asked Sam to take on the role of the dog preparing for the kill. He spoke:

> Let's get that cat. Kill it. We almost got it the other day. What a kill! I didn't know if it was a rat or a cat. You gotta do it when nobody's watching. It's not often you get to kill a cat. I can't wait. It's a boring life. What else is there to do? I like to break things up. I'm still young and strong. I like to scare people. It's very exciting. Otherwise, I feel empty. The cat's an idiot. If I was afraid of the cat, I wouldn't try to kill it. Maybe we won't kill it. Once I go, I go. If I kill the cat, then they'll bring me back and lock me up. You can't always please everybody. I shouldn't feel bad. I'm nobody's puppet. No morals or ethics. I'll do what I want. Forget it. Every dog has its day.

Following the enactment, Sam spoke of the dog as energetic, strong, territorial and brutally aggressive. 'What's the dog's purpose in life?' I asked. 'To play. Killing is the result of playing. After eating the cat, his purpose is to be man's best friend.'

Sam named the dog Pfeiffer. Pfeiffer was not angry. He was just behaving according to his nature. He was amoral, a natural born killer.

In examining Sam's story, it appeared that Pfeiffer was a desirable part of Sam. Sam referred to him as a double. Yet the larger part of Sam felt like the cat, ironically named Tiger. Even the name Pfeiffer felt ironic to Sam as 'it doesn't fit. Pfeiffer sounds like a nincompoop.'

If only Sam could play, if only he could stake out his territory and defend it, if only he could live the natural life without fearing the moral consequences of his aggression. But feeling more like the Tiger, a paradoxically weak, deformed, helpless and gentle creature, Sam had trouble holding onto the desired qualities. At the end of the session he said: 'Pfeiffer is my twin. Unfortunately, he's the one that gets put to sleep.' It could be that Sam could not hold onto the playful, aggressive, destructive qualities precisely because his moral, orthodox roles were so dominant. If, as the bible says, one trades an eye for an eye, a tooth for a tooth, then Pfeiffer, awake to his instincts, must pay for his destructive acts with his life. In Sam's world, swift, punitive biblical justice was never very far away.

## The Pastor

The church Sam joined was small, independent, and fundamentalist Christian. It was comprised, according to Sam, mostly of bright, creative people, many of whom were artists and professionals, or aspiring to be so. All were lost people in search of a meaningful and profound connection to God. Sam was recruited by Bonnie who, as a young, attractive undergraduate, embodied many of the sexual and spiritual qualities that he so desired.

The church was founded and held together by a pastor, a charismatic man who dictated a strict morality to his followers. Sam tithed ten per cent of his income to the church, like others. And like others, he sometimes spoke in tongues and prophesied the future.

In retrospect, Sam claimed that he did many things against his will – withholding sexual gratification, repressing immoral thoughts and feelings, even marrying. In that Sam was used to holding in feelings, it was not difficult to abide by the repressive dictates of the pastor, at least on the surface. When the pastor informed the men of the church that masturbation was a sin, Sam acquiesced. In therapy, he recalled that as a child he would achieve pleasure by retaining control of his bowels, cutting off the movement. But as the pastor required him to cut off his sexual pleasure, a need that he so desperately wanted to express, Sam became angry. True to form, that anger remained unexpressed.

In therapy, however, shortly after working with the role of Pfeiffer, the amoral, aggressive dog, Sam's anger surfaced. He began to re-experience the feeling of being controlled by the pastor and giving up his power to the church. For the first time, he spoke of feeling like a victim, specified in the taxonomy (Landy 1993b) as 'vulnerable, trapped, defenseless, under the control of another's will or the will of fate' (p. 194). I had noted (Landy 1993b) that many of the classical heroes begin as victims but become ultimately powerful enough to do battle with their victimizers. I shared this with Sam, along with a hope that he, too, might discover his heroic qualities.

In fact, Sam was able to take a heroic step. It was several years since the pastor left his congregation and moved to another city far away. He urged his followers to stay connected to their fundamental beliefs, but the organization immediately fell apart. Summoning up all his courage, Sam called the pastor. Hearing his voice and accusatory tone, the pastor said:

> 'You are in a great deal of pain and confusion. If I've caused you pain, I'm sorry, but you are in a dangerous place right now. Are you in fellowship [that is, are you part of a church group]?'

> 'I am, replied Sam, I'm on the phone with you.'

> 'Are you in a church now?'

> 'No.'

> 'We should be in church.'

Then Sam said: 'I am not confused right now. Are you in fellowship?'

The pastor responded: 'You are dangerous because you are not in church. Don't have any expectations of me.'

'You're missing the point,' said Sam. 'Do you want to know what the point is?'

'I'm not angry…not yet,' replied the pastor.

'The point is,' said Sam, 'that I don't want to go away from this conversation angry. I respect you. We're in different places. Pray for me but don't pray that I'll return to the church. We're not so different.'

After Sam related the conversation to me, he said: 'I faced the mythical person. I felt raped by him. Not with a penis, but with a black pole. I wanna kill him. I'm worried that he's gonna judge me. All the way from across the country. My mother has the same set of values.'

Although Sam was able to take the heroic step of calling his perceived victimizer and confronting him to some degree, he still felt unsatisfied. In fact, he was unable to stay with his anger and direct it at the pastor. Consequently, he turned it back on himself, taking on the role of one sadistically violated.

In further exploring his anger, Sam spoke of his role ambivalence. On the one hand he still felt himself to be a Christian fundamentalist whose credo was: 'Love your neighbor as yourself.' On the other hand, he recognized the need to fight those neighbors who would attempt to control him in the name of love.

The connection between pastor and mother was a significant one for Sam, as he saw both as embodying a basic contradiction, one that confused and hurt him deeply – love disguised as control, power, and judgment. I thought of the flower bomb. Like the pastor, his mother was a Christian and harshly judged those with less orthodox beliefs.

Sam was unable to make the link between pastor and father, but I intuited there was some connection. As was the case with his father, the pastor abandoned Sam when he was so much in need of moral guidance and of fathering, that is, learning what it means to be a man. Sam's father left him alone with his mother, who was ultimately looking for a substitute lover, someone to meet her own needs. She was not able to fulfill her role of mother and care for her son. The pastor left Sam alone with his wife, who was ultimately looking for a substitute father (her real father had sexually abused her), someone to make up for the pain of the past. She was unable to fulfill her role of wife and love her husband.

In reflecting upon Sam's comment of feeling raped by the pastor, I recalled his earlier comment that the pastor almost lost his penis from an infection following a vasectomy. Sex, morality, violence, and retribution were powerfully dramatic themes in Sam's therapy. Neither he nor I really understood how they connected. It was clear, though, that the pastor was a commanding and confusing moral figure for Sam, especially as he cut off his reproductive capacity and almost lost his sexual potency as a result. What did this mean? Could a man be potent and impotent at the same time? Shouldn't the judge also be judged? Could the contradictory qualities of anger and forgiveness, of power and powerlessness coexist within a person wrestling with such intense moral contradictions?

In response to these questions, Sam would later invent stories of a pastor who preached moral sermons by day and cruised the streets of the inner city at night, dressed as a transvestite prostitute. He was the embodiment of the double life.

## The Good Man Who Liked to do Bad

Sam took a further leap into the murky terrain of double life by creating a character he called Rupert Stosh. In Sam's story, Stosh was considered by his wife and children and neighbors to be an exemplary husband, father, and citizen:

> But underneath he owned a slave farm in Georgia. He had 3000 slaves. The extent of his evil was great. He was a partner in a nuclear plant. But it was the slaves underground, pushing the energy, that lit Georgia – no plutonium, just slaves. One day there was a revolt. In retaliation, Slosh killed 50 slaves. Uncertain at first what to do with the bodies, he decided to use them for experiments. He wanted to find a cure for the common cold. He had 10 slaves killed each month. His conscience was clear as he reasoned: 'They have no right to complain; they should be happy they have work!' Stosh got richer and richer. He began to feel guilty that he was the perpetrator of this mini-holocaust. During his lifetime, no one ever found out about him. They thought him to be an upstanding citizen. He died a wealthy man, discovered dead in bed with a 14-year-old nubian slave girl. He had forced her to take poison. After his death, they found out. It was a big international scandal involving collusion between the government and drug companies.

Like the obolynx, the flower, and the pastor, Rupert Stosh was a figure embodying contradiction. Sam revealed his dual nature in moral terms. He was an evil man disguised as a good man. In the taxonomy (Landy 1993b pp.185-187), the roles of disguised one and double are conceptualized as sub-types of the ambivalent one. I claim that: 'The disguised one may take on a double identity purposefully, in order to realize a moral objective' (p.186).' And further: 'The double functions to reveal a hidden part of the character's personality' (p.187).

In reflecting upon his story, which he called 'The Good Man Who Liked to Do Bad,' Sam took on the role of Rupert and said: 'I have to cover up my badness until I die. I can't get rid of my need to do bad.'

In exploring his connection to the role of Rupert, the disguised one, Sam noted:

> Rupert can't get out of this thing because he's too afraid of public image. He will not allow himself to be humiliated. I was humiliated. I felt responsible for my parent's divorce. I could never help them when they fought. I wasn't allowed to grieve when my father left or when he died. I wasn't allowed to have bad feelings. My mother was threatened by my bad feelings, by any bad feelings. She is so good on the surface. Everyone sees her as good. She gives her time and her money to moral causes. She worships the Lord. But she took from me. She took so much away.

I began to see why Sam so needed to play out a double identity. He couldn't go public with his bad, unacceptable feelings for fear of being humiliated by his mother. For Sam, she was a Rupert Stosh-like character who had the power to enslave her son, to sexualize and kill him, even while others thought her to be an upstanding pillar of morality. So he split himself in two, taking on the disguise of a jokey, smiling friend in matters of love and religion, hoping that the disguise would cover up his unacceptable feelings of depravity until the day he died.

He did all this, he said, to protect his mother from bad feelings. Looking back at the taxonomy, I came across the role of murderous mother, one who is: 'vengeful, amoral, violent, and murderous' (p.205). This type functions 'to destroy her children.' I wondered if Sam, rather than protecting his mother, was actually protecting himself from a mother whom he perceived as destructive. Maybe he was identified with the nubian slave girl in the story who offers the lesson that the seductive, powerful parent can be both abusive and murderous.

In the fullest reading of this story, I saw Sam as embodying qualities of the opposing roles of tyrant and slave, victimizer and victim, moralist and immoralist. What struck me the most was the extreme images in the story. There were implications of Nazis experimenting on dead bodies, of a megalomaniac presiding over a holocaust, of slavery and child abuse and murder, and even a massive cover-up, attesting to the immorality of institutions.

If this scenario represented, in part, the inner life of Sam, no wonder he required a disguise, an acceptable persona in which to greet the world each day as he played out his roles of son and father and husband and worker. As I was soon to realize, this inner holocaust required further expression in order to allow Sam to reconstruct these everyday roles. And as one who played guide through the scenes of horror, a Virgil to Sam's Dante, I needed to prepare myself for the mythic journey to come.

## The Trial, Execution, and Burial of Bonnie

Sam and Bonnie were at a point of hurting each other and allowing their resentments to spill over onto their son. Bonnie had a new lover and regularly blamed Sam for her previous sexual unhappiness. Sam often felt humiliation when in her presence. As much as he tried to transform his anger into forgiveness, he failed. At times he carried around a burden of unexpressed rage. He tended to experience Bonnie, alternately, in one of three roles: needy, helpless child, erotic seductress, and castrating demon. Fearful of both expressing his negative feelings and letting go, Sam was incapable of separating.

Around this time, Bonnie falsely accused Sam of hitting Gabe. Unable to control his sense of injustice and guilt, Sam struck Bonnie with the back of his hand. This temporary transformation from victim to victimizer, a role Sam could not accept, would have serious consequences on the next two years of his life. Although he would never again play out the role of brutal husband in real life, he was about to explode and needed a safety valve. Drama therapy allowed the release.

In order to cope with the reality of his extreme feelings, I urged Sam to seek a helper. I consulted the taxonomy (Landy 1993b) to see that the function of helper was 'to move the hero further along his path or to rescue another from difficult circumstances, remaining loyal throughout the many twists and turns of the journey' (p.197). I made it clear to Sam that I would serve this function in his therapy. But he also needed a powerful person in the outside world to help him negotiate a separation from Bonnie. I encouraged Sam to find a lawyer, full aware of how difficult it might be to accept the role that was so connected to his father's failure as a professional defender of the accused.

The lawyer helped Sam to separate from Bonnie. Their eventual divorce settlement provided joint custody of Gabe, and it was initially decided that Gabe would live with Sam. Bonnie needed to find her own sense of balance and was incapable around this time of responding to Gabe's need for a nurturing mother. And Sam was both committed to playing the good father and fearful of living alone.

While the lawyer was negotiating the legal terms of the separation, Sam and I worked on the psychological implications. Sam married Bonnie in the church. Sam's loss of the church was traumatic. Now Sam was about to lose Bonnie and his sense of a stable home life. He felt betrayed and forced into the separation. He also felt confused and guilty, having once before experienced the traumatic divorce of his parents. Was he, like his father, the cause of all this misery? Or was the blame to be placed on the unchaste, immoral woman? He chose the latter explanation and proceeded to create an extraordinary ritual, of biblical proportions, to rid himself of his overwhelming feelings of guilt and rage. Not incidentally, he hoped the ritual would finally allow him to sign the legal papers and accept the dreaded separation.

It occurred to me that Sam needed all the power of Old Testament morality to justify his overwhelming feelings. He could not deal with the guilt, so he chose to act out the rage.

The content of Sam's ritual, which was to be a trial and execution, was brutal, involving stylized acts of torture, humiliation, and dismemberment. The object of brutality was a naked female doll, supplied by Sam. The formal structure that he devised was notable for its built-in controls and safeguards. To distance himself from violent feelings, he created several fictional personae. The primary figure was Richard, the wronged husband seeking justice through retribution. At first, Richard appeared to me as a priest, practiced in the spiritual art of ritual sacrifice. But then, as Sam seemed to also require the moral weight of the secular legal system, he transformed Richard into lawyer and prosecutor, demanding the ultimate capital punishment, and judge, who would pass sentence to that effect. Sam would assign the actual task of execution to the lawyer who seemed to embody the contradictory morality of defender and perpetrator.

To ensure emotional distance, Richard would also provide a kind of ironic, jokey commentary, taking on the qualities of a witty master of ceremonies. In this role, Sam offered comic relief from the grisly events, allowing both he and I a reminder that this would be an act of artifice and not the real thing.

The ritual was driven by a Bible story chosen by Sam from the 'Book of Judges'. For Sam, this chapter provided a motivation for the trial and ensuing execution. Sam told the story in his own words:

> A concubine runs away from her lover and sleeps around with other men. She returns to her father's house, where her lover is waiting. The father talks the man into staying overnight. The man leaves late the next day with his concubine. They wander about and are finally taken in by a kind farmer. The townsmen, suspicious of the strangers, set out to rape and kill the man, but the farmer persuades them to take the woman instead as the Israelites were in great spiritual turmoil and needed their men. The townsmen rape the woman all night long. She makes her way back to the farmer's house, then dies. The man returns home, cuts the woman up into 12 pieces and distributes the pieces to all the tribes of Israel. When someone is dirty, it is an affront to society. However, a horrible thing is often the cause for unity, as all the men join together.

I took note of the roles of: the immoral woman who becomes a victim (victimizer as victim), the father, the victimized, cuckolded, and wronged man who becomes a victimizer (victim as victimizer), the kindly farmer, the brutal killers, and the Israelites in spiritual turmoil. It seemed significant to me that the two main characters both exemplified the types, victim and victimizer. Thus, they both lived the double life.

I had the sense that all these characters, taken together, reflected Sam's inner world. He was an Israelite in turmoil who needed a kindly helper in order to kill the object of his dis-ease. The immoral object might well be that part of himself that he perceived as bad, unworthy, seductive, false. He attributed these qualities to the concubine. In killing the female part, however, he became bad, a victimizer, himself. This killer role can only be acceptable to Sam if it is taken on for a moral purpose – a 'cause of unity.' For ultimately, Sam sought unity, a balance of his often extremely oppositional feelings. I wondered if this ritual would bring him closer to that goal.

Sam presented his ritual during a span of two weeks, meeting with me for two hours each week. Sam would play all the necessary roles himself. He began the brief trial section with a dialogue between lawyer and judge:

LAWYER:   This is a religious ritual to expel the demons. Bonnie has no defense because she is a professional victim.

JUDGE:    The verdict is death by execution.
          *(He pulls a leg off the doll).*

LAWYER:   For the benefit of society.
          *(He pulls out a sign which reads: THIS IS YOUR LAST CHANCE).*

JUDGE:    Bonnie is found guilty on 7 counts:

1.  Murder of love.

2.  Arson for burning down her relationship with her son.

3.  Theft for stealing breath from Richard and stealing the goodness from herself.

4.  Dismay and regret.

5.  Lying to everyone about who she is and what her intentions are. She must face the truth.

6.  Adultery in the body and in the mind. She was never faithful.

7.  Demon possession, having to do with her illness.

It was very difficult for me to witness the next section, the execution, and to remain unconditionally accepting in my helper role. At times I was horrified and frightened, even to the point of contemplating a halt to the enactment. But I intuited that if I had done so, Sam would have felt shamed and our therapeutic bond would have weakened. I tried to hold my judgements and fears in check. Sam had finally trusted me enough to allow me to accompany him on this dark inner journey. It was too late to turn back.

The execution proceeded as the lawyer lighted candles and heated up a stick in the flame. He held it to the doll's forehead. Richard commented: 'The purpose of this is to anesthesize.' The lawyer responded: 'This is a lobotomy, but it's not working. She will have to be aware of everything to come.' The lawyer poured hot wax and coffee grinds on the body of the doll. Richard recited a running commentary in the jokey fashion of a talk-show host. The lawyer then began to break and cut up the doll into 12 pieces with a very sharp knife, even while she theoretically remained alive and screaming. He cut out her reproductive organs to ensure that she would never again bear children. He cut out the spine and the hand 'which can still grab and strangle.'

Richard and the lawyer then spoke:

RICHARD:   The evil force has been destroyed. It's our godly ordinance to do the right thing. The burial is a distribution of the parts to the 12 people who attended the funeral.

LAWYER:   My client will give the body parts to each of the people. But first, he needs a break. He's gone off to lunch. He was in love with his wife, and he did not want to be part of the trial or the execution. I did the dirty work in his place.

RICHARD:   I didn't want to mess her up or cut her or dirty her. Why couldn't she have cut up herself? There's a part of me that still loves her. I feel what I did was wrong. I was torturing her with hot wax; it was medieval, Old Testament tortures.

For the burial, Sam put on armor which he called the breastplate of righteousness, the shield of faith, the sword of spirit, the helmet of salvation. He put on sandals 'as a preparation for peace,' and said: 'Everything on me is covered. I don't need to feel guilty.'

As Sam took off his clothes and put on pieces of theatrical costume, he looked silly to me. They were more the toys of a child then the garb of a biblical patriarch. I felt uncomfortable witnessing his disrobing and dressing up. His body appeared lean and strong. Although I was fearful that the dressing up might signal an even more grotesque act, I was calmed by the absurdity of this manly warrior in a child's Halloween costume.

As Richard, Sam offered me 'communion,' chocolate and shredded wheat, which I ate. He, too, ate the offering (his favorite chocolate). We were in this together. Then he laid out a delicate cloth napkin and placed the 12 pieces of the doll on the napkin.'They are live,' he said. He sprinkled cinnamon and sugar on the napkin 'to integrate abused women into society,' and said: 'we start with the head.' Richard wrapped up the head, then each of the other body parts, in napkins that were used at his wedding. He tied each with red thread.'I do this with a great deal of compassion for her pain. God didn't tell me to cut up the body. I acted in the moment.' Sam emptied out a bag of unshelled peanuts with painted faces. 'These are the funeral guest,' he said. 'We are all responsible for each other.' Then Sam proceeded to give voice to the 12 funeral guests, most of whom would justify his need for separation and retribution.

The first person to speak, strangely, was Bonnie, herself:

> I'm gonna resurrect. You damaged me. I wasted my hopes on you. You
> were lousy in bed. You'll never recover from your family, especially your
> mother. I reported you to the marshalls. Say good-bye to Gabe. You lied
> to me. You're my number one abuser. You'll pay for it all.

Richard responded:

> This is a letter I received from Bonnie's ghost. I thought that burying
> would be the end. I'm reminded that there are strands that run deep. This
> is one of them. Who is this ghost? This is a person who can't trust me,
> who I took into myself. She's vicious. She thinks that I am a maniac and
> I could have helped her more.

One of the last guests to appear, as a voice, was Sam's mother who said,
cryptically: 'Before you know, they see. Before you see, they know.' I sensed
the god-like omnipotence of this message. Was the mother a god for Sam? Was
she the real object of Sam's trial and execution?

Richard responded:

> She knows her matronly instinct. She's the queen of all drama. She needs
> to be propped up. I'm tired of propping her up. I've set up crutches for
> her. She needs a wheelchair now. I'm not going to be pushing her or
> guiding her. She abuses me because I'm hurt. I've been embarrassed about
> talking about her. She has a greatness and a lot of misery in her life and
> can't help herself. The voice also comes from my father's mania.

Later, Sam's father appeared to tell him:

> Go out and see a movie. Something you like. You're doing a lot. Do I
> have to go on complimenting you forever? Just know you're not a
> manic-depressive like me. Have a piece of chocolate.

And finally Bonnie reappeared as a spirit:

> Richard, this is the voice of Bonnie. I have a deep love for you. With all
> my heart, I think that you are doing the right thing and I support you.
> Find a special place to throw this away. Are you sure you don't want to
> go out one more time? Why don't you give me something.
>
> RICHARD:   I just want to bury you.
>
> BONNIE:    Do it!

To end the ritual, Richard circled a candle over the body parts which he gathered
together and placed in a plastic bag. He added to the bag: a piece of rock from
the Dead Sea, a ring from Bonnie, molten ash from his father's body, and a
T-shirt that said: 'Malcolm X: By Any Means Necessary.'

Sam spoke of the final ritual acts he needed to do: incinerate (the body parts)
and sign (the divorce papers). Before he could do either, he fell in love with an
exotic artist he met by chance. This episode still felt to me like part of the ritual.

Sam saw his love object, Maya, as a magician, a healer and visionary. She came from a foreign country and was behind on her rent. She needed help. Coincidentally, Bonnie also demanded rent money from Sam.

Following their separation, Bonnie gave Richard a present – the shellacked horns of a horseshoe crab as a token/totem of their love. She gave it to him while Gabe was present. Sam felt naked receiving this in front of his son, seeing the talisman as ugly. But he couldn't manage to throw it away. He needed another ritual to rid himself of the noxious and threatening object. Coincidentally, Maya, she for whom rituals came so easily, was going to the sea to perform a ritual of her own. She would hurl the pieces of a broken African love goddess into the ocean.

She asked Sam to accompany her. She performed the ritual effortlessly, tossing the pieces of the statue into the frigid waters while chanting passionately in a foreign language. Sam was enchanted. Maya then urged Sam to chant his own sacred words over the dreaded shellacked horns.

Sam wanted to be moved by the spirit, to speak in tongues as he had in church, to rage and howl. But he held it in, becoming cool as he tossed the horns into the ocean. His only words were those of King David to Saul: 'The lines (lots) have fallen to me in pleasant places.' And then: 'I release you.' He couldn't show his anger in front of Maya, she, so much the goddess, she who could breathe water. He always seemed to be gasping for air.

In therapy, we spoke of the horns as a symbol of his horniness, his sexual frustration and fear. He spoke of his two greatest sexual fears: that of incompetence, of not being man enough, and that of castration, of being emasculated by a violent woman. Sam was satisfied to a point with Maya as object of worship. Because there was no sex, he could remain chaste and delay his anxieties. She became a Peter Pan, an eternal child, a role with which Sam could easily identify.

Sam played out his horniness in masochistic ways. He encouraged Maya to sleep over, hugged her to sleep, but restrained from sex of any kind. They were a good match as she also demanded sexual restraint. One morning, when she was feeling ill, Sam and Gabe bathed her and gave her a massage all over her naked body. He refrained from masturbation with a vehemence displayed only when he was in fellowship. Without touch, with the moral prohibitions intact, Maya remained the goddess, unsullied by his humanity. Among other things Maya served the function of delaying the funeral of Bonnie.

I asked Sam in therapy to look at the other side of the worshipper role. I had conceived of the worshipper or fundamentalist as one who needs to unconditionally embrace an orthodox faith, resisting any new ideas which might shake his foundation (see Landy 1993b, p.233). On the other side, Sam saw the nihilist, one who rejected any sense of purpose.

## Schmarty, Havel, and the Hero: Three Self-Portraits

Sam wanted to draw and created 3 self-portraits. The first was a view of himself in the recent past.

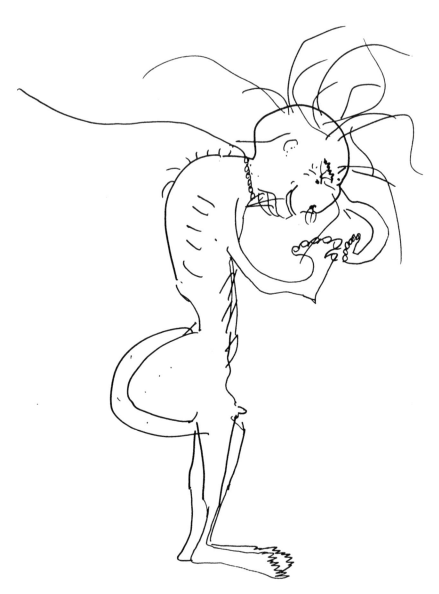

*Figure 17.2 Schmarty*

He characterized the drawing as follows:

> He is an inbred E.T., an embryo, funny and strange, demented and scary.
> His hands are feet; his whole being is alien; a chain is around his neck;
> his sparse hair protrudes wildly; he has an enlarged buttocks and a tiny
> penis. He is scrawny, with hair on his back. I'll call him Schmarty.
> Schmarty out-smarts himself. He's a genius who became a nincompoop,
> because he was always thinking too much.

About the drawing, Sam said:

> I want to destroy my dysfunctional self. I crave unity and restoration.
> 'Be still and know that He is God.' I don't want to include God in the
> equation. I just want to be still and stop clutching for my idea of God.

Sam's second drawing was a view of himself in the present. He called the figure
Havel:

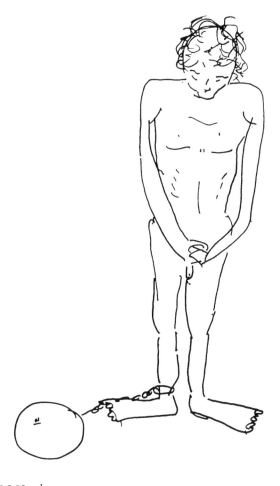

*Figure 17.3 Havel*

He is humbled, ashamed, embarrassed and awkward in taking steps. He is self-conscious and angry with himself that he was recently like Schmarty and that he could be better. He's downcast but has a sense of hope. He's a worthy man, sad, but not letting his sadness determine his course. He's waiting, alone, content with the solitude. There is a ball and chain around his ankle. His penis is still visible, but larger than Schmarty's, hanging down.

The third image was of the future, of Sam's new self, of the hero. He said:

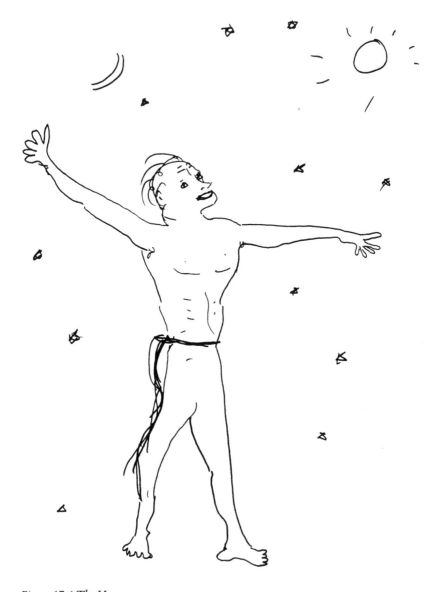

*Figure 17.4 The Hero*

The new Sam should be clothed, regal, adorned. He has his honor back and is not naked before the world anymore. In fact, the image does appear naked, except for a belt or rope around his waist. The upper torso and feet are naked. But his genitals are not exposed, his hands have the right amount of digits. His body is fuller and his arms reach out, toward the sun and moon and stars.

Upon completing these drawings, Sam exclaimed that he was ready to bury the pieces. He came face-to-face with three parts of himself. The first was Schmarty, 'the dysfunctional self,' a lost soul, a sexual misfit, barely human, chained around the neck like a dog. This alien was once smart but now ignorant because he thought too much. Schmarty reminded me of Sam's father, a genius who was outsmarted by his own intellect and died a failure. In many ways, Sam had internalized this sense of intellectual failure, which is embodied as a sub-human alien.

The second part of Sam was Havel, the humbled, the shamed one, who is still imprisoned, though this time around the leg, like a slave. Although depressed, he is hopeful. Although naked and exposed, he is more sexually developed than Schmarty and possibly smarter as he has the ability to wait and to face the future. Havel appeared to be a spiritual figure, a pre-heroic searcher. He also appeared to be a transitional figure between the alien and the hero. This could be the figure that brought Sam into the church in hopes of 'unity and restoration.' With Havel, Sam had a bridge from the failed intellectual alien to the hero, from one version of father to another. In pronouncing the name, Sam seemed to be saying: 'hovel,' literally a broken down house, a dump. I wondered if Sam saw this figure as a bridge between a homeless, hopeless being and a homebody, one who has a place on the planet.

The third creation, Sam, the new man, the heroic one, has found a way to clothe and protect his vulnerability. He is one who can reach out beyond himself into the world. This figure represented a goal for Sam. He is both grounded in the earth, mundane, and reaching for the stars, extraordinary, both dressed and undressed, protected and open. He is one who knows how to live the double life.

In order to bury the pieces of his broken marriage and, more generally, his frustrated relationships with intimates, Sam needed to free himself of the many chains that bound him to an identity as, at best, shameful and depressed, at worst, sick and sub-human. In reviewing the progression of self-images, Sam saw the possibilities of removing the 'old ball and chain.' He could envision a hopeful state, a less vulnerable sense of being. Yet he knew that he still needed to make peace with Schmarty and listen to the wisdom of Havel.

The ritual of trial and execution was over. Although it helped Sam release a degree of anger and confusion, it fell short of Sam's ultimate goals – to destroy his 'dysfunctional self' and bring unity and restoration. It did, however, bring him to the bridge, that transitional point between Schmarty, the alien, and the hero who would continue to search for ways to negotiate the double life.

## Christ in the Power Plant

Sam walked the streets for days, carrying the dismembered pieces of the doll, thinking of ways to dispose of them. It occurred to him that he needed to recycle the pieces, to transform the horrible deed into a new, useful form. On a whim he entered the main power plant in the city and met with an engineer. 'Can you take these body parts,' he said, 'and burn them in your incinerator?' The man, rather than reacting in horror, was compassionate. He listened to Sam's story of a failed marriage and ritual dismemberment and gently replied: 'I can't do it. The doll contains PCB's. It's a pollutant. Burning it in our incinerator would be a violation of the city ordinance. Why don't you go home and take it easy for awhile. Then recycle the doll with the other plastic garbage.'

For Sam, this chance meeting was an epiphany. The engineer became a kind of Christ-like figure who had the power to forgive him. Later, I asked Sam to take on the role of the engineer, whom he named Joe. He set Joe at the dinner table. He was telling his wife about the encounter with Sam:

> A funny thing happened at work today. A guy came in and wanted me to burn up something in the incinerator – his wife. It was a doll, you see. He didn't seem crazy. He wanted me to take up this cut up Barbie doll and burn it. I understand what would drive a guy to do this. You don't want to take out the violence on a real person. The anger builds up. I turned him away. It sends polycarbons in the air. I felt compassion for him. It seemed he had everything in control. I think he got rid of it. Makes me think of all the shit I've put up with. Maybe I should cut up a couple of dolls. Maybe cutting up the doll saved him. Maybe he cut up himself and got cut up by others. I feel compassion for him.

In many ways, through invoking this compassionate helper, Sam was able to help himself complete the burial, or rather cremation, of the doll. He went home, placed the doll with the rest of the plastic garbage, and recycled it. The substance of the doll, all 12 pieces, would be destroyed then re-formed into new and useful material.

## The Next Trial

Sam and Bonnie were divorced and Bonnie remarried within a very short time. Maya left Sam within an equally short time when she realized that he was not as free a spirit (neither financially nor emotionally) as he purported to be. Sam nurtured and supported Gabe, but his ability to maintain his business contacts was waning. As much as he was a loving, supportive father, he also felt too much the needy son. His several experiences with new women were failures.

He tended to choose unavailable women, endlessly searching for perfection –
for the beauty, who was, in reality, either a prostitute or exploitative beast, or
the innocent, who he could befriend or father but never love as an equal. None
were able to heal the wound left by his loss of parent, lover and god.

Sam began to retreat into a deep depression. Bonnie, now in a stable
relationship, wanted Gabe to live with her, and Sam recognized Gabe's need
for a more balanced home life than he could provide. As he brought his son to
Bonnie's house, he feared that he was losing another crucial role – that of loving,
nurturing father, a moral model for his son.

Bonnie wanted full custody of their son, and proceeded in a way that was
devastating to Sam – she signed a legal document accusing him of physically
abusing Gabe, also citing that Sam was an unfit father because he abused
cocaine. Beyond his outrage and anger, Sam feared that he was, indeed, a bad
person who simply tried to be good. Could it be true that he was responsible
for the unhappiness of his son and his wife? Could it be that he was even
responsible for his father's sickness and death, his parent's divorce, and his
mother's misery? With these thoughts spinning in his mind, he began to
decompensate. In the next trial, he would be the accused. How could he prove
his innocence when he felt so guilty?

Sam entered a manic phase. He came to therapy exclaiming that he had
found his way back to his art. He was playing music again, jamming with a
number of bands, taking classes, composing bits and pieces of ambitious works.
He brought in a list of more than 100 ideas for new musical projects, rambling
on about each one. He gathered scores of letters from friends and relatives
attesting to Bonnie's unstable mental health. He obsessively built his defense.

Again, I urged Sam to seek a lawyer, but with little money, he could only
work with a legal aid lawyer who was too busy to provide much support. He
entered a relationship with an immature and exploitative woman and experienced great highs of sexual passion. She played hard to get which kept Sam
pursuing her even more.

## The Hand

In therapy, Sam acted out a scene of a hand which had a life of its own. Separate
from the body, the hand began to choke a man. Sam acted this out in graphic,
manic detail. 'Finally,' said Sam, 'the hand kills the guy, but stays alive, itself.
The other hand comes and caresses the killer hand.' Sam was on a self-destructive path. Even his body was coming apart and rebelling. He was figuratively
choking himself, but, as much as he tried, was unable to caress, that is, to sooth
the self-destructive, suicidal impulses.

I attempted to keep playing the helper and encouraged him to stay on track.
I looked for moments of balance, of doubleness that might allow alternative
perspectives to emerge. Many months later he would say: 'The hand supports

but also sabotages. It'll pick up a bible and a gun.' But for now, he was moving too fast, losing trust in our therapeutic bond. His hand was a saboteur and seemed to be inching toward some act of self-sabotage. The trial was fast approaching and he was embracing single roles, single poles. He felt bad, alien, disembodied, out of control. He fluctuated between extreme emotional states of depression and mania.

## The Break

One night, he broke. Bonnie's accusations were cruel and relentless. Gabe was uncommunicative and confused by his mother's accusations. His lover threatened to abandon him. His arthritic condition was raging. His lawyer was unreachable. Fighting a deep depression, he became severely intoxicated, got into a fistfight with his brother, and entered the psychiatric unit of a large city hospital.

Sam's heroic journey appeared to come to an abrupt halt. For the first time in his life, he was diagnosed mentally ill, with bipolar disorder. In need of a helper, he befriended a psychiatrist in the hospital who prescribed medication to stabilize his severe mood swings. Within several days, Sam calmed down. The medication kicked in and even though it held him in a hazy bubble, his ebullient spirit returned. When I visited him, he seemed to be playing the McMurphy role in *One Flew Over the Cuckoo's Nest*. He was playing at being mentally ill. It was all a joke, a disguise to spare him from a worse incarceration. The other patients were his friends and his audience. He was there to cheer up the crazy people, to provide for them, to liberate them.

He remained hospitalized for 18 days and was sent home with a supply of psychotropic medication. His illness was no joke. Back in drama therapy, stabilized by medication, he needed to discover a way to accept his new role as a mentally ill person, who exists to: 'reveal the dark, shadowy sides of human nature and challenge the conventional notion of sanity' (see Landy 1993b, p.178). He was in denial of his newly enacted role for good reason – he didn't want to be his father.

Our first sessions were difficult, centered on his problems with the medications and fears of losing his spontaneity and passion. He remained derailed, afraid of living alone, unable to get back to the double life. The external circumstances remained: he would have to face his accuser, once his wife, and a judge and plead his innocence. Fearful of the outcome and unable to find his balance, his enactments in therapy were filled with images of the holocaust. As to his present state of being, he said: 'I feel like I've been swimming in a bath of acid and my flesh has been burned.'

I felt at this time stretched to my limits. Once before, as a young teacher of emotionally disturbed adolescents, I experienced the suicide of a gifted musician whom I had supervised and cared for. Previous to his death, he was in a highly manic phase. At the time I felt powerless and incompetent, without a helper to turn to. Sam's predicament, some 25 years later, re-stimulated some of those feelings. At least now, though, I could consult with his psychiatrist. When I did, to my dismay and delight, he deferred to me, saying: 'Sam trusts you. You know him much better than I. All I can do is adjust his medication as needed. Encourage him to take the medication. You're the key person now. You can help him more than anyone.'

Within a week, I felt quite helpless. Reminded of his responsibilities, Sam again began to decompensate. Days after his return, he took himself off the medication, experimented with a powerful psychedelic drug, and paid a prostitute a lot of money for one blissful night of pleasure. He obsessively attempted to re-connect with his former lover, but she refused to let him touch her. She would only see him if he took her to up-scale restaurants.

When he sobered up, he fell into a deep depression. During our session he said: 'I'm pushing the limits of madness and death.' Again he brought up the image of the holocaust, referring to himself as a holocaust victim, just like his father. In recognizing the connection, Sam turned a corner.

Getting back on the path of the double life, he began to look at the father role in all its fearful contradictions. The father was supposed to be strong and protective and 'provide a positive masculine role model' (Landy 1993b, p. 208) to his son. But, in fact, Sam's father was the opposite, weak and negligent, a clinical manic-depressive whose illness, compounded by physical disabilities, led to his premature death.

In finding my own direction, I imagined my task was to first help Sam accept his psychiatric illness which, in many ways, had victimized him. And in doing so, I felt the need to lead Sam into an understanding that his illness was part of a legacy from his father. If I could help Sam accept his illness and connection to his father, I hoped then to guide Sam back toward the double life – discovering his abilities in the face of his disability. In particular, I hoped that Sam could discover a way to father the part of himself that felt abandoned and alienated.

## The Worms

We moved slowly after Sam's return, meeting twice a week. As we did not proceed in a straight line, I was looking for small shifts, little movements away from extreme positions. One such moment was Sam's reference to himself as a 'holocaust survivor' rather than 'holocaust victim.' With this small shift of consciousness, I thought, Sam again had the chance to move away from the powerless position of the alien. Sam made up this story:

> A guy was 100 per cent disabled. He has worms in his brain. He's been a victim all his life. The doctors stick instruments up his butt and find worms. They shine a light in his mouth. They see the worms inside. He's

in pain. The doctor gives him medicine and says: 'You are 100 per cent disabled. You must go right away to the sanatorium.' He runs home for car fare. His throat closes up and he can't talk. He closes his door, but the cops are waiting for him. He goes to the fire escape. The born-again Christians tell him to jump. He does and falls in the snow. His head crashes open and the worms escape and vanish. The snow soothes his head. He feels relief.

Reflecting upon the story, Sam said: 'The worms were his gift of knowledge. My father didn't want to give up his illness because he thought it was his intelligence.'

Sam and I explored the implications of this thought. We questioned the connection between wisdom and sickness. Did one have to be mad in order to be creative and wise? Weren't all the great artists and musicians and geniuses mad? Is intelligence actually an emotional curse? Could one be wise and healthy at the same time? And what would that mean?

The story was significant for several reasons. For one, it allowed Sam to admit for the first time that he had 'worms in his brain.' Like his father, he had a disability, bipolar disorder. Sam also acknowledged that he was different from his father in that he allowed himself to seek help in the form of medication and drama therapy. These remedies would not erase his illness, but rather provide support for his search for balance. In the story, the characters of doctors, cops and born-again Christians also serve as potential helpers, but each has a kind of sinister quality, leading him to run, hide, and jump to his death. They do not ultimately offer the help that he needs. It could have been that Sam was doubtful that the professions of medicine, law and religion could solve his problems. Or it could have been that he doubted his own capacity to diagnose, protect, and save himself through those conventional moral systems. If he wanted to get rid of his worms (whether madness or intelligence or some combination), he seemed to imply, he must proceed at great risk, outside the law.

Perhaps most significantly, the story led Sam into an understanding that his father, if he did not bring on his own madness, also did nothing to overcome his disability. The figure of the father seemed to mock the epigram: Knowledge is power. His perverse distortion was: Knowledge is madness, or Madness is power. Going deeper, Sam became aware that his father's role of intellectual madman protected him from feeling and from intimacy, from becoming a loving father to his son and a loving husband to his wife.

Sam's growing awareness was potentially confusing. On the one hand, he was afraid to accept his disability, fearful of becoming his father. On the other hand, he was also afraid to abandon the worms of disability for two good reasons – he might, like his father, risk a loss of creativity and genius, and he might then need to commit to an intimate, loving relationship with another human being. However, I pointed out that in taking the risk, he might discover that health is not incongruous with creativity and wisdom. And he might discover that intimacy, a state of openness, soothes and provides relief from many years of torment by gnawing, parasitic demons.

To be his father or not to be – that was the question that Sam faced. In part, he realized that he had no choice. In part, he began to realize that he did.

## The Host

The image of worms and vile, dependent creatures appeared several times throughout our work together. The worms were parasites that depended upon hosts for their sustenance. In a leap, Sam spoke of feeling forced into the host role. In that role, he served others, making sure that they were comfortable, at ease, well taken care of, even as he was longing for the same. He became his mother's host when his father abandoned the family. As he grew up, he played the master of ceremonies at parties, with friends and relatives, alike, entertaining them, assuring them a good time, even as he was secretly resenting the need to serve. Even in his church, he was appointed the head of hospitality, a host for Christ.

Yet for all his hosting, Sam also felt like a parasite, attached to the very host that he was supposed to support. Was he his mother's host or her appendage? Did he have to play the fool for his pastor in order to merge with the spirit of Christ? Was he required to play the clown to his dying, manic father, or was he victim to that sick body that had inhabited his mind for so many years? Didn't he have the right to be supported, hosted, nurtured – by virtue of being a son and a celebrant? Why had the worm turned?

After Sam's hospitalization, we resumed the difficult task of separation from mother and father, from the massive objects of dependency, all the while wrestling with the paradox of parasite and host. Sam was wounded by the consequences of separating from Bonnie and moved cautiously and haltingly toward further separations. He attempted to stage a second ritual of separation, this time from his mother, but he could not follow through with his elaborate dramatic preparations. Instead, he created dialogues and poetry, which keep him on safer ground. His clearest statement came in the poem, 'My Mother is A Part of Me,' in which he said:

> Part of me is holding up my mother.

> It's my hand, thrust deep inside her,
> holding her up, like a puppet.

> she's playing dead.

> She doesn't have to get angry with me
> because I'm holding her up; she wouldn't
> jeopardize her well-being...

It doesn't matter what is used to hold her;
but the fact is, it's inside that we must go
inside to calm her, to still her while she
recoups, while she feels that someone special
is there, someone, not even her husband, but
a part of her, me, going through her, helping
her out, just like carrying the groceries,
or opening the car door, or turning off
the broiler.

Once in a while, there's an accident and she
won't let me in and I can't get my calm.

In order to get my calm, she's got to let me
inside to support her. But when she's mad
and when she's not letting me in, I know
that there's torture I must endure to end up
okay...

It's a strange sort of fun; it's fun
while it lasts. the moment of no drama,
of no talking, of having peace and relaxing
before the demons remember their rant.

In the poem, Sam is the host and his mother is the parasite. The image of the hand came strongly into play as he saw his mother as a puppet, an empty shell, that could only live when he provided life through his hand. The same hand that previously expressed a suicidal fantasy now expressed a sexual and spiritual one. This is the hand that creates and procreates by being 'thrust deep inside her.'

The reason Sam played host/puppeteer was to achieve a sense of peace and calm, to forestall his mother's rage. When his mother was enraged, she became a kind of threatening demon who could not only physically torture him, but also deprive him of his spiritual need to serve. He recalled that several years earlier, in her rage, she threatened to kill herself. The threat for Sam was twofold: if he saw himself as parasite, then he would die with his host. If he saw himself as host, then he would be lost without the thing that needed him most.

Sam recognized that in order to separate from his mother he had to counterbalance the roles of host and parasite. He had to further find a way to supply and demand, assured that he had enough to give and that he was worthy of receiving. Moving in both directions at once, seeking balance, he reflected: 'My patterns are like hers. I'm now a single parent, like her. I married someone ill, just like she did. She corrects herself through me. She sees me as half a person. It's herself that she hates and doesn't even see her disrespect toward me.'

The image of Sam as half a person, as cut off, seemed most significant to me. In the past, he could only imagine himself as whole when merged with his mother. In his attempt to actually become whole, that is, to seek an independent identity, he saw her more clearly as a half person, herself, as a mother in name only, as a puppet with no real life force of her own. To become a whole person and effectively live the double life, he clearly needed to forge a separate identity. And he needed not only to discover a way to integrate the host and parasite parts of himself, but also to search out the other sides of the roles of host (that is, not-host) and parasite (that is, not-parasite).

## The Tentacle

Further along, amidst his fantasies of beautiful yet unavailable women, Sam mentioned: 'I see a woman who is beautiful. It's like getting stung by a tentacle. I am paralyzed, out of joint. It's a physical thing, like the pleasure right before an orgasm.'

I asked Sam to take on the role of the tentacle, intuiting another opportunity to explore the host/parasite paradox. Sam obliged:

> I am a tentacle – my stink, it causes death. Things I like, I touch. I enjoy paralyzing things, making them mine, if only for a moment. I have a lonely life. But I am part of a larger body – one of many tentacles. I am controlled by a larger body. I move independent of my brethren. I am graceful. I am very vulnerable and in that, I survive. When I seek my prey, I can get my tentacle chopped off. I have to be very careful. I am waiting for the perfect victim. When I sink 'em it's like no other feeling in the whole world. It's like being transported into a life we'll never know again. It's a hard life. I think I'll make peace with my quest for pleasure. I'm hungry for touch. I'm 160 feet long, translucent. You might find it ugly. I have suction cups and strands and dark red tiny tips. As I come to my brain area, I get thicker and thicker. Very smart. It's in the length of things that difficulties occur. It takes a long time for me to unravel. I wish I was alone, but I am attached. To the big hill. He goes his own way and pulls me along. Maybe I would be satisfied with one victim. Maybe I wouldn't want to be attached. But I need to be attached. It's my nature. I'm trapped. If I found the perfect victim, I'd have to share her. With the rest of us. With the tentacles and the hill. The hill is an appetite. The hill is a consuming, faceless tyrant. He does what he wants and he takes us along. He's the leader. Named Orb. Things would be scary without him. He can see in all directions. I can see in only two. Nothing to say to the hill. I don't want to get him angry. When I'm miles away, I'll scream: 'Forget it!' I'm mad at him. He held me down. I've seen things I've wanted to touch before. But he keeps going and drags me along and makes me swim. The Orb is probably smarter than me. But

he's blind in a way. And he's got a strong survival instinct. He knows what the dangers are. I've been with him long enough. I think I can make it on my own. Now that I'm free, I'll curl up and find a new resting place. I'm going to feel myself alone, apart. Learn how to swim, to feel myself as a tentacle – not even that – as another creature. Name? I hate labels, but I think for now – Dan. Dan the Man. I think that other than stinging victims, I'll embrace them, court them, and if they want me to sting them, maybe I will. Maybe we could taste each other. I'm scared. I don't know how to do it alone. Maybe now that I've left the Orb, maybe he won't want me back. But I make the decisions. I can't concentrate on the dangers. I have to be in peace and go in peace and make peace. Maybe the waters here are too deep. Maybe I need shallower waters. Warmer, friendly creatures. I've never been in shallow waters before.

Sam felt very hopeful following this enactment. On the one hand, his tentacle was a toxic, phallic, disembodied force that is lethal to others and controlled by a more powerful entity. But on the other, it was a dependent parasite struggling for independence and willing to face the consequences of separating.

In comparing himself to the tentacle, Sam said: 'I feel long, vulnerable and attached to the Orb. But I'm resentful I have to go along with it. I'm becoming my own octopus. Now that I've broken away, I'll become my own.' Sam well recognized the problems associated with separating: 'I feel like a severed limb. Out of my depth. I feel the need to rush to make up for myself. A little lost. I'm trying to learn how to fail successfully and go on.'

Through further reflection, Sam realized that on the other side of the parasite was, potentially, a severed limb, a lost one who must find shallower waters and friendlier creatures in order to survive. In other words, when separating, one must be prepared for the consequences. If the consequences are grave, then one must find a way to change one's inner and outer circumstances. In terms of role, Sam saw his journey as a move from parasite to lost one to survivor.

On the other side of the host, whom Sam envisioned as a controlling tyrant, was the positive role type most familiar to Sam – that of the searcher, the hero, who would continue to move Sam along his spiritual path. This role type was already part of Sam's internal cast of characters. Sam ended his story of the tentacle on a practical note – looking for a very grounded way to realize his very basic needs for security and compassion. It was the survivor who would help him find the appropriate depth, warmth, and kindness both from himself and from his environment.

In concluding, I asked Sam to speak about the connection between the Orb and his own life. He mentioned, first, that Bonnie was an orb from whom he needed to separate. Then, more poignantly, he said that his mother and father were orbs. He saw his mother as a parasitic orb, controlling in her helplessness, in her pressure on Sam to deny his feelings because she could not express her own. And he saw his father as a selfish orb, exerting his power by swimming away from the family, taking an independent, albeit self-destructive path.

Playing with the word, *tentacle*, Sam realized that in response to these two powerful orbs, he had become *tentative* as he pitched a tent and hid out. 'I took the middle ground, not having to make decisions and determine when to go on my own.' Well into his therapeutic journey, having survived a loss of church and faith, a traumatic divorce, and a psychiatric breakdown, the middle ground became something other then a place of indecision and inertia. It became a bridge between several distant roles longing for connection: lost one and survivor, parasite and host, individual and social animal. This bridge was built by and for he who wishes to live the double life more effectively.

## The Father

Sam appeared at his trial well prepared. He had taken all appropriate measures to secure his innocence and trusted the reality that he was neither child abuser nor drug abuser. The judge affirmed that reality. Sam was absolved of all charges. The case was dismissed. During the pre-trial period, Sam was only permitted to visit his son, Gabe, while supervised. After the trial, he could see Gabe freely and resume the role of father. It was a difficult role to maintain, given all the turmoil stirred up by Bonnie's accusations, Sam's fears, and Gabe's confusions. But Sam persisted. He needed, more than ever, to father his son, especially as he attempted to make peace with his own dead father.

Sam and I had spent many hours exploring the legacy from his father. Sam had thought that the most notable item in the estate was bipolar disorder. As mentioned above, the role of madman protected his father from intimacy, and Sam feared that he might also be doomed to live a brief, unfulfilled, isolated existence. I wondered whether there was another side to the role of madman, a way to reconceive the frightening legacy of mental illness.

Earlier, Sam had mentioned: 'I have my father's lips.' The image of lips came up several times in our work. Sam told me that on a critical visit to the mental hospital, his father, half delirious, had said: 'I want to kiss you on the lips. Those are my lips.' Fearful of being pulled into his father in an unnatural way, Sam was horrified and backed off. I asked Sam to make up a story about the lips. He offered this:

> Once upon a time, there was a boy who had his father's lips. They were so huge that when he smiled people would touch them and love them. The father gave the son his lips so that the father would have normal lips. 'If only he could handle those lips,' people said, 'he would be a man.' But he couldn't. He decided to get a brace and brace them up. He put up a sign: 'These are not my lips! They have been given to me. I want to live a normal life!' People stopped talking to him. One day he woke up and the lips were off. He cried and stayed in his bed all day. He stroked

the lips and watched them die. He wrapped them up in a shroud and put them in a box and wrote on it: 'Dad's old lips.' He went outside and smiled and for the first time, everything was OK. At least for now.

In many ways, this was another story about separation. To live a normal life, Sam thought, he needed to get rid of his father's lips, even at the risk of being seen by others as unmanly. He needed to avoid being sucked in, merging with the sickness that appeared to emanate from his father mouth. Once, when playing his father, Sam offered the line: 'I'm sick. I have a mouth disease. Nobody knows what it is.'

Castration fears and fears of homosexuality also appeared in Sam's imagery throughout our work. But at this point in his therapy, some two and a half years into the process, many of those fears had been worked through. Sam was ready to resume his relationship with Gabe because he had discovered a way to separate from his father's inability to be intimate. Sam wished to use his lips to kiss his son in an appropriate, loving way, and to speak encouraging and caring words.

Sam did not learn to be a man from his father, or rather, Sam's education was a distorted one. The man that was his model was one who lost his power (his potency), his home, his family, and his mind. As some would deface a portrait by drawing a mustache over the lips, Sam's father attempted to de-face his son. But in claiming his face as his own and by burying that of his father, Sam asserted his independence, his manliness. At least for now, everything was OK.

Nearing his fortieth birthday, struggling to offer an alternative model to Gabe, Sam took on the role of his father one more time in therapy. I asked him, as father, to speak to his son. He couldn't speak directly to the son, so he used me as an intermediary, asking me the following:

'Can you tell him I love him. He doesn't have to be like me, the way I was. He should not have anything to do with the parts of me that were unwell. I expect him to find his own way. He is bipolar, but he has the tools.'

'What went wrong with you?' I asked the father.

'For years I blamed it on my parents. I had a disease. I was too afraid of being helped. I was afraid I might be cured. Then I wouldn't know what to do.'

'You were afraid to live a normal life?' I asked.

'Yeah. It is too demanding. I was afraid of getting involved, people things, making casseroles. I've been too irritable too long.'

Sam was indeed ready for the separation from his father. In doing so, he was rehearsing the words to say to Gabe, who saw him as stigmatized and who hesitated to trust him, in the same way that he had experienced his father. He hoped to tell him that like his father before him, he had a sickness. But unlike his father, he sought help and received it. And because he got better, he was able to live a normal life. He hoped he would be able to tell this to Gabe face-to-face, without an intermediary. He hoped his lips could form the words: 'I love you.'

## Enot

Sam was no longer in denial of his illness, his fear, and his shame. He was able to proclaim openly: 'My disability is my ability.' He was living well with his many role ambivalences. In one session, he again created an alien role, a disabled figure whom he called Enot. He described him as: on a throne, majestic, resting, feet bound, empty, meditative, calm, and benevolent. Although there was something inhuman and alien about him, Sam also said:

> He's evolved through his disability to someone of higher understanding. E-not, he's not. He's not playing music, he's not eating, he's not doing. I think Enot is, Enot is becoming. He might have gotten his name by being in denial.

Through Enot, an apparent denier of being, Sam was able to conceive of the other side, that of the loving father, that of the the non-alien, the not-not. Enot embodied both that which is hopeless and foreign and that which is hopeful and possible.

## Forty Wishes

Sam's fortieth birthday was imminent. He was leading a solitary life, needing to remain separate from people until he experienced a stronger sense of himself as a social being. He continued to experience depression and odd moments of hyperactivity, but generally, he felt in control of his moods. He had been free of all medication for many months. He found that his clients had not abandoned him and that he was able to work enough to support himself. He had not lost his abilities as an artisan.

He was again devoted to music, working at a high level, continuous hours each day, creating a number of promising pieces. Now in mid- life, he dreaded facing his 40th birthday without a family, a church, a recognition for his art. I asked if he wanted to create a ritual. He seemed very enthusiastic but was unable to come up with an acceptable idea.

In session I thought of Sam's desire to lead a normal life. One 'normal' image that came to mind was a birthday cake. I asked Sam to draw a birthday cake and add 40 candles, each one representing a wish for the coming year. We were far away from the ritual candles in the trial and execution scene that dripped wax on the naked doll. Each wish was articulated with great feeling and hope. Some of the most poignant wishes were:

> To see my mother filled in her needs for accomplishment, to be a good father/to grow as a father, to leave Gabe a legacy of honesty, self-respect, and love, to be honored by Gabe out of respect which would, in turn, provide me self-esteem and self- love, and to see my own father as not lost, as a father.

In a paradoxical linking of two wishes, Sam desired to have significant relationships and to feel unattached.

## The Double Life

Sam, while picking up his son, peeked into Gabe's notebook. He had written: 'I don't want to grow up. Old people don't play and have fun.' Could it be, thought Sam, that he was becoming one of the old people? He had always seen himself as a child, an irresponsible, spontaneous person with a great capacity to play and have fun. But in his son's eyes, he had metamorphosed. From Sam's point of view, however, the transformation was incomplete. It was not that he left one state of being for another, but that he now embodied one role and its counterpart simultaneously. If he began his heroic therapeutic journey as a child, he ended as a grown-up with child-like qualities, though severely tested, still intact.

I asked him to reflect upon the last three years of treatment. For the first time he said: 'I have been leading a double life.' He realized that his work was very much centered on the image of the double, the good man who is bad, the pastor who is immoral, the disabled one who is able. He articulated his many attempts to deny the double life by falling into extreme depressive or manic states of being, by seeking unconditional devotion to one sexual or spiritual object of worship, by desiring to be born again in a flash, washed clean of guilt and forgiven.

Then, unexpectedly, he informed me that he was ready to reduce our meetings, with the eventual goal of terminating therapy. He no longer felt fully like a client. I experienced my own double reaction at the time: a sadness of losing such an extraordinarily brave and creative client who became a screen upon which to view my own role ambivalence, and a delight that Sam was indeed ready to leave the therapeutic orb, having completed this leg of his journey.

Sam, still the client, was preparing to be not-client. Sam, the child, had found a way to be grown-up. Sam, the man who had lost his son, had discovered new depths of fathering both his son and himself. Sam, the immoralist, the bad, shameful murderer, had discovered a way to make peace with the worst of his demons and move toward the goal of living a compassionate life. Sam, the fundamentalist, had found a way to work through his nihilism. Sam, the alien, had found ways to reconnect to his intimates, his art, and his craft. Sam, the disabled one, had discovered his many abilities.

Sam created a number of demonic personae in his work through drama therapy including: Pfeiffer the killer dog, Rupert Stosh the good man who liked to do bad, the dismembered doll and its executioner, the disembodied hand and the parasitic worms. And he created a number of alien personae who were either sub-human or lost souls on this earth. Taken together, all these roles seemed to support Sam's extreme feelings of either rage or depression. Yet in his ability to view each demon and alien in the context of its counterpart, Sam discovered a way to make peace with the extremities of his existence. Sam was well aware that the demonic and alien roles would never be extinguished, but as he had invoked and named his tormenters, they would, in themselves, be less alien and thus less apt to disable his life.

Toward the end of our work together, Sam had two clarifying dreams. In one, Bonnie loses control and acts out in a psychotic fashion. Sam commented: 'I felt separation from her. Her problems are her own.' In the second, Sam rows his mother in a boat around a plush resort. She rocks the boat, falls into the water, which is shallow, and floats down to her parents. Money falls in with her. Sam scoops up the money and gives it to his mother. He pays her back everything he owes her. He helps her dry out in a caring, responsible fashion. Then he watches her walk away. 'She can take care of herself,' said Sam.

Sam and I separated gradually throughout the next year, using our meeting times to acknowledge and revisit the difficulties of separation as it became more and more of a reality. During this time, Sam became ready to take care of himself, having extricated his suckers from those real and imagined figures who would devour him. He would search for new orbs but with a new consciousness. In that he dared to cross over the murky waters that separate the two poles of his existence, he discovered that he was no stranger to either shore. Because he could survive the antipodes, he could indeed find his elusive balance and effectively live the double life.

# References

Ahsen, A. (1972) *Eidetic Parents Test and Analysis.* New York: Brandon House.

Ahsen, A. (1983) Odysseus and Oedipus Rex: Image psychology and the literary technique of consciousness. *Journal of Mental Imagery 7,* 1, 143–168.

Ahsen, A. (1984) *Rhea Complex.* New York: Brandon House.

Aldridge, D. and Brandt, G. (1991b) Music therapy and inflammatory bowel disease. *The Arts in Psychotherapy 18,* 113–121.

American Psychiatric Association (1995) *Diagnostic and Statistical Manual of Mental Disorders,* 4th edition. Washington, DC: APA.

Arbus, D. (1972) *Diane Arbus.* Millerton, NY: Aperture.

Aristotle (1954) *Poetics.* (I. Bywater, trans.) New York: Modern Library.

Artaud, A. (1958) *The Theatre and Its Double.* New York: Grove Press.

*The Arts in Psychotherapy* (1992) *Special Issue on Aesthetics.* New York: Pergamon Press.

Axline, V. (1947) *Play Therapy.* Boston: Houghton Mifflin.

Beck, J. (1972) *The Life of the Theatre.* San Francisco: City Lights.

Berger, M. (ed) (1970) *Videotape Techniques in Psychiatric Training and Treatment.* New York: Brunner Mazel.

Berne, E. (1961) *Transactional Analysis in Psychotherapy.* New York: Grove Press.

Blatner, H. (1973) *Acting-In.* New York: Springer.

Bloom, B., Krathwohl, D. and Masia, B. (1956) *The Taxonomy of Educational Objectives, Cognitive Domain.* New York: David McKay.

Blumer, H. (1962) Society as symbolic interaction. In A. Rose (ed) *Human Behavior and Social Processes.* New York: Houghton Mifflin.

Boal, A. (1979) *Theatre of the Oppressed.* New York: Urizen Books.

Bolton, G. (1979) *Towards a Theory of Drama in Education.* London: Longman.

Brecht, B. (1965) The measures taken. In E. Bentley (trans) *The Jewish Wife and Other Short Plays.* New York: Grove Press

Brecht, B. (1967) *Gesammelte Werke.* Frankfurt am Main: Suhrkamp Verlag.

Brecht, B. (1977) *Collected Plays, Volume 2.* New York: Vintage.

Breitenbach, N. (1979) Secret faces. *Dramatherapy 2,* 18–23.

Britton, J. (1970) *Language and Learning.* London: Penguin.

Buber, M. (1948) *Between Man and Man.* New York: Macmillan.

Buber, M. (1966) *The Knowledge of Man.* New York: Harper and Row.

Bullough, E. (1964) 'Psychical distance' as a factor in art and an aesthetic principle. In M. Rader (ed) *A Modern Book of Esthetics*, 3rd. ed. New York: Holt, Rinehart and Winston.

Burke, K. (1972) *Dramatism and Development*. Barre, MA: Clark University Press.

Carter, H. (1982) What is it – Research or research? *Children's Theatre Review 31*, 26–31.

Casement, P. (1985) *On Learning from the Patient*. London: Tavistock.

Chumaciero, C. (1992) What song comes to mind? induced song recall: transference/countertransference in dyadic music associations in treatment and supervision. *The Arts in Psychotherapy 19*, 325–332.

Clevenger, T. (1965) Behavioral research in theatre. *Educational Theatre Journal 17*, 118–121.

Cole, D. (1975) *The Theatrical Event*. Middletown, CT: Wesleyan University Press.

Combs, C. (1981) A Piagetian view of creative dramatics: Delimited, adaptive play and imitation. *Children's Theatre Review 30*, 25–31.

Cook, C. (1917) *The Play Way*. London: Heinemann.

Cooley, C. (1922) *Human Nature and Social Order*. New York: Scribner's.

Courtney, R. (1974) *Play, Drama, and Thought*. New York: Drama Book Specialists.

Courtney, R. (1982) *Replay: Studies in Human Drama in Education*. Toronto: Ontario Institute for Studies in Education.

Craig, E.G. (1919) *The Theatre Advancing*. New York: Blom.

Dequine, E. and Pearson-Davis, S. (1983) Videotaped improvisational drama with emotionally disturbed adolescents: A pilot study. *The Arts in Psychotherapy 10*, 15–22.

Derrida, J. (1986) *Glas*. Lincoln: University of Nebraska Press.

Dewey, J. (1934) *Art as Experience*. New York: Minton, Balch.

Dewey, J. (1966) *Democracy and Education*. New York: Free Press.

Duchartre, P. (1966) *The Italian Comedy*. New York: Dover.

Ekstein, R. and Friedman, S. (1957) The function of acting out, play action, and play acting in the psychotherapeutic process. *Journal of the American Psychoanalytical Association 5*, 581–629.

Eliade, M. (1972) *Shamanism: Archaic Techniques of Ecstasy*. Princeton, NJ: Princeton University Press.

Eliaz, E. (1988) *Transference in Drama Therapy*. Unpublished Ph.D. dissertation. New York: New York University.

Emunah, R. (1983) Drama therapy with adult psychiatric patients. *The Arts in Psychotherapy 10*, 77–84.

Erikson, E. (1952) *Childhood and Society*. New York: Norton.

Erikson, E. (1968) *Identity: Youth and Crisis*. New York: Norton.

Fox, J. (ed) (1987) *The Essential Moreno*. New York: Springer.

Freud, A. (1946) *The Psychoanalytic Treatment of Children.* London: Imago.

Freud, S. (1920) Beyond the pleasure principle. In J. Strachey (ed) *The Standard Edition of the Complete Works of Sigmund Freud, Vol. 18.* London: Hogarth.

Freud, S. (1949) *An Outline of Psychoanalysis.* James Strachey, translator. New York: Norton.

Freud, S. (1963) *General Psychological Theory.* New York: Collier.

Freud, S. and Breuer, J. (1966) *Studies in Hysteria.* New York: Avon Books.

Fryrear, J. and Fleshman, B. (eds) (1981) *Videotherapy in Mental Health.* Springfield, IL: Charles C Thomas.

Furman, L. (1981) Creative drama as a vehicle for assessing comprehension. *Children's Theatre Review 30,* 33–38.

Gardner, H. (1983) *Frames of Mind: The Theory of Multiple Intelligences.* New York: Basic Books.

Ginsberg, A. (1956) *Howl.* In A. Ginsberg *Howl and Other Poems.* San Francisco: City Lights.

Goffman, E. (1959) *The Presentation of Self in Everyday Life.* Garden City, NY: Doubleday.

Gordon, R. (1981) Humanizing offenders through acting therapy. In G. Schattner and R. Courtney (eds) *Drama in Therapy.* New York: Drama Book Specialists.

Gould, S. (1989) *Wonderful Life.* New York: Norton.

Green, R.L. (ed) (1965) *The Works of Lewis Carroll.* Feltham, Middlesex: The Hamlyn Publishing Group.

Gregoric, L. and M. (1982) Sociodrama: Video in social action. In J. Fryrear and B. Fleshman (eds) *Videotherapy in Mental Health.* Springfield, IL: Charles C. Thomas.

Grotowski, J. (1968) *Towards a Poor Theatre.* New York: Simon and Schuster.

Hare, A.P. (1985) *Social Interaction as Drama.* Beverly Hills: Sage.

Harley, G. (1950) *Masks as Agents of Social Control in Liberia.* Cambridge, MA: Peabody Museum of American Archeology.

Harris, A. (1966) *Rags to Riches.* New Orleans: Anchorage Press.

Harrop, J. and Epstein, S. (1982) *Acting with Style.* Englewood Cliffs, NJ: Prentice-Hall.

Hart, S. and Waren, M. (eds) (1983) *The Arts in Prisons.* New York: CASTA, CUNY.

Herron, R. and Sutton-Smith, B. (eds) (1971) *Child's Play.* New York: Wiley.

Hillman, J. (1983) *Healing Fiction.* Barrytown, NY: Station Hill Press.

Howells, J. and Townsend, D. (1973) Puppetry as a medium for play diagnosis. *Child Psychiatry Quarterly 6,* 9–14.

Huizinga, J. (1955) *Homo Ludens – A Study of the Play Element in Culture.* Boston: Beacon.

Huntsman, K. (1982) Improvisational dramatic activities: Key to self-actualization? *Children's Theatre Review 31,* 3–9.

Iannotti, R. (1978) Effects of role-taking experience on role-taking, empathy, altruism and aggression. *Developmental Psychology 14,* 199–224.

Irwin, E. (1975) Facilitating children's language development through play. *The Speech Teacher 24*, 15–23.

Irwin, E. (1983) The diagnostic and therapeutic use of pretend play. In C. Schaefer and K. O'Connor (eds) *Handbook of Play Therapy*. New York: Wiley.

Irwin, E. (1985) Externalizing and improvising imagery through drama therapy: a psychoanalytic view. *Journal of Mental Imagery 9*, 33–42.

Irwin, E. and Frank, M. (1977) Facilitating the play process with learning disabled children. *Academic Therapy 12*, 435–444.

Irwin, E. and Kovacs, A. (1979) Analysis of children's drawings and stories. *Journal of the Association for the Care of Children in Hospitals 8*, 39–48.

Irwin, E. and Malloy, E. (1975) Family puppet interview. *Family Process 14*, 179–191.

Irwin, E. and McWilliams, B. (1974) Play therapy for children with cleft palates. *Children Today*, May-June, 18–22.

Irwin, E. and Rubin, J. (1976) Art and drama interviews: Decoding symbolic messages. *The Arts in Psychotherapy 3*, 169–175.

Irwin, E. and Shapiro, M. (1975) Puppetry as a diagnostic and therapeutic technique. In I. Jakab (ed) *Psychiatry and Art*. Basel: Karger.

Irwin, E., Levy, P. and Shapiro, M. (1972) Assessment of drama therapy in a child guidance setting. *Group Psychotherapy and Psychodrama 25*, 105–116.

Jackins, H. (1965) *The Human Side of Human Beings*. Seattle, WA: Rational Island Press.

James, W. (1948) *Psychology*. New York: World Publishing Co.

Jennings, S. (1982) *Role flexibility: A central concept for dramatherapy*. Paper presented at the Art and Dramatherapy Conference, St. Albans, England.

Jennings, S. (1982) *The development of social identity through dramatherapy*. Paper presented at the 5th International Congress of Psychomotricite, Florence, Italy.

Jennings, S. (1987) *Dramatherapy: Theory and Practice I*. London: Routledge.

Jennings, S. (1990) *Dramatherapy with Families, Groups and Individuals*. London: Jessica Kingsley Publishers.

Jennings, S. and Minde, A. (1993) *Art Therapy and Dramatherapy: Masks of the Soul*. London: Jessica Kingsley Publishers.

Johnson, D. (1980a) *Cognitive organization in paranoid and nonparanoid schizophrenia*. Unpublished doctoral dissertation, Yale University, New Haven.

Johnson, D. (1980b) Effects of a theatre experience on hospitalized psychiatric patients. *The Arts in Psychotherapy 7*, 265–272.

Johnson, D. (1981) Drama therapy and the schizophrenic condition. In G. Schattner and K. Courtney (eds) *Drama in Therapy Vol. 2*. New York: Drama Book Specialists.

Johnson, D. (1982a) Developmental approaches in drama therapy. *The Arts in Psychotherapy 9*, 183–190.

Johnson, D. (1982b) Principles and techniques of drama therapy. *The Arts in Psychotherapy 9*, 83–90.

Johnson, D. (1991) Perspective: Taking the next step: Forming the National Creative Arts Therapies Association. *The Arts in Psychotherapy 18*, 387–393.

Johnson, D. (1994) Shame dynamics among creative arts therapies. *The Arts in Psychotherapy 12*, 173–178.

Johnson, D. and Quinlan, D. (1980) Fluid and rigid boundaries of paranoid and nonparanoid schizophrenics on a role-playing task. *Journal of Personality Assessment 44*, 523–531.

Johnson, D. and Quinlan, D. (1982) *Representational boundaries in the role portrayals among paranoid and nonparanoid schizophrenics.* Unpublished manuscript.

Jung, C.G. (1964) *Man and His Symbols.* Garden City, NY: Doubleday.

Jung, C.G. (1968) *Analytic Psychology: Its Theory and Practice.* London: Routledge and Kegan Paul.

Jung, C.G. (1971) *Psychological Types.* Princeton: Princeton University Press.

Junge, M. and Linesch, D. (1993) Our own Voices: new paradigms for art therapy research. *The Arts in Psychotherapy 20*, 61–67.

Kafka, F. (1948) *The Penal Colony.* New York: Schocken.

Keats, J. (1950) *Selected Poems.* New York: Appleton-Century-Crofts.

Kim, J. (1993) *Transformation of Korean Shamans through Enactment of Spirits in Naerim Kut.* Unpublished PhD dissertation, New York University.

Kirby, E.T. (1975) *Ur-Drama: The Origins of Theatre.* New York: New York University Press.

Klein, M. (1932) *The Psychoanalysis of Childhood.* London: Hogarth.

Knill, P. (1994) Multiplicity as a tradition: Theories for interdisciplinary arts therapies. *The Arts in Psychotherapy 21*, 319–328.

Kohlberg, L. (1976) *Recent Research in Moral Education.* New York: Holt, Rhinehart and Winston.

Krathwohl, D., Bloom, B.S. and Masia, B.B. (1964) *The Taxonomy of Behavioral Objectives, Affective Domain.* New York: David McKay.

Kundera, M. (1984) *The Unbearable Lightness of Being.* New York: Harper and Row.

Laing, R.D. (1967) *The Politics of Experience.* New York: Pantheon.

Landy, R. (1975) *Dramatic Education – An Interdisciplinary Approach to Learning.* Unpublished PhD dissertation, Santa Barbara, CA: University of California.

Landy, R. (1977) Measuring audience response to characters and scenes in theatre for children. *Children's Theatre Review 26*, 10–13.

Landy, R. (1981) An exploration of the process of learning through drama. *Children's Theatre Review, Research Edition 30*, 2, 39–44.

Landy, R. (1982a) *Handbook of Educational Drama and Theatre.* Westport CT: Greenwood Press.

Landy, R. (1982b) Training the drama therapist – a four-part model. *The Arts in Psychotherapy 9*, 2, 91–99.

Landy, R. (1983) The use of distancing in drama therapy. *The Arts in Psychotherapy 10*, 175–185.

Landy, R. (1984) Conceptual and methodological issues of research in drama therapy. *The Arts in Psychotherapy 11*, 89–100.

Landy, R. (1986) *Drama Therapy – Concepts and Practices.* Springfield, IL: Charles C. Thomas.

Landy, R. (1987) The creative arts therapy workshop as form and function. *The Arts in Psychotherapy 14,* 279–283.

Landy, R. (1990). The concept of role in drama therapy. *The Arts in Psychotherapy 17,* 223–230.

Landy, R. (1991) The dramatic basis of role theory. *The Arts in Psychotherapy 18,* 29–41.

Landy, R. (1993a) The child, the dreamer, the artist and the fool: In search of understanding the meaning of expressive therapy. *The Arts in Psychotherapy 20,* 359–370.

Landy, R. (1993b) *Persona and Performance – The Meaning of Role in Drama, Therapy, and Everyday Life.* London: Jessica Kingsley Publishers.

Landy, R. (1994) *Drama Therapy: Concepts, Theories and Practices,* 2nd edition. Springfield, IL: C.C. Thomas.

Landy, R. (1995) *Hetty Green – The Witch of Wall Street.* Unpublished play.

Langer, S. (1953) *Feeling and Form.* New York: Scribner's.

Lawrence, S. (1981) Journal: Drama therapy with severely disturbed adults. In G. Schattner and R. Courtney (eds) *Drama in Therapy.* New York: Drama Book Specialists.

Lazier, G. (1976) Scientific research in theatre. In S. Madeja (ed) *Arts and Aesthetics: An Agenda for the Future.* St. Louis, MO: CEMREL.

Lazier, G. and Karioth, E. (1972) *The Inventory of Dramatic Behavior: A Content Analysis Technique for Creative Dramatics.* Theatre Science Laboratory, Florida State University.

Leaf, L. (1980) *Identification and Classification of the Educational Objectives of Creative Dramatics when it is done with Handicapped Persons Ages Five–Eighteen in the United States.* Unpublished PhD dissertation, University of Oregon.

Linton, R. (1936) *The Study of Man.* New York: Appleton-Century.

Lowenfeld, M. (1939) The world pictures of children. *British Journal of Medical Psychology 18,* 65–101.

Lowenfeld, M. (1967) *Play in Childhood.* New York: Wiley and Sons.

Lowenfeld, M. (1970) The Lowenfeld Technique. In R. Bowyer (ed) *The Lowenfeld World Technique.* Oxford: Pergamon.

Mahler, M. (1975) *The Psychological Birth of the Human Infant: Symbiosis and Individuation.* New York: Basic Books.

Mayer, J. and McManus, D. (1988) *Landslide, The Unmasking of the President, 1984–1988.* Boston: Houghton Mifflin.

Maslow, A. (1971) *The Farther Reaches of Human Nature.* New York: Random House.

May, R. (1969) *Existential Psychology.* New York: Random House.

McNiff, S. (1993) Perspective: The authority of experience *The Arts in Psychotherapy 10,* 3–9.

McReynolds, P. and DeVoge, S. (1977) The use of improvisational techniques in assessment. In P. McReynolds (ed) *Advances in Psychological Assessment, Vol. 4.* San Francisco: Jossey-Bass.

Mead, G. (1925) Genesis of the self and social control. *International Journal of Ethics 35*, 251–273.

Mead, G. (1934, 1962) *Mind, Self and Society.* Chicago: University of Chicago Press.

Mead, M. (1928) *Coming of Age in Samoa.* New York: Morrow.

Meatyard, R. (1974) *The Family Album of Lucybelle Crater.* Millerton, NY: The Jargon Society.

Miller, G. (1972) Is saying believing? Possible effects of counterattitudinal role-playing on actors' attitudes and self-concept. *Empirical Research in the Theatre 2*, 1–9.

Milton, J. (1957, ed. M. Hughes) *John Milton Complete Poems and Major Prose.* New York: The Odyssey Press.

Moffett, J. (1968) *Teaching the Universe of Discourse.* Boston: Houghton-Mifflin.

Moreno, J. L. (1946, 1959, 1962) *Psychodrama*, three volumes. Beacon, NY: Beacon House.

Moreno, J.L. (1953) *Who Shall Survive?* Beacon, New York: Beacon House.

Moreno, J.L. (1960) *The Sociometry Reader.* Glencoe, Illinois: The Free Press.

Mossman, H. (1973) The psychological effect of counterattitudinal acting. *Empirical Research in the Theatre 3*, 18–25.

Müller, H. (1984) *Hamletmachine and Other Texts for the Stage.* New York: PAJ Publications.

Nichols, M. and Zax, M. (1977) *Catharsis in Psychotherapy.* New York: Gardner Press.

O'Toole, J. (1976) *Theatre in Education.* London: Hodder and Stoughton.

Ouspensky, P. (1971) *A New Model of the Universe.* New York: Vintage.

Paisley, W. (1969) Cited in O. Holsti, *Content Analysis for the Social Sciences and Humanities.* Menlo Park, CA: Addison-Wesley.

Perls, F. (1947) *Ego, Hunger and Aggression.* New York: Random House.

Perls, F. (1969) *Gestalt Therapy Verbatim.* Moab, Utah: Real People Press.

Perlstein, S. (1981) *A Stage for Memory, Life History Plays by Older Adults.* New York: Teacher and Writers Collaborative.

Philpott, A. (1977) *Puppets and Therapy.* Boston: Plays, Inc.

Piaget, J. (1962) *Play, Dreams and Imitation in Childhood.* New York: Norton.

Piaget, J. (1971) *The Child's Conception of the World.* London: Routledge and Kegan Paul.

Piaget, J. (1977) *The Origin of Intelligence in the Child.* London: Penguin.

Poe, E.A. (1966) William Wilson. In W. H. Auden (ed) *Edgar Allan Poe, Selected Prose and Poetry.* New York: Holt, Rinehart and Winston.

Portner, E. (1981) Drama in therapy: Experiences of a ten year-old. In G. Schattner and R. Courtney (eds) *Drama in Therapy, Vol. 1.* New York: Drama Book Specialists.

Propp, V. (1968) *Morphology of the Folktale*, 2nd ed. Austin, Texas: University of Texas Press.

Riso, D. (1987) *Personality Types*. Boston: Houghton Mifflin.

Rogers, C. (1961) *On Becoming a Person*. Boston: Houghton Mifflin.

Roheim, G. (1948) Psychoanalysis and anthropology. In S. Lorand (ed) *Psychoanalysis Today*. London: Allen and Unwin.

Rosenberg, H., Castellano, R., Chrein, G. and Pinciotti, P. (1982) Answering a research need: Developing an imagery-based theory for the field of creative drama. *Children's Theatre Review 31*, 16–21.

Roth, P. (1986) *The Counterlife*. New York: Farrar Straus Giroux.

Rubin, J. and Irwin, E. (1975) Art and drama: Parts of a puzzle. In I. Jakab (ed) *Psychiatry and Art*, Vol. 4. Basel: Karger.

Sarbin, T. (1954) Role theory. In G. Lindzey (ed) *Handbook of Social Psychology*. Cambridge, MA: Addison-Wesley.

Sarbin, T. (1962) Role enactment. In J. Dyal (ed) *Readings in Psychology: Understanding Human Behavior*. New York: McGraw-Hill.

Sarbin, T. (ed) (1986) *Narrative Psychology*. New York: Praeger.

Sarbin, T. and Allen, V. (1968) Role theory. In G. Lindzey and E. Aronson (eds) *The Handbook of Social Psychology, 2nd ed*. Reading, Mass.: Addison-Wesley.

Sarnoff, C. (1976) *Latency*. New York: Jason Aronson.

Schaefer, C. and O'Connor, K. (eds) (1983) *Handbook of Play Therapy*. New York: Wiley and Sons.

Schaper, K. (1982) Psychological research and its implication for creative drama. *Children's Theatre Review 31*, 16–18.

Schattner, G. and Courtney, R. (eds) (1981) *Drama in Therapy Vol. I and Vol. 2*. New York: Drama Book Specialists.

Schechner, R. (1985) *Between Theater and Anthropology*. Philadelphia: University of Pennsylvania Press.

Schechner, R. and Schuman, M. (eds) (1976) *Ritual, Play, and Performance: Readings in the Social Sciences / Theatre*. New York: Seabury Press.

Scheff, T. (1976) Audience awareness and catharsis in drama. *The Psychoanalytic Review 63*, 529–554.

Scheff, T. (1979) *Catharsis in Healing, Ritual and Drama*. Berkeley: University of California Press.

Scheff, T. (1981) The distancing of emotion in psychotherapy. *Psychotherapy: Theory, Research and Practice 18*, 1, 46–53.

Scheff, T. (1991) *Emotions and Violence: Shame and Rage in Destructive Conflicts*. Lexington, MA.: Lexington Books.

Selman, R. (1971) Taking another's perspective: Role-taking development in early childhood. *Child Development 42*, 1721–1734.

Shaftel, F. and G. (1967) *Role-Playing for Social Values*. Englewood-Cliffs, NJ: Prentice-Hall.

Shakespeare, W. (1953, ed. C. Sisson) *William Shakespeare – The Complete Works*. New York: Harper and Row.

Shakespeare, W. (1963) *Hamlet*. New York: Washington Square Press.

Shakespeare, W. (1966) *A Midsummer Night's Dream*. New York: Washington Square Press.

Shaw, A. (1968) *A development of a taxonomy of educational objectives in creative dramatics*. Unpublished doctoral dissertation, Columbia University.

Silverman, M. (1987) *The myth of play therapy*. Unpublished paper delivered at Symposium on Play Therapy, New York University.

Singer, J. (1966) *Daydreaming*. New York: Random House.

Singer, J. (1973) *The Child's World of Make-Believe*. New York: Academic Press.

Slade, P. (1954) *Child Drama*. London: University of London Press.

Smith, S. (1984) *The Mask in Modern Drama*. Berkeley: University of California Press.

Sophocles (1960) Philoctetes. In D. Grene and R. Lattimore *Greek Tragedies vol.III*. Chicago: University of Chicago Press.

Sorell, W. (1974) *The Other Face: The Mask in the Arts*. London: Thames and Hudson.

Stake, R. (1974) *Evaluating the Arts in Education*. Columbus, OH: Charles E. Merrill.

Stanislavski, C. (1936) *An Actor Prepares*. New York: Theatre Arts Books.

Stanislavski, C. (1949) *Building a Character*. New York: Theatre Arts Books.

Stanislavski, C. (1961) *Creating a Role*. New York: Theatre Arts Books.

Stevenson, R.L. (1986) *The Strange Case of Dr. Jekyll and Mr. Hyde*. Chester Springs, PA: Dufour Editions.

Sutton-Smith, B. and Lazier, G. (1971) Psychology and drama. *Empirical Research in the Theatre 1*,38–47.

Sutton-Smith, B., Lazier, G. and Zahn, D. (1972) *Developmental stages in dramatic improvisation. Proceedings of the American Psychological Association 79*, 421–423.

Turner, V. (1981) *From Ritual to Theatre: The Human Seriousness of Play*. New York: Performing Arts Journal Publications.

Wagner, B.J. (1976) *Dorothy Heathcote, Drama as a Learning Medium*. Washington, D.C.: National Education Association.

Ward, W. (1957) *Playmaking with Children*, second edition. New York: Appleton-Century-Crofts.

Way, B. (1967) *Development through Drama*. London: Longman.

Weitz, M. (1976) Research on the arts and in aesthetics: Some pitfalls, some possibilities. In S. Madeja (ed) *Arts and Aesthetics: An Agenda for the Future*. St. Louis, MO: CEMREL.

Werner, H. (1948) *Comparative Psychology of Mental Development*. New York: International Universities Press.

Whitman, W. (1950) Song of myself. In J. Kouwenhoven (ed) *Leaves of Grass*. New York: Modern Library.

Willett, J. (ed) (1964) *Brecht on Theatre*. New York: Hill and Wang.

Winnicott, D.W. (1971) *Playing and Reality.* London: Tavistock.

Wiseman, F. (1974) *Primate.* Boston, MA: Zipporah Films.

Witkin, R. (1974) *The Intelligence of Feeling.* London: Heinemann.

Wolpe, J. (1990) *The Practice of Behavior Therapy*, 4th edition. New York: Pergamon Press.

Woltmann, A. (1951) The use of puppetry as a projective method in therapy. In W. Anderson and G. Anderson (eds) *An Introduction to Projective Techniques.* New York: Prentice Hall.

Woltmann, A. (1971) Spontaneous puppetry by children as a projective method. In A. Rubin and M. Haworth (eds) *Projective Techniques With Children.* New York: Grune and Stratton.

Woodruff, M. (1982) Erikson's theory of psychosocial development: The socialization of developmental drama. *Children's Theatre Review 31*, 22–25.

Wordsworth, W. (1807/1965) Intimations of immortality. In C.Baker (ed) *The Prelude, Selected Poems and Sonnets.* New York: Holt, Rinehart and Winston.

Yeats, W.B. (1921) The second coming. *Collected Poems of W. B.Yeats.* New York: Macmillan.

# Subject Index

*Note: Page numbers in bold
type refer to figures*

abuse, treatment for 195,
    196
acting
    'as if' 4
    workshops 46
actor
    Greek 105–6
    and role 170
Actor's Studio 15
*A.D. 1952* 62–4
adolescent, role type
    117–18
aesthetic distance 32,
    86–9, 104
aggression 186
    genesis 184
    play 184
    roles 185
agnostic, role type 129
AIDS 214
aims 3
    aesthetic aims 3
    affective 3
    therapeutic and
        dramatic 2
albinism 181
alienation 14–15
alter ego, of protagonist
    23, 213–51
American Society of
    Group Psychotherapy
    and Psychodrama 10
anger 221–2
anthropology 4, 11

artist 157
    performing 152
    role type 131
assessment, through role
    method 199–201
Assessment of Dramatic
    Involvement Scale 38
atheist, role type 129
awareness, psychological 6

baby role 177, 178, 182
basketball 84
beauty, role type 118–19
behavioral approaches
    41, 194
bigot, role type 122
bipolar disorder 216–51
    definition 217–18
Bread and Puppet
    Theatre 58
bride
    image 175
    role 175
bridges 175
brother, role type 124
bureaucrat, role type 125

case studies 34
    Doris 80–1
    Georgie 171–9, 183–8
    Herb 197–8
    June 199
    Mackey 180–3, 183–8
    Michael 111–16
        revisited 132–6
    Sam 216–51
        as Havel *235*, 236–7
        as a hero *236*, 237
        as Schmarty *234*,
            234–5
    *see also* Hetty Green play
catharsis 2, 16–17, 22–3,
    32, 48
    notion of 26–7
    in sociodrama 25

and story–telling 19
    within distancing
        model 91–2
Chicago 167
childhood, dramatic
    conception 169
child(ren) 76–7, 140,
    141, 156
    development 169
    guidance 37
    role type 117
*Children's Theatre Review* 35
chorus, role type 113, 126
class roles 126
cleric, role type 129
client
    –therapist relationship
        87–9
    role in individual drama
        therapy 90–1
    understanding for 76–9
clinical state scale 37
cognition 3
collaboration, and
    isolation 202–6
Collaboration in the
    Creative Arts
    Therapies course,
    New York University
    166, 205
*commedia dell'arte* 106
competencies
    drama/theatre 5
    therapeutic 5
content analysis 39
counseling 9–10
    definition 1
*Counterlife, The* (Roth) 103
countertransference, and
    role seduction 92–4
coward, role type 122
crankie 19–20, 54
creative arts 75–6
    therapies 143, 165, 166

isolation and collaboration in 202–6
research agenda 137–9

daughter, role type 124
death, role of 187
deceiver, role type 121
demon, role type 130–1
depression 218
development
  stage 141
  theory 29–31
devoted worshipper, role of 197–8
diagnostic role–playing test 37
disabled groups 9
  awareness and understanding of 6–7
  drama/theatre practice with 8
  role 181
distancing ix, 13–27, 32, 47–8, 83, 91–2
  aesthetic 32, 86–9, 104
  and story-telling 19–20
  techniques 18–19, 80–1
dolls 20, 48–9
domains 192
double (or alter ego) 23, 150
  Sam's life 216–51
drama, definition 1
drama therapist see therapists
Drama in Therapy (Schattner and Courtney) 34
dreamer 149, 157
  role type 131
dreams, interpretation 150

eater role 188
educational drama 11
  theory 31
educational objectives, taxonomy in creative dramatics 37–8
elderly 19, 76, 77
emotionally disturbed 23
  children 37
Empirical Research in the Theatre 35
England 12
epic theatre 15–16, 54–5
  and story-telling 19–20
eunuch, role type 118
evocateur role 96
ex-offenders 8
existential approach 85
Expressive Therapies Program, Lesley College 85
expressive therapy 85, 140, 140–58, 165

facilitator, therapist as 195
fairy, role type 130
fairytale 108–9
Family Album of Lucybelle Crater, The (Meatyard) 62
family legacies 174
father, image/role 176
field studies 34
Fluid Boundary and Rigid Boundary Scales 35, 37
follower, drama therapist as 94–5
fool 154, 157
  role type 120

game-playing 8
genetics, role 183
Gesalt therapy 3, 7, 9

god/goddess role type 129–30
grandparent, role type 124
Greek theatre 57
  actors in 105–6
groom 176
group therapy 80–1, 153
  role of drama therapist 85–6
guide, therapist as 195
guru role 97
gypsy role 173

Hamlet 46, 66–7, 87, 146
head of state, role type 124–5
healer role 187
health care plan 166
helper, role type 122
hero, role type 128–9
Hetty Green play 208–15
  New York version 209–10, 211–12
Hoboken (New Jersey) 62–4, 209
hospitalization, of psychiatric patients 37
Hunger Artist (Landy) 60

imagery 44–5, 46, 175
  murderer 90
  use of puppets, dolls and objects 48–53
  see also therapeutic dramatization
immoralist, role type 121
incest, survivor of 196
individual treatment 84–98
  role of client 90–1
  role of drama therapist 86–9
innocent, role type 121
inspiration 208

instruments, drama
   therapy 37–8, 39
internship 7
interview, drama and
   puppetry 35–6
Inventory of Dramatic
   Behavior 38
invocateur role 96
isolation, and
   collaboration, in
   creative arts therapies
   202–6

killer, role type 127
*King Lear* 159, 160, 161
lamb, role of 197–8
*Landslide, the Unmasking of*
   *the President* (Mayer
   and McManus) 103–4
language arts 11
lawyer
   role of 113–14, 135
   role type 125
Lesley College 85
Linnaean taxonomy 115
Little Prince role 199
Living Theatre 34
lost one role 221
lover, role type 123
lower class, role type 126

madman/woman, role
   type 119
magician, role type 131
make-up 21–2, 51–3, *52*
malcontent, role type 122
*Mask-maker* (Marceau) 92
masks 2, 20, 21, 49–51
   image of 54–69
   in photography 58–64
   significance in theatre
     and therapy 67–9
   in theatre 54–8
   in therapy 64–7
matricide 45, 51–2, *52*

media, dramatic 99
mentally ill, role type 119
mentor system 161
middle class, role type
   126
*Midsummer Night's Dream,*
   *A* 89, 157, 158
models, theoretical 29–33
moment, spontaneous 4
*Mondo Wiley* (Sam's
   drawing) 218, *219*
*Money Is An End In Itself*
   (Landy) 210
moralist, role type 121
mother
   narcissistic 174
   role 113, 174
   role type 123
   *see also* Oedipal conflict
mother-in-law, role type
   123
murderer image 90
muse 207–15
music 75

narcissistic mother 174
narrative psychology 105
National Association for
   Drama Therapy
   (NADT) 159, 161,
   162
National Coalition of
   Arts Therapy
   Associations (NCATA)
   166, 203
National Theatre of the
   Deaf 9
New York University *ix*,
   166, 166 205
nurturing roles 185

objects 48–9
Oedipal conflict *42*, 45,
   51–2
one-on-one 84–98

Open Theatre 34
opportunist, role type 122
orthodox, role type 129
overdistancing 17, 104

pantomime 8
parent role 183
pariah, role type 126
pastor 224–6
performance 46
   theory 11, 32, 41
   therapeutic 41–2
Performing Arts in Crisis
   Training (PACT) 3
personal creativity,
   development of 5–6
personality 193
Philistine, role type 122
philosophy 11
photography, mask in
   58–64
play 5, 31, 40
   aggressive 184
   function of 4
   sand 30, 88
   theory 30–1
   therapy 20, 30, 71–2
   use of puppets, dolls
     and objects 48–9
Pocahontas 58–9
practicum 7
*Presentation of Self in*
   *Everyday Life, The*
   (Goffman) 102–3
presidential role 103–4,
   105
*Primate* (Wiseman) 40–1
prison, theatre in 8
professional organizations
   12
programs *see* training
projection 40
   techniques 64, 81–2
   use in drama therapy
     48–53

protagonist, double or
    alter ego of 23
provocateur role 95–6
psychiatric patients,
    short-term adult 76,
    77–9
psychoanalysis 67, 71–4,
    84–5
    theory 30–1, 32
psychoanalysts 193
psychodrama 10, 102,
    161, 194
    techniques 64, 81
    theory 38
    to balance distance
    22–3
psychodramatists 3
psychology 1, 11, 164,
    165
    narrative 105
psychotherapy 2, 67–8
    definition 1
puppetry 7, 20–1, 48–9,
    94
    interview 35–6, 48

quantitative methods
    33–4

Rags to Riches (Harris)
    55–6
reactionary, role type 124
recreation, and
    supervision 98
reflection 192
regression 178
reliving 17
remembering 17
Renaissance
    England 106
    Italy 106
representation 4
research
    agenda for creative arts
    therapies 137–9

behavioral 41
    conceptual and
    methodological
    issues 28–43
    data and results analysis
    36–9
    empirical quantitative
    35, 39, 40
    experiential 34
    methodologies 33–6
    qualitative 40–1
    questions 33
    reflective 34
    role of 42–3
revolutionary, role type
    124
ritual, aesthetically-based
    142
role ix, 1–2, 88, 115,
    144, 145
    artist 151
    behaviour 183
    concept of 99–110
    definition 111
    dramatic model 111
    early development 170
    genetics 183
    imbalance 195
    model 181
    play 141
    seduction, and
    countertransference
    92–4
    and Self 102–4,
    109–10
    taking 169
    taxonomy 111–36
    theatrical archetype
    system 116–31
    theory 29–30, 174
    type 149
role method 113–14,
    131–6
    for short-term treatment
    190–201
    appropriateness 193–4

assessment through
    199–201
    specific characteristics
    195–6
    what is it? 191–3
    who best benefits?
    196–9
role-playing 29–30, 40
    as destitute beggar
    woman 93
role-reversal 182, 184
Rorschach Index of
    Repressive Style
    (RIRS) 35, 37
Rumpelstiltskin 99–100,
    108–9

sandplay 30, 88
schizophrenics 33, 37,
    41, 77–9, 82
    expression through
    puppetry 94
Self ix, 76, 115, 145
    and Role 102–4,
    109–10
self-development 74–6
self-seduction 93
sexual masculine role
    112–13
shaminism 142
    ritual healings 142
short-term model see role
    method
sick role 181
simpleton, role type 120
sister, role type 124
social contact scale 37
social modeling 193
social sciences 40
sociodrama 23–5, 102
sociology 11
    theory 32–3
soldier, role type 125
son
    role of 113
    role type 124

story 99–100
-telling as technique in
distancing 19–20
*Beat of Black Wings, The*
(Michael) 133–5
*Rupert Stosh* (Sam) 226–7
*Wooden Clogs and the
Rubber Boots, The*
(Michael) 112
structural role model
(Johnson) 29–30
supervision, and
recreation 98
survivor role 179
of incest or torture 196
symbolic interactionism
1–2, 11, 31–2

taxonomy
of educational
objectives in creative
dramatics 37–8
role 111–36
teacher
role 97
therapist as 195
techniques 3, 9–10
distancing 18–19, 80–1
drama therapy 25–6,
79–80
interdisciplinary 7–8
theatre 11, 142, 162
definition 1
masks in 54–8
significance 67–9
performance 8–9
role in 105–6
theatre-in-education (TIE)
9
theory 10–11
therapeutic dramatization
45–7
therapist
as follower and witness
94–5

role
in group treatment
85–6
in individual
treatment 86–9
therapists 195
certain/uncertain 73–4
conventional/unconventi
onal 74
professional/unprofession
al 72–3
TIE (theatre-in-education)
9
tiger, role of 197–8, 203
*To Kill a Mockingbird*
(Lee) 114
torture, survivor of 196
training 193–4
four-part model 1–12,
74–5, 76–80
programs *ix*, 7, 12, 85,
161, 166, 205
Masters Degree 162,
165
reflections upon 70–83
transference 4, 91–2
transformation 29
transitional object 181
treatment 7–8
*see also* role method

underdistancing 17, 87,
104
United States 85
university courses *ix*, 10,
12, 85, 161, 162,
166, 205
upper class role type 126
Utah Shakespeare Festival
160

Verfremdungs-Effect 47
victim, role type 121–2,
184

video, therapeutic use of
22, 41
visionary, role type 129

warrior, role type 127
'Winds of Change'
(NADT 14th
Conference speech)
159
wise person, role type 121
witness, drama therapist
as 94–5
*Wizard of Oz, The* 98, 106
working class, role type
126

zombie, role type 122

# Names Index

Ahsen, A. 44, 46, 53, 64–5
Alger, H. *xi*, 8
Arbus, D. 61
Artaud, A. 2, 107
Axline, V. 85

Blake, W. *xi*, 203
Blumer, H. 31
Bly, R. 114
Boal, A. 26–7
Bolton, G. 30–1, 45
Brecht, B. *xi*, 2–3, 14, 15–16, 31, 47, 75, 107
Breitenbach, N. 21
Britton, J. 11
Burke, K. 40

Carter, J. 105
Casement, P. 87
Cole, D. 4, 107
Cooley, C. 1–2, 31, 100
Courtney, R. 31, 34
Craig, E.G. 58, 68, 107

Eliot, T.S. 45–6
Erickson, E. 68

Fox, J. 101
Freud, S. 30, 67, 75, 110, 149

Gardner, H. 144
Ginsberg, A. 207, 208
Goffman, E. 30, 40, 102–3
Gould, S.J. 114–15
Green, H. 208–15
Grotowski, J. 2

Harley, G. 69
Heathcote, D. 30
Hoffman, A. 168
Hoffman, D. 68
Homer 207

Irwin, E. 30, 35–6, 40, 48, 193
    Levy, P. and Shapiro, M. 37
    and Shapiro, M. 34

James, W. 100
Johnson, D. 29–30, 34, 40, 41, 166
    and Quinlan, D. 30, 37
Jung, C.G. 2, 67, 75, 85, 185

Kafka, F. *xi*, 60
Karioth, E., and Lazier, G. 38
Kirby, E.T. 142
Klein, M. 68
Kohlberg, L. 31

Landy, R.J. 30–1, 97–8, 109, 111, 190
Lazier, G. 39
    and Karioth, E. 38
    and Sutton-Smith, B. 38
Leaf, L. 38
Lee, H. 114
Levy, P., Shapiro, M. and Irwin, E. 37

Linton, R. 100
Lowenfeld, M. 30, 68, 85, 88

McManus, D., and Mayer, J. 103–4
McNiff, S. 144
Mantle, M. 153
Marceau, M. 92
Maslow, A. 85
Mayer, J., and McManus, D. 103–4
Mead, G.H. 1–2, 30, 31, 40, 59, 100–1
Meatyard, R.E. 61–2, 63, 64
Melville, H. *xi*
Milton, J. 207
Moffett, J. 11
Moreno, J.L. 16–17, 24, 68, 85, 101–2, 116
Moyer, W. 165
Muller, H. 107

O'Neill, E. 19
Ouspensky, P. 39

Paisley, W. 39
Perls, F. 68, 85
Piaget, J. 31, 40
Pinero, M. 8
Poe, E. A. *xi*
Portner, E. 34, 193

Quinlan, D., and Johnson, D. 30, 37

Reagan, R. 103–4
Roth, P. 103, 110

Sarbin, T. *ix*, 30, 76, 102, 104–5, 110

Schechner, R. 143
Scheff, T. 14, 16–18, 27,
    32, 47–8, 87, 143
Schumann, P. 58
Selman, R. 30, 31
Shakespeare, W. 207
Shapiro, M.
  and Irwin, E. 34
  Irwin, E. and Levy, P. 37
Shaw, A. 37–8
Silverman, M. 71–2
Sophocles *xi*
Stanislavski, C. 2, 3, 15,
    32, 106–7
Sutton-Smith, B., and
    Lazier, G. 38


Walcott, J. 114–15
Weitz, M. 42
Whitman, W. 207, 208
Wilson, R. 107
Winnicott, D.W. 85, 175
Wiseman, F. 40–1
Witkin, R. 87


Zefman, W.F. 160–1,
    166, 167

# Drama and Healing
## The Roots of Drama Therapy
*Roger Grainger*
ISBN 1 85302 337 X pb

'The Rev. Roger Grainger's new book is undoubtedly an important contribution to the growing body of literature on the theory of drama therapy. It is at once a Scholarly and an unusually personal discussion of the place of drama in the treatment of severe mental illness.'

*– British Journal of Occupational Therapy*

'This is by far the most thoughtful book on dramatherapy that I have come across… This book is strongly recommended for creative arts therapists and psychotherapists alike.'

*– Group Analysis*

'extremely thought provoking…the links made between different theoretical and creative streams are extremely interesting.'

*– Counselling*

# The Glass of Heaven
## The Faith of the Dramatherapist
*Roger Grainger*
ISBN 1 85302 284 5 200 pb

# Dramatherapy with Families, Groups and Individuals
## Waiting in the Wings
*Sue Jennings*
ISBN 1 85302 144 X pb
ISBN 1 85302 014 1 hb

'Not only is it extremely well written, but the theoretical models and issues outlined are worked through with the use of detailed and clear examples…deserves to be widely read by specialists and non-specialists alike.'

*– Counselling*

'She shows an impressive knowledge of myths and dramatic literature and demonstrates their therapeutic validity. The case examples are wonderful.

*– Dramascope*

'This is a clear, well-written text that reflects a dramatherapist who is clinically astute and well-grounded in drama, theatre, and ritual processes… There is no doubt that Jennings is a trailblazing pioneer whose journey makes ours a little easier.'

*– The Arts in Psychotherapy*

**Jessica Kingsley Publishers**
116 Pentonville Road, London N1 9JB

# Storymaking in Bereavement
## Dragons Fight in the Meadow
*Alida Gersie*

ISBN 1 85302 176 8 pb ISBN 1 85302 065 6 hb

'Gersie is intuitive, sensitive and wise as she guides her readers into the territory of bereavement, love and loss... Each storymaking structure is exciting and brimming with potential... Alida Gersie has succeeded in brilliantly finding ways to empower individuals coming to grips with mortality...her work *Storymaking in Bereavement: Dragons in the Meadow* empowers us as helping professionals. Now we have a tool that gives us a little more courage compassion and insight so that we too are better armed to fight dragons in the meadow.'

*— The Arts in Psychotherapy*

'This is a fascinating book which may reunite readers with stories of their childhood and provide new insights into their meaning. It presents an innovative approach to bereavement counselling which reflects the wise counsel of some of the original story tellers and the oral tradition which we have lost. There are poignant stories and no avoidance of "difficult" feelings encountered during the grief process. This book is a delight to read on account of its descriptive qualities. It is also a source, in an accessible form, of a wealth of information. It addresses an area which is of concern to all occupational therapists.'

*— British Journal of Occupational Therapy*

'This is an erudite, imaginative book by an author who is deeply involved in her topic and is an enjoyable and absorbing read. The book would be of value to course leaders and students on courses covering loss, separation and divorce, abortion, terminal illness and death and to anyone who gives support to the dying and bereaved.'

*— Nursing Times*

'This book is beautifully written. It is immensely rich in its use of story, metaphor and literary allusion to illustrate the process of grief and healing...moving and deeply compassionate. In addition to its overt theme, a book which touches its reader so deeply provides a subtle lesson in how a counsellor may allow herself to be deeply touched by her client.'

*— Counselling*

'Anyone interested in story as a form of therapy or in bereavement or the existential adaption to the idea of death will find this book overflowing with exciting concepts and powerful healing images... There is a well constructed balance between psychological conception and folk story in this book. This material is a rich collection of ideas which can be used in both the classroom and the counselor's office.'

*— Religious Studies Review*

Jessica Kingsley Publishers
116 Pentonville Road, London N1 9JB

# Dramatherapy for People with Learning Disabilities
## A World of Difference
*Anna Chesner, Foreword by Sue Emmy Jennings*

ISBN 1 85302 208 X pb

'This is an excellent book with which to approach the Millenium. It is the first book to address the contemporary issues in the application of dramatherapy with people who have learning disabilities... Anna Chesner's thoughtful writing moves the theory and practice forward in an accessible way... It is well illustrated with client pictures and explains how the dramatherapist enables the client 'to find a form for the feelings', which may include fury and revenge...the final chapter, breaks unique ground with a psychodramatic approach to dramatherapy for people with learning disabilities. The strength of this book is in its up-to-date, 'user-friendly' mode of writing which includes dialogues, vignettes as well as client illustrations. Chesner has broken new ground in building bridges between dramatherapy and music therapy as well as dramatherapy and psychodrama.'

*– From the foreword by Sue Emmy Jennings*

'a clear and detailed exploration of the uses of dramatherapy for people with learning disabilities...a fascinating and stimulating mixture of theory and practice...of value to anyone concerned with enriching the lives of people with learning disabilities.

*– Down's Syndrome Association Newsletter*

# Movement and Drama in Therapy, 2nd edition
## A Holistic Approach
*Audrey G. Wethered*
*Foreword by Chloë Gardner*

ISBN 1 85302 199 7 pb

'[Readers] may find, in these pages, a theory connecting the inner world with practical daily living... I wish this book every success. I hope it will reach many people and light sparks, answer quests, strengthen endeavour and broaden horizons.'

*– from the Foreword*

**Jessica Kingsley Publishers**
116 Pentonville Road, London N1 9JB

## Post Traumatic Stress Disorder and Dramatherapy
### Treatment and Risk-Reduction
*Linda Winn, Foreword by Alida Gersie*
ISBN 1 85302 183 0 pb

'This publication will be purchased by trainers and those new to this kind of work for its lucid approach to defining PTSD and the situations where it may be found. Parts of the book would be useful to people involved in personnel or management as information for those working alongside a therapist or dramatherapist or those involved in establishing or promoting such a therapeutic approach. It has helpful chapters on prevention, debriefing and supervision which are applicable to an institutional context.'

*– British Journal of Guidance and Counselling*

'Although written for a specialized minority, the book is clearly presented, so that the reality of what is being described is brought home to those of us who are strangers to PTSD and its clinical problems. For people who are involved in drama it is completely fascinating, however, because it shows how essential dramatic awareness is to our mental well-being.'

*– Radius*

'It is a book that stays close to the daily reality of life in our hospitals, clinics and social services centres. At times the author speaks a language of tough care as well as substantial tenderness. Through straightforward description of her own practice she encourages other mental health practitioners to bear emotional and imaginative witness, thereby to help people to work through their terrible experiences.'

*– From the Foreword*

## Dramatherapy
### Clinical Studies
*Edited by Steve Mitchell*
ISBN 1 85302 304 3 pb

**Jessica Kingsley Publishers**
**116 Pentonville Road, London N1 9JB**

# Art Therapy and Dramatherapy
## Masks of the Soul
*Sue Jennings and Åse Minde*

ISBN 1 85302 181 4 pb
ISBN 1 85302 027 3 hb

'The creativity of the authors is testified to by their production of a new form. In addition to being a 'how to' manual for art and dramatherapy, this book is a melange of autobiography, anthropology, psychoanalysis, case reports, cross-cultural analysis, art reproduction, poetry, literary quotation, and mythology.'
*– The Lancet*

'There is energy, creativeness and richness of imagery in this book… The book is well referenced and relevant theoretical concepts are explained…there is some very good sound advice…on many different issues.' – Inscape
'…this book would enrich any occupational therapy department library.'
*– British Journal of Occupational Therapy*

'will prove useful to both beginning and advanced art therapists… The authors, whose passion for their work is obvious, are creative and generous in providing a text rich in methodology for arts therapists interested in expanding their practice.'
*– American Journal of Art Therapy*

'…the links between theory and practice are shown in detail…this book will be useful to students and exponents of these therapies alike.'
*– Nursing Times*

'This is a well researched study for the serious therapist. But it is also intelligible and stimulating for the non-specialist…there is a generous sprinkling of black and white illustrations well placed within the text to which they closely relate… It is a reference book for inspiration as well as information.'
*– Reform*

'…an interesting book, relevant to those of us who work in multi-disciplinary contexts or who wish to do such collaborative work. The scope for collaborative inter-disciplinary work is evidenced in part 2 with examples of work greatly adding to the coherency and purpose of the book in its entirety.'
*– Counselling*

'This book is an excellent and concise summation of the notions of dramatherapy and a detailed guide to it's application… Jennings's book will appeal to a broad multidisciplinary readership, with many of the notions encountered of great interest and value for the developing and practising psychiatric nurse. Further, this represents an excellent resource book for those who are engaged in dramatic activities with clients, peers or students.'
*– Australian Journal of Mental Health Nursing*

**Jessica Kingsley Publishers**
116 Pentonville Road, London N1 9JB

# Storymaking in Education and Therapy

*Alida Gersie and Nancy King*

ISBN 1 85302 519 4 hb  ISBN 1 85302 520 8 pb

'The myths themselves are veritable jewels that evoke an immediate response in the reader, and they stand on their own as a valuable asset to any library... This is in essence a 'How to' book replete with instructions for achieving personal growth and facilitating creativity in just about every avenue of expression... This book contains many exciting and compelling ideas'

*— The Arts in Psychotherapy*

'It is intended primarily for professionals in mental health and education who are interested in using traditional myths and folk tales in conducting group counseling and education classes. However, the stories in themselves are fascinating to read.'

*— Contemporary Psychology*

'This is a lovely book... There is something for everyone here... The practical exercises suggest ways in which these stories can be used in a group setting. People involved in counselling and therapy will also find valuable insights into the lives of people they help through the common language of myth. Moreover, the book will appeal to anyone interested in literature and story-telling in general. The quality of the presentation of the book adds to its appeal...this is a book to keep, use and refer back to again and again... In short, this is a publication for nurse teachers, psychiatric nurse therapists, counsellors and anyone interested in exploring the universal heritage that is handed down through story-telling and the sharing of myths. Buy it.'

*— Nursing Times*

'The book contains a strong introduction to this particular approach to storymaking, and has within it enough source materials and reflective advice to inspire and guide any group facilitator or teacher... The book contains a rich variety of thought provoking and inspiring material. Within the area of dramatherapy's use of narrative, myth and story form this is easily the most substantial and significant piece of work to date...a core text for dramatherapists to acquire.'

*— Dramatherapy*

'This is an essential and wonderful book for anyone interested in working with stories in education or therapy... It is a true discovery'

*— Dr Ofra Ayalon, Haifa University*

**Jessica Kingsley Publishers**
**116 Pentonville Road, London N1 9JB**

## Play Therapy with Abused Children
*Ann Cattanach*
ISBN 1 85302 193 8 pb ISBN 1 85302 120 2 hb

'…a welcome addition to the sparse literature in this area. I would recommend the book to anyone working in this field but especially to beginners… This is a well presented, clear and easy-to-read book, providing a balanced mixture of factual information and case material.'
— *British Journal of Occupational Therapy*

'Her accounts of the way in which play is used to make sense of traumatic experiences are full of insight and often moving. All aspects of the work are covered… This is an exceptional volume…goes far beyond a mere text book.'
— *Therapy Weekly*

## Play Therapy
### Where the Sky Meets the Underworld
*Ann Cattanach*
ISBN 1 85302 211 X pb

'…an excellent, stimulating read with a manageable style and numerous sensitive insights into the world of play for the child and how it can become a therapeutic process where children 'play out' their perception of their own experi-ences…uses clear, straightforward language to discuss the theoretical basis for play therapy… The book does not make great claims as to its powers of healing, but it seems to offer a means towards constructively working through traumatic experiences for children.'
— *Nursery World*

'Cattanach packs a large amount of theory into this easy-to-read volume, together with practical guidelines on how to be a safe companion for the child's journey.'
— *Professional Social Work*

'This is an excellent introduction to an activity whose relevance is increasingly recognised and used, not least in the communication of good health practices.'
— *Institute of Health Education*

**Jessica Kingsley Publishers**
116 Pentonville Road, London N1 9JB

## The Metaphoric Body
### Guide to Expressive Therapy Through Images and Archetypes

*Leah Bartal and Nira Ne'eman*

*Foreword by Professor Harris Chaiklin*

ISBN 1 85302 152 0

'A rich confluence of Eastern and Western influences shape the content of this expressive arts resource book...provides numerous movement ideas and themes suitable for educational workshops, body awareness classes as well as for work with individuals...a rich source of developmental material for professionals in fields such as movement education, the expressive arts or expressive art therapies...an important practical supplement to professionals working through the expressive arts.

*– The Arts in Psychotherapy*

'This well-researched book...offers creative arts therapists, educators and artists a wealth of resources on myth, metaphor and the creative process... Personal stories, poems, drawings and photos vividly report the imaginative responses these tasks evoke... Photos and diagrams help focus the directions for the movement experiences that follow... The authors, with their extensive background in Hebrew literature, give us a new dimension of mythic exploration through Biblical Stories... Certain selected Greek myths...also provide rich experiences in visualization and improvisation... *The Metaphoric Body* is a book to be read carefully. It opens many doors to creativity and will appeal to everyone interested in the creative process, especially teachers and dancers...'

*– American Journal of Dance Therapy*

'This book is a beautiful and timely gift to all expressive therapists, and indeed to verbal therapists as well. It expands the traditional art therapy repertoire...'

*– American Journal of Art Therapy*

'This excellent resource book links the mystery and movement of the body to the psychological process of transformation... Starting with a powerful and sensitive awareness of the body, readers can explore relationships with the world and nature, communication with others and themselves and set out on allegorical journeys through the great truths of being as set out in ancient myths and symbols.'

*– Caduceus*

'...a very important book and is highly recommended both for teachers and students. The book is abundant with creative ideas...takes the reader step-by-step to understanding the subject. As the book is on a high academic level, it is also understandable and pleasant reading.'

*– Director, Israel Dance Library*

**Jessica Kingsley Publishers**
**116 Pentonville Road, London N1 9JB**